Clinical
Electrocardiography

A Simplified Approach

Clinical Electrocardiography

A Simplified Approach

ARY L. GOLDBERGER, M.D.

Assistant Professor of Medicine, Harvard Medical School;
Co-Director of Electrocardiography
Beth Israel Hospital
Boston, Massachusetts

EMANUEL GOLDBERGER, M.D., F.A.C.P.

Clinical Associate Professor of Medicine
New York Medical College
Valhalla, New York

THIRD EDITION

With **446** illustrations

The C. V. Mosby Company

ST. LOUIS • TORONTO • PRINCETON   1986

MOSBY

A TRADITION OF PUBLISHING EXCELLENCE

Editor: Carol Trumbold
Assistant editor: Anne Gunter
Editing supervisors: Elaine Steinborn, Max Weaver
Manuscript editor: George B. Stericker, Jr.
Book design: Kay M. Kramer
Cover design: John Rokusek
Production: Ginny Douglas

THIRD EDITION

The C.V. Mosby Company
11830 Westline Industrial Drive, St. Louis, Missouri 63146

Library of Congress Cataloging-in-Publication Data

Goldberger, Ary Louis, 1949-
  Clinical electrocardiography.

  Bibliography: p.
  Includes index.
  1. Electrocardiography.   2. Arrhythmia.
I. Goldberger, Emanuel, 1913-   . II. Title.
[DNLM: 1. Electrocardiography.   WG 140 G616c]
RC683.5.E5G593   1986   616.1′207547   86-2525
ISBN 0-8016-1916-5

C/VH/VH 9 8 7 6 5 4 3 2 1   01/A/043

For
Ellen, Zachary, and Lexy
with love

Preface

This book is an introduction to electrocardiography. It is written particularly for medical students, nurses, and paramedical assistants and assumes no previous instruction in ECG reading. Physicians wishing to review basic electrocardiography have also found the material useful. The text derives from the cumulative experience of both authors in the field of electrocardiography, beginning in 1944 with the invention of the aV_R, aV_L, and aV_F leads by one of us (E.G.). The text itself is closely based on a series of lectures given over the past decade by the other (A.G.) to physician's associates, medical students, nurses, house officers, and emergency room physicians.

We have divided the book into three sections. Part I covers the basic principles of electrocardiography, normal ECG patterns, and the major abnormal P-QRS-T patterns. Part II describes the major abnormalities of heart rhythm and conduction. Part III is an extensive collection of practice questions and problems for review. In addition, we have interspersed practice questions throughout the text. In reading ECGs, as in learning a new language, fluency is attained only with repetition and review.

The clinical applications of ECG reading have been stressed throughout the book. Each time an abnormal pattern is mentioned, there is a brief discussion of the conditions that might have produced it. Although this is not intended as a manual of therapeutics, general principles of treatment and clinical management are briefly discussed. In addi-

tion, students are encouraged to approach ECGs in terms of a rational simple differential diagnosis, rather than through the tedium of rote memorization. It is comforting for most students to discover that the number of possible arrhythmias that can produce a heart rate of 170 beats per minute is limited to just a handful of choices. Only three basic ECG patterns are found with cardiac arrest. Similarly, there are only a few causes of low-voltage patterns, of patterns in which the QRS complex is abnormally wide, etc.

In approaching any given ECG, there are always three essential questions. First, what does the ECG show; second, what are the possible causes of this pattern; and, third, what if anything should be done about it? Most conventional ECG books focus on the first question, emphasizing pattern recognition. However, it is only a first step, for example, to note the premature ventricular contractions (PVCs) on an ECG. The more important question is what could have produced these abnormal beats: excessive caffeine intake, digitalis toxicity, hypoxemia, myocardial ischemia, hypokalemia, or something else? Treatment, of course, will depend on the answers to these questions.

The aim of this book, therefore, is to present the ECG as it is used on the hospital wards, in the outpatient clinics, and in the intensive and coronary care units, where recognition of normal and abnormal patterns is only the starting point in patient care and management.

The third edition contains new information on multiple topics, including arrhythmias, conduction disturbances, myocardial ischemia and infarction, and pacemakers. A new section on common pitfalls in ECG interpretation has been added (Chapter 19). Furthermore, the self-assessment problems in Part III have been expanded.

This project was sponsored by the trustees of the Dr. Louis B. and Anna H. Goldberger Memorial Foundation for Medical Research.

Finally, we would like to thank Blanche and Ellen Goldberger for their encouragement and support. Ellen Goldberger contributed both artwork and editorial assistance and, once again, endured the karmic clutter of ECG clippings.

Ary L. Goldberger
Emanuel Goldberger

Contents

PART ONE

Basic Principles and Patterns

1 Introductory Principles

DEFINITION

An *electrocardiogram* (ECG)* records cardiac electrical currents (voltages, potentials) by means of metal *electrodes* placed on the surface of the body. As described in Chapter 3, these metal electrodes are placed on the arms, legs, and chest wall (precordium).

BASIC CARDIAC ELECTROPHYSIOLOGY

Before discussing the basic ECG patterns, we will review some elementary aspects of cardiac electrophysiology. Fortunately, only certain simple principles are required for clinical interpretation of ECGs. In addition, it is worth mentioning now that no special knowledge of electronics or electrophysiology is necessary despite the connotations of the term "electrocardiography."

In simplest terms the function of the heart is to contract and pump blood to the lungs for oxygenation and then to pump this oxygenated blood into the general (systemic) circulation. The signal for cardiac contraction is the spread of electrical currents through the heart muscle. These currents are produced both by specialized nervous conducting tissue within the heart and by the heart muscle itself. The ECG records the currents produced by the heart muscle.

*The abbreviation *EKG* is sometimes used.

ELECTRICAL STIMULATION OF THE HEART

The electrical "wiring" of the heart is outlined in Fig. 1-1. Normally the signal for cardiac electrical stimulation starts in the *sinus node* (also called the sinoatrial or SA node). The sinus node is located in the right atrium near the opening of the superior vena cava. It is a small collection of specialized cells capable of spontaneously generating electrical stimuli (signals). From the sinus node, this electrical stimulus spreads first through the right atrium and then into the left atrium. In this way the sinus node functions as the normal *pacemaker* of the heart.

The first phase of cardiac activation consists of the electrical stimulation of the right and left atria. This electrical stimulation, in turn, signals the atria to contract and to pump blood simultaneously through the tricuspid and mitral valves into the right and left ventricles respectively. The electrical stimulus then spreads to specialized conduction tissues in the *atrioventricular* (AV) *junction* (which includes the *AV node* and *bundle of His*) and then into the *left and right bundle branches,* which carry the stimulus to the ventricular muscle cells.

The AV junction, which functions as an electrical "bridge" connecting the atria and ventricles, is located at the base of the interatrial septum and extends into the ventricular septum (as shown in Fig. 1-1). It has two subdivisions: The upper (proximal) part is

3

CONDUCTION SYSTEM OF THE HEART

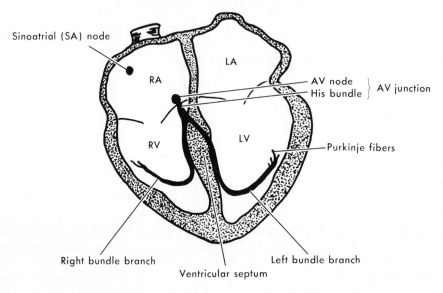

Fig. 1-1. Normally the cardiac stimulus is generated in the *SA node* (located in the right atrium, *RA*). It then spreads through the *RA* and *LA* (right and left atria). Next, it spreads through the *AV node* and *His bundle,* which comprise the *AV junction*. It then passes into the left and right ventricles (*LV* and *RV*) by way of the *left* and *right bundle branches,* which are continuations of the His bundle. Finally, it spreads to the ventricular muscle cells through the *Purkinje fibers.*

the AV node. (In older texts the terms "AV node" and "AV junction" are used synonymously.) The lower (distal) segment of the AV junction is called the bundle of His, after the physiologist who described it. The bundle of His then divides into two main branches: the right bundle branch, which brings the electrical stimulus to the right ventricle, and the left bundle branch,* which brings the electrical stimulus to the left ventricle (Fig. 1-1).

The electrical stimulus spreads simultaneously down the left and right bundle branches into the ventricular muscle itself *(ventricular myocardium)*. The stimulus spreads itself into the ventricular myocardium by way of specialized conducting cells, called *Purkinje fibers,* located in the ventricular muscle.

Under normal circumstances, when the sinus node is pacing the heart (normal sinus rhythm), the AV junction appears to function primarily as a shuttle, directing the electrical stimulus into the ventricles. However, under some circumstances (described later) the AV junction can also function as an independent pacemaker of the heart. For example, if the sinus node fails to function properly, the AV junction may act as an *escape* pacemaker. In such cases an AV junc-

---

*The left bundle actually divides into two subbranches called *fascicles* (which are discussed on pp. 219 to 221).

tional rhythm (and *not* sinus rhythm) is present. This produces a distinct ECG pattern (described in Chapter 12).

Just as the spread of electrical stimuli through the atria leads to atrial contraction, so the spread of the electrical stimuli through the ventricles leads to ventricular contraction with pumping of blood to the lungs and into the general circulation.

In summary, the electrical stimulation of the heart normally follows a repetitive sequence of five steps:

1. Production of a stimulus from pacemaker cells in the sinus node (in the right atrium)
2. Stimulation of the right and left atria
3. Spread of the stimulus to the AV junction (AV node and bundle of His)
4. Spread of the stimulus simultaneously through the left and right bundle branches
5. Stimulation of the left and right ventricular myocardium

CARDIAC CONDUCTIVITY AND AUTOMATICITY

The speed with which the electrical impulses are conducted through different parts of the heart varies. For example, conduction speed is *slowest* through the AV node and *fastest* through the Purkinje fibers. The relatively slow conduction speed through the AV node is of functional importance because it allows the ventricles time to fill with blood before the signal for cardiac contraction arrives.

In addition to *conductivity* the other major electrical feature of the heart is *automaticity*. Automaticity refers to the capacity of certain myocardial cells to function as pacemakers, to spontaneously generate electrical impulses that spread throughout the heart. Normally, as mentioned earlier, the sinus node is the pacemaker of the heart because of its inherent automaticity. Under special conditions other cells outside the sinus node (in the atria, the

AV junction, or the ventricles) can also act as independent pacemakers. For example, as mentioned before, if the automaticity of the sinus node is depressed, the AV junction may function as an escape pacemaker. In other conditions the automaticity of pacemakers outside the sinus node may become abnormally increased, and these *ectopic* (non-sinus) pacemakers may compete with the sinus node for control of the heartbeat. *Ectopy* is discussed in detail in Part II of this book (in the section on cardiac arrhythmias).

If you understand the normal physiologic stimulation of the heart, you have the basis for understanding the abnormalities of heart rhythm (arrhythmias) and conduction that produce distinctive ECG patterns. For example, failure of the sinus node to stimulate the heart properly may result in various rhythm disturbances, such as sinoatrial block (SA block), discussed in Chapter 11. Similarly, blockage of the spread of the stimulus through the AV junction produces various degrees of AV heart block (Chapter 15). Disease of the bundle branches may produce left or right bundle branch block (Chapter 7). Finally, any disease process that involves the ventricular muscle itself (for example, destruction of the heart muscle by myocardial infarction) also produces marked changes in the normal ECG patterns.

The first part of this book therefore is devoted to explaining the basis of the normal ECG, followed by a detailed look at major conditions causing abnormal P, QRS, and T* patterns. The second part of the book is devoted to describing the various abnormal rhythms (arrhythmias) and AV conduction disturbances that can occur. The third part of the book is a collection of review questions and examples. A short selective bibliography is provided at the end of the text.

---

*P, QRS, and T are defined in Chapter 2.

REVIEW OF CHAPTER 1

An ECG records the electrical voltages (potentials) produced in the heart. It does this by means of metal electrodes (connected to an electrocardiograph) placed on the patient's extremities and chest wall.

The electrical voltages of the heart are produced by specialized conduction fibers within the heart and by the heart muscle fibers themselves.

Normally a stimulus starts in the sinus (SA) node, located high in the right atrium near the superior vena cava. From here the stimulus spreads downward and to the left through the right and left atria and reaches the AV node, located at the beginning of the interventricular septum (Fig. 1-1). After a delay, the stimulus spreads through the AV junction (AV node and bundle of His). The bundle of His then subdivides into right and left branches. The right bundle branch runs down the interventricular septum and into the right ventricle. From there, small fibers, the Purkinje fibers, bring the stimulus outward into the main muscle mass of the right ventricle. Simultaneously, the left main bundle branch carries the stimulus down the interventricular septum to the muscle mass of the left ventricle, also by way of the Purkinje fibers.

This sequence of stimulation of the heart is the normal basic process. Disturbances of this sequence may produce abnormalities in the rhythm of the heart (the cardiac arrhythmias) or abnormalities in cardiac conduction (SA block, AV heart block, or bundle branch block).

Review Question—Chapter 1

1. Label the major parts of the cardiac conduction system in this diagram and then trace the spread of the normal cardiac stimulus from atria to ventricles.

Answer

1. See Fig. 1-1.

2 Basic ECG Waves

DEPOLARIZATION AND REPOLARIZATION

In Chapter 1 we used the general term "electrical stimulation" to refer to the spread of electrical stimuli through the atria and ventricles. The technical term for this cardiac electrical stimulation is *depolarization*. The return of heart muscle cells to their resting state following stimulation (depolarization) is called *repolarization*. These terms are derived from the fact that the normal myocardial cells (atrial and ventricular) are *polarized;* that is, they carry electrical charges on their surface. Fig. 2-1, *A,* shows the resting polarized state of a normal heart muscle cell. Notice that the outside of the resting cell is positive and the inside of the cell is negative (about $-90\,mV$).

When a heart muscle cell is stimulated, it

POLARIZED RESTING CELL

DEPOLARIZING CELL

DEPOLARIZED CELL

REPOLARIZING CELL

Fig. 2-1. Depolarization and repolarization. The resting heart muscle cell, **A,** is polarized; that is, it carries an electrical charge, with the outside of the cell positively charged and the inside negatively charged. When the cell is stimulated *(S),* as in **B,** it begins to depolarize *(stippled area).* The fully depolarized cell, **C,** is positively charged on the inside and negatively charged on the outside. Repolarization, **D,** occurs when the stimulated cell returns to the resting state. The direction of depolarization and repolarization is represented by *arrows.* Depolarization (stimulation) of the atria produces the P wave on the ECG, whereas depolarization of the ventricles produces the QRS complex. Repolarization of the ventricles produces the ST-T complex.

depolarizes. As a result, the outside of the cell, in the area where the stimulation has occurred, becomes negative, while the inside of the cell becomes positive. This produces a difference in electrical voltage on the outside of the cell between the stimulated depolarized area and the unstimulated polarized area (Fig. 2-1, *B*). As a result, a small electrical current is formed. This electrical current spreads along the length of the cell as stimulation and depolarization occur until the entire cell is depolarized (Fig. 2-1, *C*). The path of depolarization can be represented by an arrow, as shown in Fig. 2-1. For individual myocardial cells (fibers) depolarization and repolarization proceed in the same direction. However, for the entire myocardium depolarization proceeds from innermost layer (endocardium) to outermost layer (epicardium) while repolarization proceeds in the opposite direction. The mechanism of this difference is not well understood.

This depolarizing electrical current is recorded by the ECG as a *P wave* (when the atria are stimulated and depolarize) and as a *QRS complex* (when the ventricles are stimulated and depolarize).

After a period of time, the fully stimulated and depolarized cell begins to return to the resting state. This is known as repolarization. A small area on the outside of the cell becomes positive again (Fig. 2-1, *D*). The repolarization spreads along the length of the cell until the entire cell is once again fully repolarized. Ventricular repolarization is recorded by the ECG as the *ST segment, T wave,* and *U wave.* (Atrial repolarization is usually obscured by ventricular potentials, as will be discussed later.)

The ECG records the electrical activity of a large mass of atrial and ventricular cells, not just the electrical activity of a single cell. Since cardiac depolarization and repolarization normally occur in a synchronized fashion, the ECG is able to record these electrical currents as specific waves (P wave, QRS complex, ST segment, T wave, and U wave).

To summarize, regardless of whether the ECG is normal or abnormal, it merely records two basic events: (1) depolarization, the spread of a stimulus through the heart muscle, and (2) repolarization, the return of the stimulated heart muscle to the resting state.

BASIC ECG COMPLEXES: P, QRS, ST, T, AND U WAVES

This spread of a stimulus through the atria and ventricles and the return of the stimulated atrial and ventricular muscle to the resting state produce, as noted previously, the electrical currents recorded on the ECG. Furthermore, each phase of cardiac electrical activity produces a specific wave or complex (shown in Fig. 2-2). These basic ECG waves are labeled alphabetically and begin with the P wave.

P wave: atrial depolarization (stimulation)
QRS complex: ventricular depolarization (stimulation)
ST segment
T wave } ventricular repolarization
U wave (recovery)

The P wave represents the spread of a stimulus through the atria (atrial depolarization). The QRS complex represents the spread of a stimulus through the ventricles (ventricular depolarization). The ST segment and T wave represent return of the stimulated ventricular muscle to the resting state (ventricular repolarization). The U wave is a small deflection sometimes seen just after the T wave. It represents the final phase of ventricular repolarization, although its exact significance is not known.

You are probably wondering why there is no wave or complex representing the return of the stimulated atria to the resting state. The atrial ST segment (STa) and atrial T wave (Ta) are generally not observed on the normal ECG because of their low amplitudes.

(An important exception is discussed on p. 147.) Similarly the routine ECG is not sensitive enough to record any electrical activity during the spread of the stimulus through the AV junction (AV node and bundle of His). The spread of the electrical stimulus through the AV junction occurs between the beginning of the P wave and the beginning of the QRS complex. This interval, which is known as the PR interval, is a measure of the time it takes for the stimulus to spread through the atria and pass through the AV junction.

To summarize, the P-QRS-ST-T-U sequence represents the repetitive cycle of the electrical activity in the heart, beginning with the spread of a stimulus through the atria (P wave) and ending with the return of the stimulated ventricular muscle to the resting state (ST-T-U sequence). As shown in the rhythm strip in Fig. 2-3, this cardiac cycle repeats itself again and again.

ECG PAPER

The P-QRS-T sequence is recorded on special ECG paper (shown in Figs. 2-3 and 2-4). This paper is divided into gridlike boxes. Each of the small boxes is 1 millimeter square (1 mm²). The paper usually moves out of the electrocardiograph at a speed of 25 mm/sec. Therefore, horizontally, each millimeter of the ECG paper is equal to 0.04 second (25 mm/sec × 0.04 sec = 1 mm). Notice also that between every five boxes there are heavier lines, so each of the 5 mm units horizontally corresponds to 0.2 second (5 × 0.04 = 0.2).

BASIC ECG COMPLEXES

Fig. 2-2. The P wave represents atrial depolarization. The PR interval is the time from initial stimulation of the atria to initial stimulation of the ventricles. The QRS represents ventricular depolarization. The ST segment, T wave, and U wave are produced by ventricular repolarization.

Fig. 2-3. Cardiac cycle. The basic cycle (P-QRS-T) repeats itself again and again.

The ECG can therefore be regarded as a moving graph, which horizontally corresponds to time, with 0.04 and 0.2 second divisions. Vertically, the ECG graph measures the voltage, or amplitudes, of the ECG waves or deflections. The exact voltage can be measured because the electrocardiograph is so standardized that 1 millivolt (1 mV) produces a deflection of 10 mm amplitude (1 mV = 10 mm). (In most electrocardiographs, the standardization can also be set at one-half or two times normal sensitivity.)

BASIC ECG MEASUREMENTS AND SOME NORMAL VALUES
Standardization Mark

As just noted, the electrocardiograph must be properly standardized so a 1 mV signal produces a 10 mm deflection. Therefore every electrocardiograph has a special standardization button that produces a 1 mV wave. As shown in Fig. 2-5, the standardization mark (St) produced when the machine is correctly calibrated is a square wave 10 mm tall. If the machine is not standardized correctly, the 1

Fig. 2-4. ECG paper is a graph divided into millimeter squares. Time is measured on the horizontal axis. Each small millimeter box equals 0.04 second, and each larger (5 mm) box equals 0.2 second with a paper speed of 25 mm/sec. The amplitude of any wave is measured on the vertical axis in millimeters.

A   B   C

Fig. 2-5. Standardization mark. Before taking an ECG, the operator must calibrate the machine so the standardization mark is 10 mm tall, **A.** Electrocardiographs can also be set at half standardization, **B,** or 2 × standardization, **C.**

mV signal will produce a deflection either more or less than 10 mm, and the amplitudes of the P, QRS, and T deflections will be larger or smaller than they should. The standardization deflection is also important because the standardization can be varied in the newer electrocardiographs (Fig. 2-5). When very large deflections are present (as occurs, for example, in some patients who have an electronic pacemaker that produces very large spikes), it may be advisable to take the ECG at half standardization to avoid damaging the stylus and to get the entire tracing on the paper. If the ECG complexes are very small, it may be advisable to double the standardization (for example, to study a small Q wave more thoroughly). The standardization need be set only once on an ECG—just before the first lead is recorded.

Because the ECG is standardized, we can describe any part of the P, QRS, and T deflections in two ways. We can measure the amplitude (voltage) of any of the deflections, and we can also measure the width (duration) of any of the deflections. We can therefore measure the amplitude and width of the P wave, the amplitude and width of the QRS complex, the amplitude of the ST segment deviation (if present), and the amplitude of

Fig. 2-6. Positive and negative complexes. The P wave here is positive (upward), and the T wave is negative (downward). The QRS complex is biphasic (partly positive, partly negative), and the ST segment isoelectric (neither positive nor negative).

the T wave. For clinical purposes, if the standardization is set at 1 mV = 10 mm, the height of a wave is usually recorded in millimeters and not in millivolts. For example, in Fig. 2-3, the P wave is 1 mm in amplitude, the QRS complex is 8 mm, and the T wave is about 3.5 mm.

In describing the amplitude of any wave or

Fig. 2-7. Measurement of the PR interval. See text.

deflection, it is also necessary to specify if it is positive or negative. By convention, an *upward* deflection or wave is called *positive*. A *downward* deflection or wave is called *negative*. A deflection or wave that rests on the baseline is said to be *isoelectric*. A deflection that is partly positive and partly negative is called *biphasic*. For example, in Fig. 2-6 the P wave is positive, the QRS complex is biphasic (initially positive, then negative), the ST segment is isoelectric (flat on the baseline), and the T wave is negative.

In this chapter we shall describe the P, QRS, ST, T, and U waves in a general way and the measurement of the heart rate, the PR interval, the QRS width, the QT interval, and their normal values in detail.

P wave

The P wave, which represents atrial depolarization, is a small deflection before the QRS complex. The normal values for P wave amplitude and width are described in Chapter 6.

PR Interval

The PR interval is measured from the beginning of the P wave to the beginning of the QRS complex (Fig. 2-7). The PR interval may vary slightly in different leads, and the

shortest PR interval should be noted. The PR interval represents the time it takes for the stimulus to spread through the atria and to pass through the AV junction. (This physiologic delay allows the ventricles to fill fully with blood before ventricular depolarization occurs.) *In adults the normal PR interval is between 0.12 and 0.2 second (three to five small boxes).* When conduction through the AV junction is impaired, the PR interval may become prolonged. Prolongation of the PR interval above 0.2 second is called *first-degree heart block* and is discussed in Chapter 15.

QRS Nomenclature

One of the most confusing aspects of electrocardiography for the beginning student is the nomenclature of the QRS complex. The QRS complex, as noted previously, represents the spread of a stimulus through the ventricles. However, not every QRS complex contains a Q wave, an R wave, and an S wave; hence the confusion. This bothersome but unavoidable nomenclature becomes understandable if you remember the following (Fig. 2-8): If the initial deflection of the QRS complex is negative (below the baseline), it is called a Q wave. The first positive deflection in the QRS complex is called an R

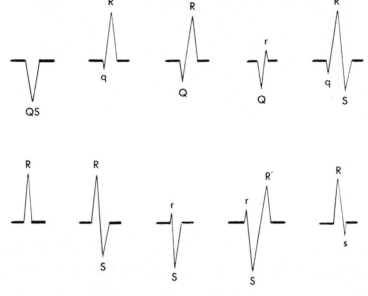

Fig. 2-8. QRS nomenclature. See text.

wave. A negative deflection following the R wave is called an S wave. Thus this QRS complex $\left(\begin{smallmatrix} R \\ \wedge \\ Q \; S \end{smallmatrix}\right)$ contains a Q wave, an R wave, and an S wave. This one $\left(\begin{smallmatrix} R \\ \wedge \end{smallmatrix}\right)$ does not. If the entire QRS complex is positive, it is simply called an R wave. However, if the entire complex is negative, it is termed a QS wave (not just a Q wave as you might expect). Occasionally the QRS complex will contain more than two or three deflections, and in such cases the extra waves are called R' (R prime) waves if they are positive and S' (S prime) waves if they are negative. Fig. 2-8 shows the various possible QRS complexes and the nomenclature of the respective waves. Note that the capital letters (QRS) are used to designate waves of relatively large amplitude while small letters (qrs) are used to label relatively small waves (Fig. 2-8).

This nomenclature is confusing at first, but it allows you to describe any QRS complex over the phone and to evoke in the mind of the trained listener an exact mental picture of the complex named. For example, in describing an ECG you might say that lead V_1 showed an rS complex $\left(\begin{smallmatrix} r \\ \vee \\ S \end{smallmatrix}\right)$ ("small r, capital S") while lead aV_F showed a QS wave $\left(\begin{smallmatrix} \vee \\ QS \end{smallmatrix}\right)$.

QRS Width (Interval)

The QRS width (Fig. 2-9) represents the time required for a stimulus to spread through the ventricles (ventricular depolarization) and is normally 0.1 second or less. If the spread of stimulus through the ventricles is slowed, for example, by a block in one of the bundle branches, the QRS width will be prolonged. (The full differential diagnosis of a wide QRS is discussed on p. 155.)

Fig. 2-9. Measurement of the QRS width. See text.

Fig. 2-10. Characteristics of the normal ST segment and T wave. *J*, junction, marks the beginning of the ST segment.

ST Segment

The ST segment is the portion of the ECG cycle from the end of the QRS complex to the beginning of the T wave (Fig 2-10). It represents the beginning of ventricular repolarization. The normal ST segment is usually *isoelectric* (that is, flat on the baseline, neither positive nor negative), but it may be slightly elevated or depressed normally (usually by less than 1 mm). Some pathologic conditions, such as myocardial infarction, produce characteristic abnormal deviations of the ST segment. The very beginning of the ST segment (actually the junction between the end of the QRS complex and the beginning of the ST segment) is sometimes called the J point. Fig. 2-10 shows the J point and the normal shape of the ST segment. Fig. 2-11 compares a normal isoelectric ST segment with abnormal ST segment elevation and ST segment depression.

T Wave

The T wave represents part of ventricular repolarization. A normal T wave has an asymmetric shape; that is, its peak is closer to the end of the wave than to the beginning (Fig. 2-10). When the T wave is positive, it normally rises slowly and then abruptly returns to the baseline.* When the T wave is negative, it descends slowly and abruptly rises to the baseline (Fig. 2-10). The *asymmetry* of the normal T wave contrasts with the symmetry of T waves in certain abnormal conditions, such as myocardial infarction (Chapters 8 and 9) and high serum potassium (hyperkalemia) (Chapter 10).

---

*The exact point at which the ST segment ends and the T wave begins is arbitrary and sometimes impossible to define.

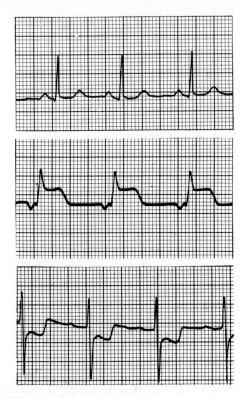

Fig. 2-11. ST segments. *Top,* Normal. *Middle,* Abnormal elevation. *Bottom,* Abnormal depression.

Table 1. QT Interval: Upper Limits of Normal

Measured RR Interval (sec)	Heart Rate (per min)	QT Interval Upper Normal Limits(sec)
1.50	40	0.50
1.20	50	0.45
1.00	60	0.42
0.86	70	0.40
0.80	75	0.38
0.75	80	0.37
0.67	90	0.35
0.60	100	0.34
0.50	120	0.31
0.40	150	0.25

perceptibly with the U wave. As a result you may be measuring the QU interval rather than the QT interval.

Table 1 shows the upper normal limits for the QT interval with different heart rates. Unfortunately, there is no simple rule for calculating the normal limits of the QT interval.

Because of this problem, another index of the QT has been devised. It is the *rate-corrected* QT or QT$_c$. The rate-corrected QT is obtained by dividing the QT that you actually measure by the square root of the RR interval:

$$\frac{QT}{\sqrt{RR}}$$

Normally the QT$_c$ is less than 0.44.

QT Interval

The QT interval is measured from the beginning of the QRS complex to the end of the T wave (Fig. 2-12). The QT interval primarily represents the return of the stimulated ventricles to their resting state (ventricular repolarization). The normal values for the QT interval depend on the heart rate. As the heart rate increases (RR interval shortens), the QT interval normally shortens; as the heart rate decreases (RR interval lengthens), the QT interval lengthens.

You should measure several QT intervals and use the average value. The QT interval is often difficult to measure when it is long because the end of the T wave may merge im-

There are a number of factors that can abnormally prolong the QT interval (Fig. 2-13). For example, certain drugs, such as quinidine and procainamide (Pronestyl, Procan SR), and electrolyte disturbances, such as a low serum potassium (hypokalemia) or low serum calcium (hypocalcemia), can prolong the QT interval. The QT interval may also be prolonged with myocardial ischemia and infarction and with subarachnoid hemorrhage.

Fig. 2-12. Measurement of the QT interval. *RR* is the interval between two consecutive QRS complexes. See text.

QT prolongation may predispose patients to potentially lethal ventricular arrhythmias (see p. 210).

The QT interval may also be shortened, for example, by digitalis in therapeutic doses or by hypercalcemia (high serum calcium concentration). The lower limits of normal for the QT interval have not been well defined, so only the upper normal values are given in Table 1.

U Wave

The U wave is a small rounded deflection sometimes seen after the T wave (Fig. 2-2). As noted previously, the exact significance of the U wave is not known. Functionally U waves represent the last phase of ventricular repolarization. Prominent U waves are characteristic of hypokalemia (low serum potassium, Chapter 10). Very prominent U waves may also be seen in other settings, for example, in patients taking drugs such as quinidine or one of the phenothiazines, or sometimes after cerebrovascular accidents. The appearance of very prominent U waves in such settings, with or without actual QT prolongation, may also predispose patients to ventricular arrhythmias (p. 210).

Fig. 2-13. Abnormal QT prolongation in a patient taking quinidine. The QT interval (0.6 sec) is markedly prolonged for the heart rate (65/min). See Table 1. The rate-corrected QT (normally less than 0.44) is also prolonged (0.63).*

---

*In Fig. 2-13, find the QT_c:

$$\frac{QT}{\sqrt{RR}} = \frac{0.60}{\sqrt{0.92}} = 0.63$$

Normally the direction of the U wave is the same as the direction of the T wave. Negative U waves sometimes appear with positive T waves. This is abnormal and has been noted in left ventricular hypertrophy and myocardial ischemia.

Calculation of Heart Rate

There are two simple methods for measuring the heart rate (number of heartbeats per minute) from the ECG.

1. The easier way, when the heart rate is regular, is to count the number of large (0.2 sec) boxes between two successive QRS complexes and divide the constant (300) by this. (The number of large time boxes is divided into 300, because 300 × 0.2 = 60 and we are calculating the heart rate in beats per minute or 60 seconds.)

For example, in Fig. 2-14 the heart rate is 100 beats/min, since there are three large time boxes between two successive R waves (300 ÷ 3 = 100). Similarly, if there are two large time boxes between two successive R waves, the heart rate is 150 beats/min. If there are five intervening large time boxes, the heart rate is 60 beats/min.

If it is necessary to measure the heart rate very accurately from the ECG, you can use the following modification of the above rule: Count the number of small (0.04 sec) boxes between two successive R waves and divide the constant (1500) by this number. For example, in Fig. 2-14 there are 15 small time boxes between two successive QRS complexes. Therefore the heart rate is 1500 ÷ 15 = 100 beats/min. (The constant 1500 is used since 1500 × 0.04 = 60 and the heart rate is calculated in beats per 60 seconds.)

2. If the heart rate is irregular, the first method will not be accurate since the intervals between QRS complexes will vary from beat to beat. In such cases an average rate can be determined simply by counting the number of cardiac *cycles* every 6 seconds and multiplying this number by 10 (Fig. 2-15). (A cardiac cycle is the interval between two successive R waves.) Counting the number of cardiac cycles every 6 seconds can be easily done because the top of the ECG paper, as

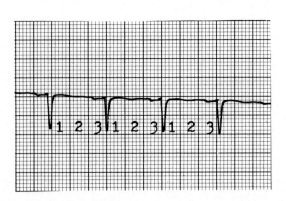

Fig. 2-14. Measurement of heart rate (beats per minute) by counting the number of large (0.2 sec) time boxes between two successive QRS complexes and dividing 300 by this number. In this example the heart rate is 300 ÷ 3 = 100 beats/min.

shown in Fig. 2-14, is generally scored with vertical marks every 3 seconds.

By definition, a heart rate exceeding 100 beats/min is termed "tachycardia" (*tachys,* Greek, swift) while one slower than 60 beats/min is called "bradycardia" (*bradys,* slow). Thus, during exercise you probably develop a sinus tachycardia but during sleep or relaxation your pulse rate may drop into the 50s, or even lower, indicating a sinus bradycardia.

THE ECG AS A COMBINATION OF ATRIAL AND VENTRICULAR ELECTROCARDIOGRAMS

The ECG we have been discussing really consists of two separate but normally related parts: an atrial ECG, represented by the P wave, and a ventricular ECG, represented by the QRS-T-U sequence. With normal sinus rhythm, when the sinus node is pacing the heart, the P wave (atrial stimulation or depolarization) will always precede the QRS complex (ventricular stimulation or depolarization) because the atria are first to be elec-

trically stimulated. Therefore we normally consider the P-QRS-T cycle as a unit. However, as we shall see later on, in some abnormal conditions the atria and the ventricles can be stimulated by separate pacemakers. For example, suppose that the AV junction is diseased and stimuli cannot pass from the atria to the ventricles. In such cases a new (subsidiary) pacemaker located below the level of the block in the AV junction may take over the task of pacing the ventricles while the sinus node continues to pace the atria. In this case, stimulation of the atria is independent of stimulation of the ventricles, and the P waves and QRS complexes have no relation to each other. This type of arrhythmia is called *complete heart block* and is described in detail in Chapter 15. Fig. 15-5 shows an example of this abnormal condition, in which the atrial and ventricular ECGs are independent of each other.

THE ECG IN PERSPECTIVE

Up to this point we have described the basic components of the ECG. Several general

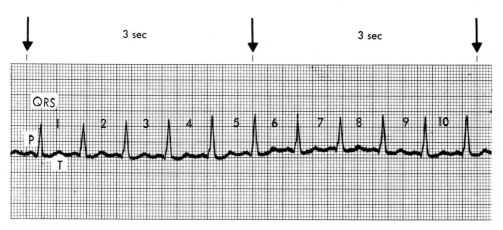

Fig. 2-15. Measurement of heart rate (beats per minute) by counting the number of cardiac cycles in a 6-second interval and multiplying by 10. In this example there are 10 cardiac cycles/6 sec. Therefore the heart rate is 10 × 10 = 100 beats/min.

points should be emphasized before proceeding with our discussion of actual ECG patterns.

First, it is always necessary to remember that the ECG is a recording of cardiac *electrical* acitivity. It does not directly measure the *mechanical* function of the heart, that is, how well the heart is contracting and performing as a pump. Thus a patient with acute pulmonary edema may have a normal ECG. Conversely, a patient with a grossly abnormal ECG may have normal cardiac function.

Furthermore, the ECG does not directly depict abnormalities in cardiac structure, such as ventricular septal defects, or abnormalities of the heart valves. The ECG only records the electrical changes produced by structural defects. However, in some cases it is possible to infer a specific structural diagnosis such as mitral stenosis, pulmonary embolism, or myocardial infarction from the ECG because typical electrical abnormalities may develop in such patients.

Finally, it is necessary to remember that the ECG does not record all the heart's electrical activity. The electrodes placed on the surface of the body record only those currents transmitted to the area of electrode placement. Therefore there are actually "silent" electrical areas of the heart. For example, repolarization of the atria (as noted earlier) is generally not recorded by the conventional electrocardiograph; also the spread of stimulus through the AV junction is not detected by the conventional ECG. The electrical activity of the AV junction can be recorded using a special apparatus and a special electrode placed in the heart (*His bundle electrogram*). In addition, remember that the ECG records the summation of electrical potentials produced by innumerable cardiac muscle cells. Therefore the presence of a normal ECG does not necessarily mean that all these heart muscle cells are being depolarized and repolarized in a normal way.

For these reasons, the ECG must be regarded as any other laboratory test, with proper consideration for both its uses and its limitations (see Chapter 19).

In Chapter 3 we shall describe the 12 ECG leads and then proceed with a discussion of normal and abnormal ECG patterns.

REVIEW OF CHAPTER 2

The ECG, whether normal or abnormal, records the following two basic physiologic processes: (1) *Depolarization* (the spread of a stimulus through the heart muscle) produces the P wave from the atria and the QRS complex from the ventricles. (2) *Repolarization* (the return of stimulated muscle to the resting state) produces the atrial ST segment and T wave (which are ordinarily not seen on the ECG) and the ventricular ST segment, T wave, and U wave.

ECGs are recorded on special paper that is divided into gridlike boxes (Fig. 2-4). Each small box is 1 mm². Each millimeter horizontally represents 0.04 second. Each 0.2 second is noted by a heavier vertical line. ECG deflections are usually standardized so a 1 mV signal produces a 10 mm deflection. Therefore, each millimeter vertically represents 0.1 mV. Each 5 mm interval is noted by a heavier horizontal line.

Basic measurements of an ECG should include the following:

1. *Standardization mark.* The ECG needs to be standardized only before the first lead is recorded.
2. *PR interval.* The PR interval is measured from the beginning of the P wave to the beginning of the QRS complex. The normal PR interval varies from 0.12 to 0.2 second.
3. *QRS width.* The normal QRS width is 0.1 second or less. Description of the QRS complex is shown in Fig. 2-8.
4. *QT interval.* The QT interval is measured from the beginning of the QRS complex to the end of the T wave. It varies with the heart rate, becoming shorter as the heart rate increases.
5. *Heart rate.* The heart rate can be calculated in two ways:
   METHOD 1. Count the number of large (0.2 sec) time boxes between two successive R waves and divide the constant, 300, by this number (Fig. 2-14). If you want a more accurate measurement of the rate, divide the constant, 1500, by the number of small (0.04 sec) time boxes between two successive R waves.
   METHOD 2. Count the number of cardiac cycles that occur every 6 seconds and multiply this number by 10 (Fig. 2-15). A vertical mark appears on the top of the ECG paper every 3 seconds. A cardiac cycle is the interval between two successive R waves.

A heart rate slower than 60 beats/min is called *bradycardia;* a heart rate faster than 100 beats/min is called *tachycardia*.

Review Questions—Chapter 2

1. Calculate the heart rate in each of the following examples.

2. Name the major abnormality in each example.

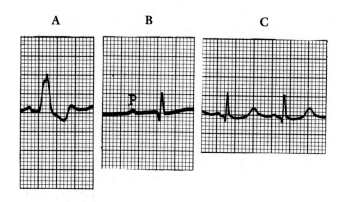

3. A block in the AV node is most likely to
   a. Prolong the PR interval
   b. Prolong the QRS width
   c. Prolong the QT interval
   d. None of the above
4. A block in the left or right bundle branch is most likely to
   a. Prolong the PR interval
   b. Prolong the QRS width
   c. Shorten the QT interval
   d. None of the above
5. Name the component waves of the QRS complexes shown below.

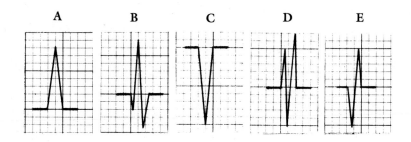

Answers

1. a. 50 beats/min.
   b. 150 beats/min.
   c. 60 beats/min.
   d. Approximately 160 beats/min. There are 16 QRS cycles in 6 seconds.*
2. a. Abnormally wide QRS complex (0.14 sec).
   b. Abnormally long PR interval (approximately 0.3 sec).

   c. Abnormally long QT interval (0.4 sec). The RR interval measures 0.6 second, and the heart rate is 100/min. (See Table 1, p. 17.)
3. a.
4. b.
5. a. R.
   b. qRS.
   c. QS.
   d. RSR′.
   e. QR.

---

*Notice the irregularity of the QRS complexes and the absence of P waves. The rhythm here is *atrial fibrillation* (Chapter 13).

3 ECG Leads

In Chapter 1 we pointed out that the heart produces electrical currents similar to the familiar dry cell battery. The strength or voltage of these currents and the way they are distributed throughout the body can be measured by a suitable recording instrument, such as an electrocardiograph.

The body acts as a conductor of electricity. Therefore, recording electrodes placed at some distance from the heart, such as on the arms, legs, or chest wall, are able to detect the voltages of the cardiac currents conducted to these locations. The usual way of recording these voltages from the heart is with the 12 standard ECG *leads*. The leads actually show the *differences* in voltage (potential) between electrodes placed on the surface of the body.

Taking an ECG is like drawing a picture or taking a photograph of a person. If we want to know what a person's face really looks like, for example, we have to draw it or take photographs from the front, side, and back. One view is not enough. Similarly, it is necessary to record multiple ECG leads to be able to describe the electrical activity of the heart adequately. Fig. 3-1 shows the various ECG patterns that are obtained when electrodes are placed at varying points on the chest. Notice that each lead presents a different pattern.

A sample ECG is shown in Fig. 3-2, illustrating the 12 leads. The 12 leads can be subdivided into two groups: the six *extremity* (limb) leads (shown in the top rows) and the six *chest (precordial)* leads (shown in the bottom rows).

The six extremity leads—I, II, III, aV_R, aV_L, and aV_F—show voltage differences by means of electrodes placed on the limbs. They can be further divided into two subgroups: the *bipolar* extremity leads (I, II, and III) and the *unipolar* extremity leads (aV_R, aV_L, and aV_F).

The six chest leads—V_1, V_2, V_3, V_4, V_5, and V_6—present voltage differences by means of electrodes placed at various positions on the chest wall.

Fig. 3-1. Multiple chest leads give a three-dimensional view of cardiac electrical activity.

Fig. 3-2. Sample ECG mounted for interpretation showing the 12 standard leads.

The 12 ECG leads can also be viewed as 12 "channels." However, in contrast to television channels (which can be tuned to different events), the 12 ECG channels (leads) are all tuned to the *same* event (the P-QRS-T cycle), with each lead viewing the event from a different angle.

EXTREMITY (LIMB) LEADS
Bipolar Leads (I, II, and III)

We will begin with the extremity leads, since they are recorded first. In connecting a patient to an electrocardiograph, first place metal electrodes on the arms and legs. The

right leg electrode functions solely as an electrical ground, so you need concern yourself with it no further. As shown in Fig. 3-3, attach the arm electrodes just above the wrist and the leg electrodes above the ankles.

The electrical voltages of the heart are conducted through the torso to the extremities. Therefore an electrode placed on the right wrist will detect electrical voltages equivalent to those detected below the right shoulder. Similarly, the voltages detected at the left wrist or anywhere else on the left arm will be equivalent to those detected below the left shoulder. Finally, voltages detected by the left leg electrode will be comparable to those at the left thigh or near the groin. In clinical practice the electrodes are attached to the wrists and ankles simply for convenience.*

As mentioned, the extremity leads consist of two groups: the bipolar (I, II, and III) and the unipolar (aV_R, aV_L, and aV_F) leads. The bipolar leads are so named because the differences in electrical voltage between two extremities are recorded by them.

From lead I, for example, the difference in voltage is recorded between the left arm (LA) and the right arm (RA).

$$Lead\ I = LA - RA$$

From lead II the difference is recorded between the left leg (LL) and the right arm (RA).

$$Lead\ II = LL - RA$$

From lead III the difference is recorded between the left leg (LL) and the left arm (LA).

$$Lead\ III = LL - LA$$

Consider then what happens when you turn on the electrocardiograph to lead I. The LA electrode detects the electrical voltages of the heart transmitted to the left arm. The RA electrode detects the voltages transmitted to the right arm. Inside the electrocardiograph the RA voltages are subtracted from the LA voltages and the difference appears at lead I. When lead II is recorded, a similar situation occurs between the voltages of LL and RA. When lead III is recorded, the same occurs between the voltages of LL and LA.

Leads I, II, and III can be represented schematically in terms of a triangle, called *Einthoven's triangle* (after the Dutch physician who invented the electrocardiograph). At first the ECG consisted only of recordings

---

*Obviously, if you are taking an ECG on an amputee or someone with a cast, you will have to place the electrodes below or near the shoulders or groin depending on the circumstance.

Fig. 3-3. Metal electrodes placed on the patient to take an ECG. The right leg *(RL)* electrode functions solely as ground to prevent alternating current interference.

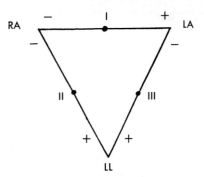

Fig. 3-4. Orientations of leads I, II, and III. Lead I records the difference in electrical potentials between the left arm and the right arm. Lead II records it between the left leg and the right arm. Lead III records it between the left leg and left arm.

from leads I, II, and III. Einthoven's triangle (Fig. 3-4) shows the spatial orientation of the three bipolar extremity leads (I, II, and III). As you can see, lead I points horizontally. Its left pole (LA) is positive and its right pole (RA) is negative. Therefore lead I = LA − RA. Lead II points diagonally downward. Its lower pole (LL) is positive and its upper pole (RA) is negative. Therefore lead II = LL − RA. Lead III also points diagonally downward. Its lower pole (LL) is positive and its upper pole (LA) is negative. Therefore lead III = LL − LA.

Einthoven, of course, could have hooked the leads up differently; but because of the way he arranged them, the bipolar leads are related by the following simple equation:

$$\text{Lead I} + \text{Lead III} = \text{Lead II}$$

In other words, add the voltage in lead I to that in lead III and you get the voltage in lead II.* You can test this equation by look-

ing at the ECG in Fig. 3-2. Add the voltage of the R wave in lead I (+ 6 mm) to the voltage of the R wave in lead III (+ 5 mm) and you get +11 mm, the voltage of the R wave in lead II. You can do the same with the voltages of the P waves and T waves.

It is a good custom to scan leads I, II, and III rapidly when you first look at a mounted ECG. If the R wave in lead II does not seem to be the sum of the R waves in leads I and III, this may be a clue that the leads have been either recorded incorrectly or mounted improperly.

Einthoven's equation is simply the result of the way the bipolar leads are recorded. (The LA is positive in lead I and negative in lead III and thus cancels out when the two leads are added.)

$$\frac{\begin{array}{l} \text{I} = \cancel{\text{LA}} - \text{RA} \\ \text{III} = \text{LL} - \cancel{\text{LA}} \end{array}}{\text{I} + \text{III} = \text{LL} - \text{RA} = \text{II}}$$

In electrocardiography, therefore, one plus three equals two.

To summarize, the first three leads (I, II, and III) are bipolar extremity leads, which historically were the first invented. These leads record the differences in electrical voltage between extremities.

In Fig. 3-5, we have redrawn the Einthoven triangle so leads I, II, and III all in-

---

*This rule is only approximate. It is exact when the three bipolar extremity leads are recorded simultaneously, using a three-channel electrocardiograph, because the peaks of the R waves in the three leads do *not* occur simultaneously. The exact rule is as follows: the voltage at the peak of the R wave (or at any point) in lead II equals the sum of the voltages in leads I and III at points occurring simultaneously.

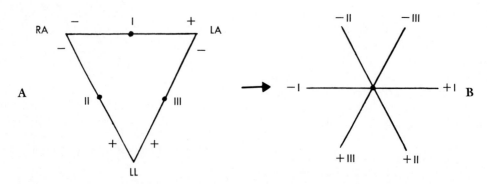

Fig. 3-5. Einthoven's triangle, **A,** has been converted to a triaxial diagram, **B.** This is done simply by shifting leads I, II, and III so they intersect at a common point.

tersect at a common central point. This was done simply by sliding lead I downward, sliding lead II rightward, and sliding lead III leftward. The result is the *triaxial* diagram in Fig. 3-5, *B*. This triaxial diagram is simply a useful way of representing the three bipolar leads and will be used later (in Chapter 5).

Unipolar Extremity Leads (aV$_R$, aV$_L$, and aV$_F$)

Following the invention of the three bipolar extremity leads nine additional leads were added. In the 1930s Dr. Frank N. Wilson and his colleagues at the University of Michigan invented the unipolar limb leads and introduced the six unipolar chest leads, V$_1$ through V$_6$. Shortly after this, one of the authors of this text (E.G.) invented the three augmented unipolar extremity leads, aV$_R$, aV$_L$, and aV$_F$. The abbreviation *a* refers to *augmented; V, voltage; R, L,* and *F, right arm, left arm,* and *left foot* (leg) respectively. So, today, 12 leads are routinely employed.

A unipolar lead records the electrical voltages at one location relative to zero potential, rather than relative to the voltages at another extremity, as in the case of the bipolar extremity leads. The zero potential is obtained inside the electrocardiograph by joining the three extremity leads to a central terminal. Since the sum of the voltages of RA, LA, and LL equals zero, the central terminal has a zero voltage. The aV$_R$, aV$_L$, and aV$_F$ leads are derived in a slightly different way, because the voltages recorded by the electrocardiograph have been augmented 50% over the actual voltages detected at each extremity. This augmentation is also done electronically inside the electrocardiograph.*

Just as we used Einthoven's triangle to represent the spatial orientation of the three bipolar extremity leads, so we can use the diagram in Fig. 3-6 to represent the spatial orientation of the three unipolar extremity leads. Note that each of the unipolar leads can be represented by a line (axis) with a positive and a negative pole. Since the diagram has three axes, it is also called a *triaxial* diagram.

The positive pole of lead aV$_R$, the right arm lead, points upward and to the patient's right arm as you would expect. The positive pole of lead aV$_L$ points upward and to the patient's left arm. The positive pole of lead aV$_F$ points downward toward the patient's left foot.

Furthermore, just as leads I, II, and III are

---

*Augmentation was developed to make the complexes more readable.

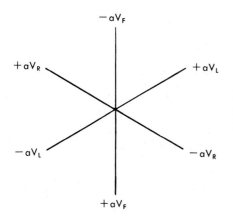

Fig. 3-6. Triaxial lead diagram showing the relationship of the three augmented unipolar leads: aV$_R$, aV$_L$, and aV$_F$.

related by Einthoven's equation, so leads aV_R, aV_L, and aV_F likewise are related:

$$aV_R + aV_L + aV_F = 0$$

In other words, when the three unipolar extremity leads are recorded, they should total zero. Thus the sum of the P wave voltages is zero, the sum of the QRS voltages is zero, and the same holds for the T wave voltages. Go back to Fig. 3-2 and test this equation by adding the sum of the QRS voltages in the three unipolar extremity leads, aV_R, aV_L, and aV_F.

It is also a good custom to scan leads aV_R, aV_L, and aV_F rapidly when you first look at a mounted ECG. If the sum of the waves in these three leads does not equal zero, this may also be a clue that these leads have either been recorded incorrectly or mounted improperly.

The ECG leads, both bipolar and unipolar, have two major features, which we have already described. They have both a specific *orientation* and a specific *polarity*.

Thus the axis of lead I is oriented horizontally while the axis of lead aV_R points diago-

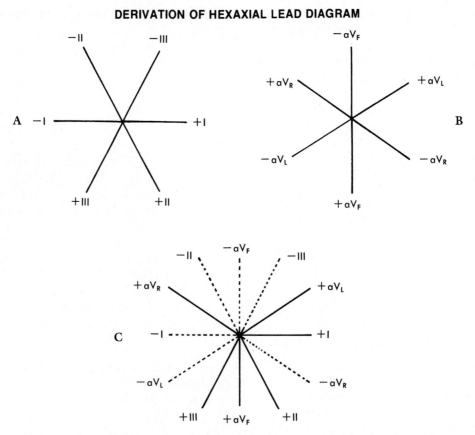

DERIVATION OF HEXAXIAL LEAD DIAGRAM

Fig. 3-7. Triaxial diagrams of the bipolar leads (I, II, and III), **A,** and the unipolar leads (aV_R, aV_L, and aV_F), **B,** can be combined into a hexaxial diagram, **C,** showing the relationship of all six extremity leads.

nally downward. The orientation of the bipolar leads is shown in Einthoven's triangle (Fig. 3-5) while that of the unipolar extremity leads is diagrammed in Fig. 3-6.

The second major feature of the ECG leads, their polarity, can be represented by a line (axis) with a positive and a negative pole, as shown before. The polarity and spatial orientation of the leads are discussed further in Chapters 4 and 5 (when we describe the normal ECG patterns seen in each of the leads and the concept of electrical axis).

Do not be confused by the difference in meaning between ECG electrodes and ECG leads. An *electrode* is simply the metal plate used to detect the electrical currents of the heart in any location. An ECG *lead*, as we have been discussing, shows the differences in voltage detected by these electrodes. (For example, lead I presents the differences in voltage detected by the left and right arm electrodes.) Therefore, a lead is simply a means of recording the differences in cardiac voltages obtained by different electrodes.

Relationship Between Unipolar and Bipolar Extremity Leads

The Einthoven triangle (Fig. 3-4) shows the relationship of the three bipolar extremity leads (I, II, and III). Similarly the triaxial diagram in Fig. 3-7 shows the relationship of the three unipolar extremity leads (aV_R, aV_L, and aV_F). For convenience, we can combine these two diagrams so the axes of all six extremity leads intersect at a common point. The result is the *hexaxial* lead diagram shown in Fig. 3-7. The hexaxial diagram shows the spatial orientation of the six extremity leads (I, II, III, aV_R, aV_L, and aV_F).

The exact relationships among the three unipolar extremity leads and the three bipolar extremity leads can also be described mathematically. However, for present purposes, the following simple guidelines allow you to get an overall impression of the similarities between these two sets of leads.

As you might expect by looking at the hexaxial diagram, the pattern in lead aV_L usually resembles that in lead I. Lead aV_R and lead II, on the other hand, point in opposite directions. Therefore, the P-QRS-T pattern recorded by lead aV_R is generally the reverse of that recorded by lead II. (For example, when lead II shows a qR $\left(\begin{smallmatrix} R \\ \wedge \\ \end{smallmatrix}\right)$ pattern lead aV_R usually shows an rS $\left(\begin{smallmatrix} r \\ \vee \\ S \end{smallmatrix}\right)$ pattern.) Finally, the pattern shown by lead aV_F usually but not always resembles that shown by lead III.

CHEST (PRECORDIAL) LEADS

The chest leads (V_1 to V_6) show the electrical currents of the heart detected by electrodes placed at different positions on the chest wall. The chest leads used today are also unipolar leads in that they measure the voltage in any one location relative to zero potential. By convention the six leads are placed as follows*:

  Lead V_1 is recorded with the electrode in the fourth intercostal space just to the right of the sternum.
  Lead V_2 is recorded with the electrode in the fourth intercostal space just to the left of the sternum.
  Lead V_3 is recorded on a line midway between leads V_2 and V_4.
  Lead V_4 is recorded in the midclavicular line in the fifth interspace.
  Lead V_5 is recorded in the anterior axillary line at the same level as lead V_4.
  Lead V_6 is recorded in the midaxillary line at the same level as lead V_4.

The chest leads are recorded simply by means of electrodes (usually attached to suction

---

*Sometimes, in special circumstances, additional leads are placed on the right side of the chest. For example, lead V_{3R} is equivalent to V_3 but the electrode is placed to the right of the sternum.

cups to hold them in place on the chest) at six designated locations on the chest wall (Fig. 3-8).

Two points are worth mentioning here:

First, how do you locate the fourth intercostal space? Start by placing your finger at the top of the sternum and moving it slowly downward. After moving down about 1½ inches, you will feel a slight horizontal ridge. This is called the *angle of Louis* (Fig. 3-8), where the manubrium joins the body of the sternum. The second intercostal space is just below and lateral to this point. Move down two more spaces and you are in the fourth interspace and ready to place lead V_1.

Second, in females the situation is complicated by breast tissue, which may result in misplacement of the chest leads. In taking ECGs on women you must remember to place the electrode *under* the breast for leads V_4 to V_6. If, as so often happens, the electrode is placed *on* the breast, you will be recording electrical voltages from higher interspaces.

(*Never* use the nipples to locate the position of any of the chest lead electrodes, even in men, because nipple location varies greatly in different persons.)

The chest leads, like the six extremity leads, can be represented diagrammatically as shown in Fig. 3-9. Like the other leads, each of the chest leads has a positive and a negative pole. The positive pole of each chest lead points anteriorly, toward the front of the chest. The negative pole of the chest leads points posteriorly, toward the back (*dotted lines* in Fig. 3-9).

TAKING AN ECG

Now you are ready to take an ECG. The extremity electrodes are attached to the patient. First, the machine is standardized (p. 11). Then the dial on the electrocardiograph is turned to lead I. Several P-QRS-T cycles are run. Next, the dial is advanced to lead II and the ECG records a few more cycles. This is repeated for leads III, aV_R, aV_L, and aV_F.

CHEST LEAD PLACEMENT

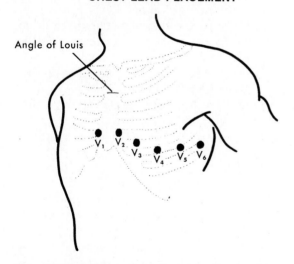

Fig. 3-8. Locations of the electrodes for the chest (precordial) leads.

ORIENTATION OF CHEST LEADS

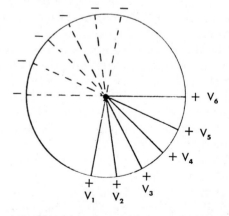

Fig. 3-9. Note that the positive poles of the chest leads point anteriorly and the negative poles (indicated by *dotted lines*) point posteriorly.

Next the dial is turned to the V position for the chest leads. The suction cup is placed in the V_1 position, and so on until the six V leads have been recorded. The result is a long ECG strip showing the 12 leads recorded sequentially.* The ECGs in this book have been cut and mounted in the usual way for interpretation (Fig. 3-2).

THE 12-LEAD ECG: FRONTAL AND HORIZONTAL PLANE LEADS

You may now be wondering why we use 12 leads in clinical electrocardiography; why not 10 or 22? The reason for exactly 12 leads is partly historical, a matter of the way the ECG has evolved over the years since Einthoven's original three bipolar extremity leads. There is nothing sacred about the electrocardiographer's dozen. In some cases, for example, we do record additional leads by placing the chest electrode at different positions on the chest wall. There are good reasons for using multiple leads. The heart, after all, is a three-dimensional structure, and its electrical currents spread out in all directions across the body. Recall that we described the ECG leads as being like photographs by which we can see the electrical activity of the heart from different locations. To a certain extent, the more points we record from the more accurate will be our representation of the heart's electrical activity.

The importance of multiple leads is illustrated in the diagnosis of myocardial infarction (MI). An MI typically affects one localized portion of either the anterior or the inferior portion of the left ventricle. The ECG changes produced by an anterior MI are usually best shown by the chest leads, which are close to and face the injured ante-

rior surface of the heart, while the changes seen with an inferior MI usually appear only in leads such as II, III, and aV_F, which face the injured inferior surface of the heart. (We discuss this further in Chapters 8 and 9.) The 12 leads therefore provide a three-dimensional view of the electrical activity of the heart.

Specifically, the six extremity leads (I, II, III, aV_R, aV_L, aV_F) will show electrical voltages transmitted onto the *frontal* plane of the body (Fig. 3-10) (while the six precordial leads show voltages transmitted onto the horizontal plane). For example, if you walk up

FRONTAL PLANE LEADS

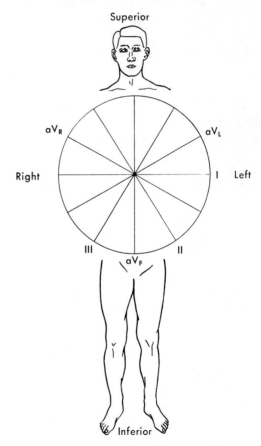

Fig. 3-10. Note the spatial relationships of the six extremity (frontal plane) leads.

---

*Many of the modern electrocardiographs have been designed to record three ECG leads simultaneously; thus leads (I, II, III), (aV_R, aV_L, aV_F), (V_1 to V_3), and (V_4 to V_6) can be recorded at the same time. (For example, see Fig. 10-6.)

HORIZONTAL PLANE LEADS

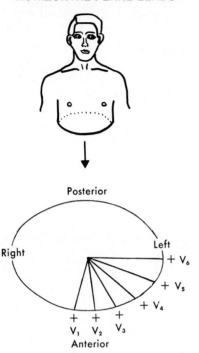

Fig. 3-11. Note the spatial relationships of the six chest (horizontal plane) leads.

to and face a large window, the window will be parallel to the frontal plane of your body. Similarly heart voltages directed upward and downward and to the right and left will be presented by the frontal plane leads. A figure with the frontal plane leads superimposed would contain the electrocardiographic relationships illustrated in the diagram on the preceding page (Fig. 3-10).

The chest leads (V_1 through V_6) present heart voltages from a different viewpoint, on the *horizontal* plane of the body, as shown in Fig. 3-11. The horizontal plane cuts your body into an upper and a lower half. Similarly the chest leads present heart voltages directed anteriorly (front), posteriorly (back), and to the right and left.

We therefore have two sets of ECG leads: six *extremity* leads (three unipolar and three bipolar), which record voltages on the frontal plane of the body, and six *chest* (precordial) leads, which record voltages on the horizontal plane. Together these 12 leads provide a three-dimensional picture of atrial and ventricular depolarization and repolarization.

CARDIAC MONITORS AND MONITOR LEADS
Bedside Cardiac Monitors

Up to now, we have described only the standard 12 lead ECG. However, it is not always necessary or feasible to record a full 12-lead ECG. For example, patients in coronary care units require continuous monitoring. In such settings special cardiac monitors are used to give a continuous beat-to-beat record of cardiac activity from one monitor lead.

Fig 3-12 shows an example of a rhythm strip obtained from a monitor lead. The monitor lead is obtained by means of three disk electrodes pasted on the chest wall. As shown in Fig. 3-13, one of these (the positive electrode) is usually pasted in the V_1 position. The other two are placed near the right and left shoulders. One serves as the negative electrode, the other as ground.

When the location of the electrodes on the chest wall is varied, the resultant ECG patterns will also vary. In addition, if the polarity of the electrodes changes (for example, connecting the negative electrode to the V_1 position and the positive electrode to the right shoulder), the ECG will show a completely opposite pattern (Fig. 3-12).

Cardiac monitors are built with electronic filters that may distort the ST-T complex. Therefore cardiac monitors should not be relied on to diagnose ST-T abnormalities. However, at times, important *changes* in the ST segment caused by ischemia (intermittent ST elevation or depression) may be shown in

Fig. 3-12. Rhythm strips from a cardiac monitor taken moments apart. Notice that **A** is completely the opposite of **B.** This is because the polarity of the electrodes in **B** was reversed.

Fig. 3-13. Monitor lead. A chest electrode (+) is placed at the V_1 position. The right shoulder acts as a negative (−) electrode. A ground electrode *(G)* is placed at the left shoulder.

Fig. 3-14. Effect of filters on the monitor leads. **A** and **B** were taken a few seconds apart. In **B** the electronic filter settings of the monitor were changed. Notice that the S waves are deeper and that ST-T changes suggesting myocardial ischemia (Chapter 8) have appeared.

bedside monitor leads. Fig. 3-14 illustrates some of the distortions produced by cardiac monitors.

Ambulatory (Holter) Monitors

The cardiac monitors described above are useful in patients confined to bed or chair, but sometimes it is essential to record the heartbeat in ambulatory patients over longer periods. A special portable ECG system, designed in 1961 by N.J. Holter, records the cardiac activity of patients as they go about their daily activities. The Holter monitor consists of electrodes placed on the chest wall and a special portable tape recorder to record the ECG. The patient can then be monitored over a long period (for example, 24 hours). The tape is played back, and the P-QRS-T complexes are displayed on a special screen. Printouts of any portion of the ECG can be obtained for further study and permanent records.

Holter monitors are invaluable in many settings. For example, in evaluating patients with unexplained syncope (fainting), the Holter monitor may reveal serious arrhythmias that are intermittent and may not be seen on a routine ECG. Holter monitors are also useful for establishing the diagnosis of the brady-tachy syndrome (p. 255), in which periods of bradycardia alternate with periods of tachycardia.

Special ECG Recordings

To help diagnose arrhythmias, special ECG electrodes have been developed for recording inside the esophagus (esophageal leads) or inside the right atrium and right ventricle (intracardiac leads). Discussion of these topics however, is beyond the scope of this introductory text.

REVIEW OF CHAPTER 3

The electrical currents produced during atrial and ventricular depolarization and repolarization are detected by electrodes placed on the extremities and chest wall.

Twelve leads are usually recorded.

The six *extremity* (limb) leads record voltages from the heart directed onto the frontal plane of the body. (This divides the body into front and back halves.) These six leads consist of the three bipolar extremity leads (I, II, and III) and three augmented unipolar extremity leads (aV_R, aV_L, and aV_F).

A *bipolar* lead records the difference between voltages from the heart detected at two extremities. A *unipolar* lead records voltages at one point relative to zero potential. The bipolar extremity leads can be represented by Einthoven's triangle (Fig. 3-4). They are related by the equation $II = I + III$. The unipolar extremity leads can also be represented by a triaxial diagram (Fig. 3-6). They are related by the equation $aV_R + aV_L + aV_F = 0$.

The three unipolar extremity leads and the three bipolar extremity leads can be shown on the same diagram, so the axes of all six leads intersect at a common point, producing the *hexaxial lead diagram.*

As a general rule, the P-QRS-T pattern in lead I resembles that in lead aV_L. Leads aV_R and II usually show reverse patterns. Lead aV_F usually resembles lead III.

Six *chest* (precordial) leads (V_1 to V_6) record voltages from the heart directed onto the horizontal plane of the body (which divides the body into an upper and a lower half). The chest (precordial) leads are taken with electrodes in specific anatomic locations (Fig. 3-8).

In addition to the 12 conventional leads, ECGs can be taken in special ways: In cardiac care units (CCUs), monitor leads, in which electrodes are placed on the chest, are generally used. Fig. 3-13 shows the usual location of the chest electrodes for a monitor lead. Continuous ECGs are often recorded using the Holter apparatus, for a period of 12 to (preferably) 24 or more hours in ambulatory patients who have transient or unpredictable arrhythmias.

Review Questions—Chapter 3

1. Leads I and II are shown below. Draw the P-QRS-T pattern in lead III.

2. Leads I, II, and III are shown below. What is wrong with these leads?

3. Draw the hexaxial lead diagram showing the six frontal plane (extremity) leads.

Answers

1. Since lead II = lead I + lead III, then according to Einthoven's equation lead III = lead II − lead I as shown below:

III

   Notice that the voltages of the P wave, QRS complex, and T wave in lead II are equal to the sum of the P wave, QRS complex, and T wave voltages in leads I and III

2. The voltages in lead II here do *not* equal those in leads I and III. The reason is that leads II and III were mislabeled. If you reverse the labels of leads II and III, you will find that the voltage in II equals the voltages in I and III.
3. See Fig. 3-7, *C.*

4 The Normal ECG

We have reviewed the cycle of atrial and ventricular depolarization and repolarization recorded by the ECG as well as the 12 lead system used to record this electrical activity. This chapter describes the P-QRS-T patterns seen normally in each of the 12 leads. Fortunately, this does not require memorization of 12 or more separate patterns. Rather, knowledge of a few basic ECG principles and understanding of the sequence of atrial and ventricular depolarization will enable us to predict the normal ECG patterns in each lead.

As you can see from the sample ECG in Fig. 3-2, each of the 12 leads appears to be different from the next. In some leads, for example, the P waves are positive (upward); in others they are negative (downward). In some leads the QRS complexes are represented by an rS wave; in other leads they are represented by qR or QS waves. Finally, in some leads the T waves are positive, and in others negative. What determines this variety in the appearance of ECG complexes in the different leads, and how does the repetitive cycle of cardiac electrical activity produce such different patterns in these leads?

THREE BASIC "LAWS" OF ELECTROCARDIOGRAPHY

Answering the preceding questions requires understanding of the following three basic ECG "laws" (Fig. 4-1):

1. A *positive* (upward) *deflection* will appear in any lead if the wave of depolarization spreads toward the positive pole of that lead. Thus, if the path of atrial stimulation is directed downward and to the left, toward the positive pole of lead II, a positive (upward) P wave will be seen in lead II (Figs. 4-2 and 4-3). Similarly, if the ventricular stimulation path is directed to the left, a positive deflection (an R wave) will be seen in lead I (Fig. 4-1, *A*).

2. A *negative* (downward) *deflection* will appear in any lead if the wave of depolarization spreads toward the negative pole of that lead (or away from the positive pole). Thus, if the atrial stimulation path spreads downward and to the left, a negative P wave will be seen in lead aV$_R$ (Figs. 4-2 and 4-3). If the ventricular stimulation path is directed entirely away from the positive pole of any lead, a negative QRS complex (QS deflection) will be seen (Fig. 4-1, *B*).

3. If the mean depolarization path is directed at right angles (perpendicular) to any lead, you will usually see a small *biphasic deflection* (consisting of positive and negative deflections of equal size). If the atrial stimulation path spreads at right angles to any lead, you will see a biphasic P wave in that lead. If the ventricular stimulation path spreads at right angles to any lead, then the QRS complex will be biphasic (Fig. 4-1, *C*). A biphasic QRS complex may consist of either an RS pattern or a QR pattern.

• • •

To summarize, when depolarization spreads toward the positive pole of any lead it produces a positive (upward) deflection. When depolarization spreads toward the neg-

40

THREE BASIC LAWS OF ELECTROCARDIOGRAPHY

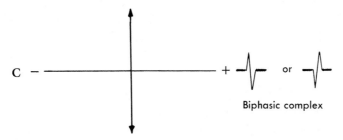

Fig. 4-1. A, A positive complex will be shown in any lead if the wave of depolarization spreads toward the positive pole of that lead. **B,** A negative complex will be shown if the depolarization wave spreads toward the negative pole (away from the positive pole) of the lead. **C,** A biphasic (partly positive, partly negative) complex will be seen if the mean direction of the wave is at right angles (perpendicular) to the lead. These three basic laws apply to both the P wave (atrial depolarization) and the QRS complex (ventricular depolarization).

ative pole (away from the positive pole) of any lead, it produces a negative (downward) deflection. When depolarization spreads at right angles to any lead axis, it produces a biphasic deflection.

We have deliberately omitted mention of repolarization—the return of the stimulated muscle to the resting state—and will touch upon this subject later in this chapter in the discussion of the normal T wave.

With these three basic ECG laws in mind, all you need to know is the direction in which depolarization spreads through the heart at any time to predict what the P waves and the QRS complexes will look like in any lead.

DIRECTION OF ATRIAL DEPOLARIZATION
WITH NORMAL SINUS RHYTHM

Fig. 4-2. With normal sinus rhythm the atrial depolarization wave will spread from the right atrium downward toward the AV, junction and left leg.

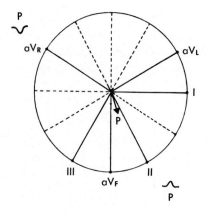

Fig. 4-3. With sinus rhythm the normal P wave will be negative (downward) in lead aV_R and positive (upward) in lead II. Recall that with normal atrial depolarization the arrow points down toward the patient's left (Fig. 4-2), away from the positive pole of lead aV_R and toward the positive pole of lead II.

DIRECTION OF ATRIAL DEPOLARIZATION
WITH AV JUNCTIONAL RHYTHM

Fig. 4-4. When the AV junction acts as the cardiac pacemaker (junctional rhythm), the atria will be depolarized in a retrograde (backward) fashion. An *arrow* representing atrial depolarization in such cases will point upward toward the right atrium, just opposite the pattern seen with sinus rhythm.

ORIENTATION OF P WAVES WITH AV
JUNCTIONAL RHYTHM

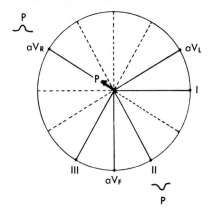

Fig. 4-5. With AV junctional rhythm the P waves will be upward (positive) in lead aV$_R$ and downward (negative) in lead II.

THE NORMAL P WAVE

Let us begin our description of the normal ECG with the first waveform seen in any cycle, the P wave, which represents atrial depolarization. Atrial depolarization is initiated by the sinus node, in the right atrium (Fig. 1-1). The atrial depolarization path therefore spreads from right to left and downward toward the AV junction. Therefore we can represent the spread of atrial depolarization by an arrow* that points downward and to the patient's left (as shown in Fig. 4-2).

Now go back to the diagram we drew in Chapter 3 showing the spatial relationship of the six frontal plane (extremity) leads. This diagram is redrawn in Fig. 4-3. Notice that the positive pole of lead aV_R points upward in the direction of the right shoulder. The normal path of atrial depolarization, as described, spreads downward toward the left leg (away from the positive pole of lead aV_R). *Therefore, with normal sinus rhythm, lead aV_R will always show a negative P wave.* Conversely, lead II is oriented with its positive pole pointing downward in the direction of the left leg (Fig. 4-3). Therefore the normal atrial depolarization path will be directed toward the positive pole of lead II. *When normal sinus rhythm is present, lead II will always record a positive (upward) P wave.*

To summarize, when normal sinus rhythm is present, the P wave will always be negative in lead aV_R and positive in lead II.

Using the same principles of analysis, can you predict what the P wave will look like in leads II and aV_R if the heart is being paced not by the sinus node but by the AV junction (AV junctional rhythm)? When the AV junction is pacing the heart, atrial depolarization will have to spread up the atria in a *retrograde* direction, just the opposite of what happens in normal sinus rhythm. Therefore an arrow representing the spread of atrial depolarization in AV junctional rhythm will point upward and to the right (Fig. 4-4), just the opposite of normal sinus rhythm. Spread of atrial depolarization upward and to the right will result in a positive P wave in lead aV_R, since the stimulus is spreading toward the positive pole of lead aV_R (Fig. 4-5). Conversely, lead II will show a negative P wave. We will discuss AV junctional rhythms in detail in Part II. The topic was introduced here simply to show how the polarity of the P wave in lead aV_R and lead II depends on the direction of atrial depolarization and how the patterns can be predicted using simple basic principles.

You need not be concerned with the polarity of the P waves in the other 10 leads. You can get all the clinical information you need to determine whether or not the sinus node is pacing the atria by simply looking at the P wave in leads II and aV_R. The size and shape of the P waves in other leads may be of importance in determining whether left or right atrial enlargement is present (which will be discussed in Chapter 6).

THE NORMAL QRS COMPLEX

The same principles as those used above can be applied in deducing the shape of the QRS waveform in the various leads. The QRS, which represents ventricular depolarization, is somewhat more complex than the P wave, but the same basic ECG rules apply to both.

To predict what the QRS will look like in the different leads, you must first know the direction of ventricular depolarization. Although the direction of atrial depolarization can be represented by a single arrow, the spread of ventricular depolarization consists of two major sequential phases:

The *first* phase is of relatively brief duration (shorter than 0.04 sec) and small amplitude;

---

*The arrows used to represent cardiac electrical potentials have both specific direction and specific magnitude and are, therefore, "vectors." The details of *vectorcardiography* lie outside the scope of this book, although vectorial principles are used throughout the discussions.

it results from the spread of stimulus through the ventricular septum. The ventricular septum is the first part of the ventricles to be stimulated. Furthermore, the left side of the septum is stimulated first (by a branch of the left bundle of His); thus the depolarization spreads from the left ventricle to the right across the septum. Phase one of ventricular depolarization, the phase of septal stimulation, can therefore be represented by a small

arrow pointing from the left septal wall to the right (Fig. 4-6, *A*).

The *second* phase of ventricular depolarization involves the simultaneous stimulation of the main mass of both the left and right ventricles from the inside (endocardium) to the outside (epicardium) of the heart muscle. In the normal heart the left ventricle is electrically predominant. In other words, it electrically overbalances the right ventricle. There-

NORMAL VENTRICULAR DEPOLARIZATION

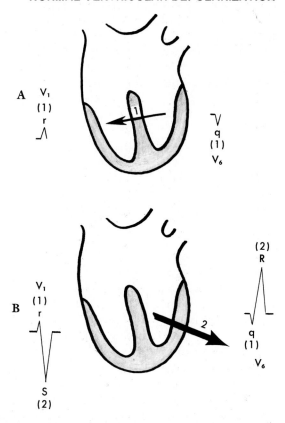

Fig. 4-6. Ventricular depolarization consists of two sequential phases. Phase one, **A,** proceeds from the left wall of the septum to the right. An *arrow* representing this phase points through the septum from the left to the right side. Phase two, **B,** is depolarization of the main bulk of the ventricles. The *arrow* points to the left ventricle, because this is normally electrically predominant. The two phases will produce an rS complex in the right chest lead (V_1) and a qR complex in the left chest lead (V_6).

fore an arrow representing phase two of ventricular stimulation will point toward the left ventricle (Fig. 4-6, *B*).

To summarize, the ventricular depolarization process can be divided into two main phases: The first phase, stimulation of the ventricular septum, is represented by a short arrow pointing to the right septal wall. The second phase, representing simultaneous left and right ventricular stimulation, is represented by a larger arrow pointing toward the left ventricle.

Now that we have outlined the ventricular stimulation sequence, we can begin to predict what types of QRS patterns this sequence will produce in the different leads. For the moment, we will discuss only the QRS patterns normally seen in the chest leads (the horizontal plane leads). We will talk first about leads V_1 and V_6.

Chest Leads

As discussed in Chapter 3, lead V_1 shows voltages detected by an electrode placed on the right side of the sternum (fourth intercostal space). Lead V_6, a left chest lead, shows voltages detected in the left midaxillary line (as shown in Fig. 3-8). What will the QRS complex look like in these leads (Fig. 4-6)?

The first phase of ventricular stimulation, septal stimulation, will produce a small positive r wave in lead V_1, reflecting the left-to-right spread of stimulus through the septum (Fig. 4-6, *A*). The arrow representing septal stimulation will point toward lead V_1. What will lead V_6 show? The left-to-right spread of septal stimulation will produce a small negative deflection (q wave) in lead V_6. Thus the same electrical event, septal stimulation, will produce a small positive deflection (or r wave) in lead V_1 and a small negative deflection (q wave) in a left precordial lead like V_6. (This situation is analogous to the one described for the P wave, which is normally positive in lead II but always negative in lead aV_R.)

The second phase of ventricular stimula-

tion is represented by an arrow pointing in the direction of the left ventricle (Fig. 4-6, *B*). The spread of stimulation to the left during the second phase will result in a negative deflection in the right precordial leads and a positive deflection in the left precordial leads. Lead V_1 will therefore show a deep negative (S) wave while lead V_6 shows a tall positive (R) wave.

Let us summarize what we have learned about the normal QRS pattern in leads V_1 and V_6. Normally lead V_1 will show an rS type of complex. The small initial r wave represents the left-to-right spread of septal stimulation. This wave is sometimes referred to as the *septal r wave* because it reflects septal stimulation. The negative (S) wave reflects the spread of ventricular stimulation forces during phase two, away from the right and toward the dominant left ventricle. Conversely, the same electrical events, septal and ventricular stimulation, viewed from an electrode in the V_6 position will produce a qR pattern. The q wave is a *septal q wave*, reflecting the left-to-right spread of the stimulus through the septum away from lead V_6. The positive (R) wave reflects the leftward spread of ventricular stimulation voltages toward the left ventricle.

Once again, we reemphasize, the same electrical event, whether depolarization of the atria or depolarization of the ventricles, will produce very different-looking waveforms in different leads because the spatial orientation of the leads is different.

We have described the patterns normally seen in leads V_1 and V_6. What happens between these leads? The answer is that as you move across the chest (in the direction of the electrically predominant left ventricle) the R wave tends to become relatively larger and the S wave becomes relatively smaller. This increase in height of the R wave, which usually reaches a maximum around lead V_4 or V_5, is called *normal R wave progression*. Fig. 4-7 shows several examples of normal R wave progression.

NORMAL CHEST LEAD PATTERNS

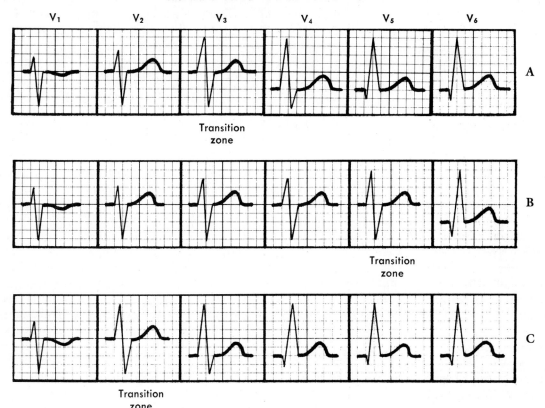

Fig. 4-7. Normally R waves in the chest leads become relatively taller from lead V_1 to the left chest leads. **A,** Note the transition in lead V_3. **B,** Somewhat delayed R wave progression, with the transition in lead V_5. **C,** Early transition in lead V_2.

At some point, generally around the V_3 or V_4 position, the R/S ratio becomes 1. This point, where the amplitude of the R wave equals that of the S wave, is called the *transition zone* (Fig. 4-7). In some normal people the transition may be seen as early as lead V_2. This is called *early transition*. In other cases the transition zone may be delayed to leads V_5 and V_6, and is called a *delayed transition*.

Examine the set of normal chest leads in Fig. 4-8. Note the rS complex in lead V_1 and the qR complex in lead V_6. The R wave tends to get gradually larger here as you

move toward the left chest leads. The transition zone, where the R wave and S wave are about equal, is in lead V_4. In normal chest leads the R wave voltage need not get literally larger as you go from leads V_1 to V_6. However, the overall trend should show a relative increase. For example, notice that in this example there is not much difference between the complexes in leads V_2 and V_3, and that the R wave in lead V_5 is taller than the R wave in lead V_6.

In summary, the normal chest lead ECG shows an rS-type complex in lead V_1 with a

Fig. 4-8. Normal chest leads. The transition is in lead V_4.

steady increase in the relative size of the R wave toward the left chest and a decrease in S wave amplitude. Leads V_5 and V_6 generally show a qR-type complex.*

The concept of *normal R wave progression* is of key importance in distinguishing normal and abnormal ECG patterns. For example, imagine the effect that an anterior wall myocardial infarction would have on normal R wave progression. Anterior wall infarction will result in the death of myocardial cells and the loss of normal positive (R wave) voltages. Therefore, one of the major ECG signs of an anterior wall infarction will be the loss of normal R wave progression in the chest leads. (The topic of myocardial infarction is discussed in detail in Chapters 8 and 9.)

Understanding the normal R wave progression in the chest leads also sets the basis for recognizing other basic ECG abnormalities. For example, consider the effect of left or right ventricular hypertrophy (enlarged muscle mass) on the chest lead patterns. As mentioned before, the left ventricle is normally electrically predominant, and left ventricular depolarization produces the deep (negative) S waves in the right chest leads and tall (positive) R waves in the left chest leads. With left ventricular hypertrophy, these left ventricular voltages will be further increased, resulting in very tall R waves in the left chest leads and very deep S waves in the right chest leads. On the other hand, right ventricular hypertrophy would be expected to shift the balance of electrical forces to the right, producing tall, positive (R) waves in the right chest leads. (These patterns of left and right ventricular hypertrophy are described in detail in Chapter 6.)

Extremity Leads

We have discussed the normal QRS patterns in the chest leads. All that remains is to describe the normal QRS patterns in the extremity leads: I, II, III, aV_R, aV_L, and aV_F.

We will begin with lead aV_R, which is the easiest to visualize. The positive pole of lead aV_R is oriented upward and toward the right shoulder. The ventricular stimulation forces are oriented primarily toward the left ventricle. Therefore, lead aV_R normally shows a predominantly negative QRS complex. You may see any of the QRS-T complexes shown in Fig. 4-9 in lead aV_R. In all cases, the QRS is predominantly negative. The T wave in lead aV_R is also normally negative.

---

*Normal chest lead patterns may show slight variation from the normal patterns we have been discussing. For example, some normal people will show a QS pattern and not an rS pattern in lead V_1. In other cases, the septal q wave in the left chest leads may not be seen and thus leads V_5 and V_6 will show an R wave and not a qR complex. On other normal ECGs, leads V_5 and V_6 may show a narrow qRs complex as a normal variant, and lead V, may show a narrow rSr'.

LEAD aV$_R$: NORMAL PATTERNS

Fig. 4-9. Normally lead aV$_R$ shows one of three basic negative patterns: an rS complex, a QS complex, or a Qr complex. The T wave also is normally negative.

NORMAL HORIZONTAL QRS AXIS

| I | II | III | aV$_R$ | aV$_L$ | aV$_F$ |

Fig. 4-10. With a horizontal QRS position (axis) leads I and aV$_L$ show qR complexes while lead II shows RS and leads III and aV$_F$ show rS complexes.

NORMAL VERTICAL QRS AXIS

| I | II | III | aV$_R$ | aV$_L$ | aV$_F$ |

Fig. 4-11. With a vertical QRS position (axis) leads II, III, and aV$_F$ show qR complexes while lead aV$_L$ (and sometimes lead I) shows RS complexes. This is just the reverse of the pattern with a normal horizontal axis.

The QRS patterns in the other five extremity leads are somewhat more complicated. The reason is that there is considerable normal variation in the QRS patterns seen in the extremity leads. For example, some normal people have an ECG that shows one pattern (Fig. 4-10) in the extremity leads. In this case, leads I and aV_L show qR-type complexes while leads III and aV_F show rS-type complexes. In other normal people the extremity leads may show just the reverse picture (Fig. 4-11). Here, leads II, III, and aV_F show qR complexes while lead aV_L and sometimes lead I show RS complexes.

How can we account for this marked normal variability in the QRS patterns shown in the extremity leads? The patterns seen depend on the *electrical position* of the heart. The term "electrical position" is virtually synonymous with *"mean QRS axis,"* which is described in greater detail in Chapter 5.

In simplest terms, the electrical position of the heart may be described as either *horizontal* or *vertical*.

1. When the heart is electrically horizontal *(horizontal QRS axis)*, ventricular depolarization is directed mainly horizontally and to the left in the frontal plane.

Looking at the frontal plane diagram (Fig. 3-10), you can see that leads I and aV_L are oriented horizontally and to the left. Therefore, when the heart is electrically horizontal, the QRS voltages will be directed toward leads I and aV_L, producing a tall R wave (usually as part of a qR complex) in these leads.

2. When the heart is electrically vertical *(vertical QRS axis)*, ventricular depolarization is directed mainly downward. Looking at the frontal plane diagram (Fig. 3-10), you can see that leads II, III, and aV_F are oriented downward. Therefore, when the heart is electrically vertical, the QRS voltages will be directed toward leads II, III, and aV_F, producing a tall R wave (usually a part of a qR complex) in these leads.

The concepts of electrically horizontal and electrically vertical heart positions can be expressed in another way. When the heart is electrically horizontal, leads I and aV_L will show qR complexes similar to the qR complexes seen normally in the left chest leads (V_5 and V_6). Leads II, III, and aV_F will show rS complexes similar to those seen in the right chest leads normally. Therefore, when

NORMAL INTERMEDIATE QRS AXIS

Fig. 4-12. Sometimes extremity leads show patterns that are hybrids of vertical and horizontal variants, with R waves in leads I, II, III, aV_L, and aV_F. This represents an intermediate QRS axis and is also a normal variant.

the heart is electrically horizontal, leads I and aV_L resemble leads V_5 and V_6 while leads II, III, and aV_F resemble the right chest leads. Conversely, when the heart is electrically vertical, just the opposite patterns will be seen in the extremity leads. With a vertical heart, leads II, III, and aV_F will show qR complexes, similar to the pattern seen in the left chest leads, while leads I and aV_L will show rS-type complexes, resembling those in the right chest leads.

Dividing the electrical position of the heart into vertical and horizontal variants is obviously an oversimplification. For example, look at Fig. 4-12. Here leads I, II, aV_L, and aV_F all show positive QRS complexes. Therefore, this tracing has features of *both* the vertical and the horizontal variants. (Sometimes this pattern is referred to as an "intermediate" heart position.)

For present purposes, however, you can regard the QRS patterns in the extremity leads to be basically variants of either the horizontal or the vertical QRS patterns described.

In summary, the extremity leads in normal people can show a variable QRS pattern. Lead aV_R normally always shows a predominantly negative QRS complex (Qr, QS, or rS). The QRS patterns in the other extremity leads will vary depending on the "electrical position" (QRS axis) of the heart. With an electrically vertical axis, leads II, III, and aV_F show qR type complexes. With an electrically horizontal axis, leads I and aV_L show qR waves. Therefore, there is no single normal ECG pattern; rather, there is a normal variability. Students and clinicians must familiarize themselves with the normal variants we have described both in the chest leads and in the extremity leads.

THE NORMAL ST SEGMENT

As noted in Chapter 2, the normal ST segment, representing the early phase of ventricular repolarization, is usually isoelectric (flat on the baseline). Slight deviations of the ST segment (usually less than 1 mm) may be seen normally. As described in Chapter 10, certain normal subjects will show more marked ST segment elevations as a normal variant (early repolarization pattern). Finally, examine the ST segments in the right chest leads (V_1 to V_3) of Figs. 3-2 and 6-10. Notice that in these examples the ST segment is short and the T wave appears to take off almost from the J point (junction of QRS complex and ST segment). This pattern of an early takeoff of the T wave in the right chest leads is not an uncommon finding in normal subjects.

THE NORMAL T WAVE

Up to this point, we have deferred discussion of ventricular repolarization—the return of stimulated muscle to the resting state, which produces the ST segment, T wave, and U wave. Deciding whether the T wave in any lead is normal or not is generally straightforward. As a rule, the T wave follows the direction of the main QRS deflection. Thus, when the main QRS deflection is positive (upright), the T wave is normally positive. We can also make some more specific rules about the direction of the normal T wave.

The normal T wave in lead aV_R is always negative, while in lead II it is always positive. Left-sided chest leads, such as V_4 to V_6, normally always show a positive T wave.

The T wave in the other leads may be variable. In the chest leads the T wave may be normally negative, isoelectric, or positive in leads V_1 and V_2. In most normal adults, the T wave becomes positive by lead V_3.* Furthermore, if the T wave is positive in any chest lead, it must remain positive in all chest

---

*In children and in some normal adults, a downward T wave may extend as far left as V_3 or V_4. This is known as the *juvenile T wave pattern.*

leads to the left of that lead. Otherwise, it is abnormal. For example, if the T wave is negative in chest leads V_1 and V_2 and becomes positive in lead V_3, it should normally remain positive in leads V_4 to V_6.

The polarity of the T wave in the extremity leads depends on the electrical position of the heart. With a horizontal heart, the main QRS deflection is positive in leads I and aV_L, and the T wave is also positive in these leads. With an electrically vertical heart, the QRS complex is positive in leads II, III, and aV_F, and the T wave is also positive in these leads. However, in some normal ECGs with a vertical axis, the T wave may be negative in lead III.

REVIEW OF CHAPTER 4

The three basic "laws" of electrocardiography are as follows:

1. A positive *(upward)* deflection will be seen in any lead if depolarization spreads toward the positive pole of that lead.
2. A negative *(downward)* deflection will be seen if depolarization spreads toward the negative pole (or away from the positive pole) of any lead.
3. If the mean depolarization path is directed at right angles *(perpendicular)* to any lead, a small biphasic (RS or QR) deflection will be seen.

Atrial depolarization starts in the sinus node and spreads downward and to the left, toward lead II and away from lead aV_R. Therefore, with normal sinus rhythm, the P wave is always positive in lead II and negative in lead aV_R.

Ventricular depolarization consists of two sequential phases:

1. The first phase of ventricular depolarization is stimulation of the ventricular septum from left to right. This produces a small (septal) r wave in the right chest leads and a small (septal) q wave in left chest leads.
2. During the second major phase of ventricular depolarization, the stimulus spreads simultaneously outward through the right and left ventricles. Since the mass of the normal left ventricle overbalances the mass of the right ventricle, the spread of depolarization through the left ventricle predominates on the normal ECG. This spread of stimulus through the left ventricle produces a tall R wave in the left chest leads (such as V_5 and V_6) (in association with a small q wave) and a deep S wave in the right chest leads (such as V_1 and V_2) (in association with a small initial r wave).

Chest leads between these extreme positions show a transitional pattern with tall R waves and deep S waves.

In the extremity leads the shape of the QRS complex varies with the electrical position of the heart:

1. When the heart is electrically horizontal, leads I and aV_L show a qR pattern.
2. When the heart is electrically vertical, leads II, III, and aV_F show a qR pattern.

The normal T wave generally follows the direction of the main deflection of the QRS complex in any lead. In the chest leads the T wave may normally be negative in leads V_1 and V_2. In most adults the T wave becomes positive by lead V_2 and remains positive in the left chest leads. In the extremity leads the T wave is always positive in lead II and negative in lead aV_R. When the heart is electrically horizontal, the QRS complex and T wave are positive in leads I and aV_L. When the heart is electrically vertical, the QRS complex and T wave are positive in leads II, III, and aV_F.

Review Questions—Chapter 4

1. Answer the following questions about the ECG below:
   a. Is it properly standardized?
   b. Examine the extremity leads. Is the QRS axis electrically vertical or electrically horizontal?
   c. Examine the chest leads. Where is the transition zone?

    d. Is the PR interval normal?

    e. Is the QRS interval normal?

    f. Are the T waves in the chest leads normal?

2. Answer the following questions about the ECG below:

    a. Is the heart electrically vertical or horizontal?

    b. What is the approximate heart rate?

    c. Examine the QRS complexes in the chest leads. What is the major abnormality?

    d. Are the T waves in leads I and aV_L normal?

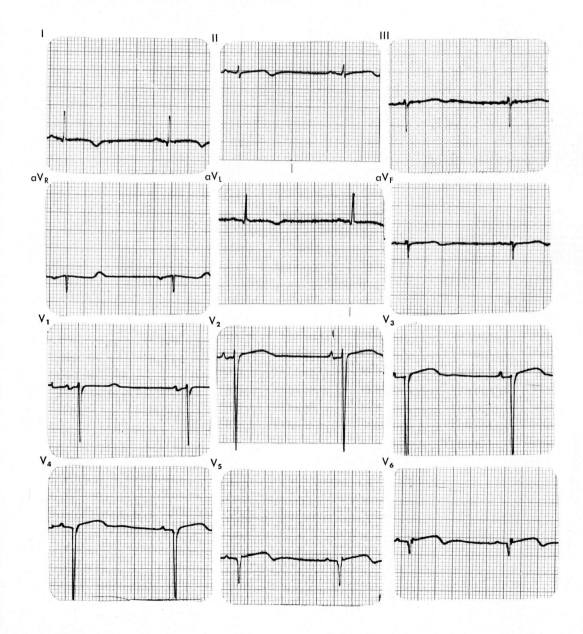

Answers

1. a. Yes. The standardization mark in lead I is 10 mm tall.
    b. Electrically horizontal. Notice that leads I and aV_L show qR complexes while leads II, III, and aV_F show RS or rS complexes.
    c. Transition zone in leads V_2 and V_3, which show RS complexes with the R wave approximately equal to the S wave.
    d. PR interval approximately 0.16 second (most readily measured in lead II here). This is within normal (0.12 to 0.2 sec).
    e. QRS width approximately 0.09 second. This is normal (less than or equal to 0.1 sec).
    f. T waves in chest leads are normal. Recall that normally T waves are upright from lead V_3 to the left in most adults. Occasionally, T waves are normally inverted in leads V_1 and V_2.

2. a. Electrically horizontal. See 1 (b) above.
    b. 50 beats/min.
    c. Loss of R wave progression. Normally, there is steady increase in R wave amplitude as you move from lead V_1 to the left. On this ECG there are small r waves in leads V_1 and V_2 with complete loss of R waves in leads V_2 to V_6. Loss of R wave progression in this case was caused by extensive anterior wall infarction (Chapter 8).
    d. No. T waves are abnormally inverted (negative) in leads I and aV_L. Recall that with an electrically horizontal heart the T waves are normally upright in leads I and aV_L.

5 Electrical Axis and Axis Deviation

In the previous chapter we described the normal ECG patterns in the chest and extremity leads. The general terms "horizontal heart" (or horizontal QRS axis) and "vertical heart" (or vertical QRS axis) were used to describe the normal variations in QRS patterns seen in the extremity leads. In this chapter we will refine this concept of electrical axis and show how you can determine the electrical axis of the QRS pattern in a simple way.

MEAN QRS AXIS

The depolarization stimulus spreads through the ventricles in different directions from instant to instant. For example, the depolarization wave may be directed toward lead I at one moment and toward lead III at the next. We can also talk about the mean direction of the QRS complex, or *mean QRS electrical axis*. If you could draw an arrow to represent the general, or mean, direction in which the QRS complex is pointed *in the frontal plane* of the body, you would be drawing the electrical axis of the QRS complex.

The term *"mean QRS axis,"* therefore, describes the general direction in the frontal plane toward which the QRS complex is predominantly pointed.

Since we are defining the QRS axis in the frontal plane, we are describing the QRS only in reference to the six extremity leads (the six frontal plane leads). (See Fig. 5-1.) Therefore the scale of reference used to measure the mean QRS axis is the diagram of the frontal plane leads (described in Chapter 3).

We also described the Einthoven triangle in Chapter 3, and we showed how the triangle can easily be converted into a triaxial lead diagram by simply having the three axes (leads I, II, and III) radiate from a central point (Fig. 5-1, *A*). Similarly we showed how the axes of the three unipolar extremity leads (aV$_R$, aV$_L$, and aV$_F$) also form a triaxial lead diagram (Fig. 5-1, *B*). These two triaxial lead diagrams were combined to produce a hexaxial lead diagram (Fig. 5-1, *C*). This is the lead diagram we shall use in determining the mean QRS axis and in describing axis deviation.

As noted in Chapter 3, each of the leads has a positive and a negative pole (Fig. 5-1, *C*). As a wave of depolarization spreads toward the positive pole, an upward (positive) deflection occurs. As a wave of depolarization spreads toward the negative pole, a downward (negative) deflection is inscribed.

Finally, in order to determine or calculate the mean QRS axis, we need a scale. By convention, the positive pole of lead I is said to be at 0°; all points below the lead I axis are positive; all points above lead I axis are negative (Fig. 5-2). Thus, as we move toward lead aV$_L$ ($-30°$), the scale becomes negative; and as we move downward toward leads II, III, and aV$_F$, the scale becomes more positive—lead II at $+60°$, lead aV$_F$ at $+90°$, lead III at $+120°$.

Fig. 5-2 shows the completed hexaxial diagram used to measure the QRS axis. By convention again, we can say that an electrical

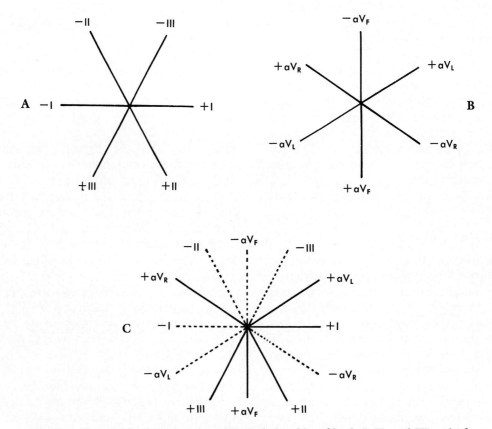

Fig. 5-1. Hexaxial lead system. **A** and **B,** Relationship of leads I, II, and III and of aV$_R$, aV$_L$, and aV$_F$. **C,** These diagrams have been combined to form a hexaxial lead diagram. Note that each lead has both a positive and a negative pole (the latter designated by *dotted lines*).

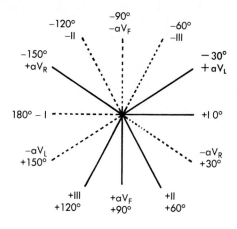

Fig. 5-2. Hexaxial lead diagram. Note that each lead has an angular designation—with lead I at 0° and all leads above it having negative angular values while those below it have positive values.

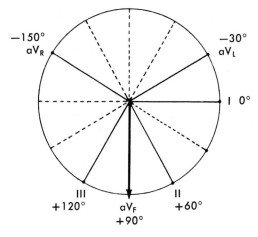

Fig. 5-3. Mean QRS axis of +90°. See text.

axis that points toward lead aV_L is *leftward* or *horizontal*. An axis that points toward leads II, III, and aV_F is *rightward* or *vertical*.

Calculation

In calculating the mean QRS axis you are answering the question: in what general direction or toward which lead axis is the QRS complex predominantly oriented? For example, consider the tracing in Fig. 5-3. Notice that there are tall R waves in leads II, III, and aV_F, indicating that the heart is electrically vertical (vertical electrical axis). Furthermore, the R wave is equally tall in leads II and III.* Therefore, by simple inspection, the mean electrical QRS axis can be seen to be directed between leads II and III and toward lead aV_F. Lead aV_F on the hexaxial diagram is at $+90°$.

As a general rule *the mean QRS axis will point midway between any two leads that show tall R waves of equal height*.

In the preceding example the mean electrical axis could have been calculated a second way. Recall from Chapter 3 that if a wave of depolarization is oriented at right angles to any lead axis a biphasic complex (RS or QR) will be recorded in that lead. Reasoning in a reverse manner, if you find a biphasic complex in any of the extremity leads, then the mean QRS axis must be directed at 90° to that lead. Now look at Fig. 5-3 again. Are there any biphasic QRS complexes? Obviously lead I is biphasic and shows an RS pattern. Therefore, the mean electrical axis must be directed at right angles to lead I. Since lead I on the hexaxial lead scale is at 0°, the mean electrical axis must be at right angles to 0° or at either $-90°$ or $+90°$. If the axis were $-90°$, then the depolarization

forces would be oriented away from the positive pole of lead aV_F and lead aV_F would show a negative complex. In this case lead aV_F shows a positive complex (tall R wave), so the axis must be $+90°$.

Fig. 5-4 shows another example. In this case, by inspection, the mean QRS axis is obviously horizontal since leads I and aV_L are positive and leads II, III, and aV_F are predominantly negative. The precise electrical axis can be calculated by looking at lead II, which shows a biphasic RS complex. Therefore, using the same logic as before, we can say that the axis must be at right angles to lead II. Since lead II is at $+60°$ on the hexaxial scale (Fig. 5-2), the axis must be either $-30°$ or $+150°$. If the axis were $+150°$, then leads II, III, and aV_F would be positive. Clearly in this case the axis is $-30°$.

Another example is presented in Fig. 5-5. The QRS complex is positive in leads II, III, and aV_F. Therefore we can say that the axis is relatively vertical. Since the R waves are of equal magnitude in leads I and III, the mean QRS axis must be oriented between these two leads, or at $+60°$.

Alternatively, we could have calculated the axis by looking at lead aV_L (in Fig. 5-5), which shows a biphasic RS-type complex. The axis must be at right angles to lead aV_L ($-30°$), that is either $-120°$ or $+60°$. Obviously, in this case, the answer is $+60°$. The electrical axis must be oriented toward lead II, which shows a tall R wave.

We now describe a second general rule: *the mean QRS axis will be oriented at right angles to any lead showing a biphasic complex. In such cases the mean QRS axis will point in the direction of leads showing tall R waves*.

Still another case is illustrated in Fig. 5-6. By inspection, the electrical axis can be seen to be oriented away from leads II, III, and aV_F and toward leads aV_R and aV_L, which show positive complexes. Since the R waves are of equal magnitude in leads aV_R and aV_L, the axis must be oriented precisely between

---

*In this case there are actually three leads (II, III, and aV_F) with R waves of equal height. In such cases the electrical axis will point toward the middle lead, that is, toward aV_F or at $+90°$.

these leads, or at $-90°$. Alternatively, look at lead I, which shows a biphasic RS complex. In this case the axis must be directed at right angles to lead I ($0°$); that is, it must be either $-90°$ or $+90°$. Since the axis is oriented away from the positive pole of lead aV_F and toward the negative pole of lead aV_F, it must be $-90°$.

Still another case can be noted (Fig. 5-7). There are two ways of approaching the calculation of the mean QRS axis in this case. Since lead aV_R shows a biphasic RS-type complex, the electrical axis must be right angles to the axis of lead aV_R. Since the axis of

lead aV_R is at $-150°$, the electrical axis in this case must be either $-60°$ or $+120°$. Clearly it must be $-60°$ in this case since lead aV_L is positive and lead III shows a negative complex.*

These basic examples should establish the ground rules for estimating the mean QRS axis. It is worth emphasizing that such calcu-

---

*The QRS axis can also be calculated by looking at lead I, which shows an R wave of equal amplitude with the S wave in lead II. The mean QRS axis must be oriented between the axis of lead I ($0°$) and the negative axis of lead II ($-120°$). Therefore it must be $-60°$.

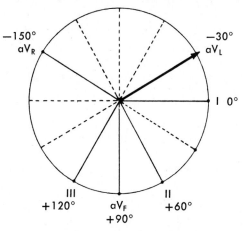

Fig. 5-4. Mean QRS of $-30°$. See text.

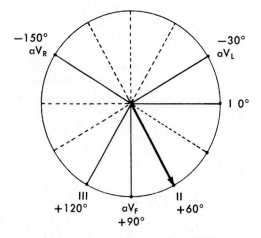

Fig. 5-5. Mean QRS axis of +60°. See text.

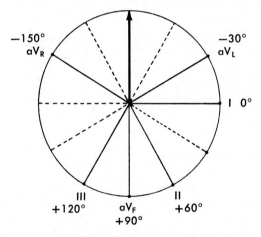

Fig. 5-6. Mean QRS axis of −90°. See text.

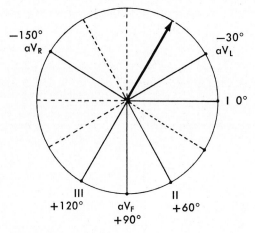

Fig. 5-7. Mean QRS axis of −60°. See text.

lations are generally only an estimate or a near approximation. An error of 10° or 15° is not significant. Therefore, it is perfectly acceptable to calculate the axis from leads in which the QRS is nearly biphasic or from two leads where the R (or S) waves are approximately equal in amplitude.*

To summarize, the mean QRS axis can be determined simply by using one or both of the following rules.

1. The mean QRS axis will point midway between the axes of two extremity leads that show tall R waves of equal amplitude.

---

*For example, when the R (or S) waves in two leads have similar but not identical voltage, the mean QRS axis will not lie exactly between these two leads. Instead, the axis will point more toward the lead with the larger amplitude.

Similarly, if a lead shows a biphasic (RS or QR) deflection where the R and S (or Q and R) waves are *not* of identical amplitude, then the mean QRS axis will *not* be pointed exactly perpendicular to that lead. If the R wave is larger than the S (or Q) wave, the axis will point slightly less than 90° away from the lead. However, if the R wave is smaller than the S (or Q) wave, the mean QRS axis will be pointed slightly more than 90° away from that lead.

2. The mean QRS axis will point at 90° (right angles) to any extremity lead that shows a biphasic (QR or RS) type complex. The mean QRS axis in such cases will be pointed in the direction of leads showing tall R waves.

AXIS DEVIATION

The mean QRS axis is a basic measurement that should be made in every ECG you read. In most normal individuals the mean QRS axis will lie between −30° and +100°. An axis of −30° or more negative is described as *left axis deviation (LAD)*. The term *right axis deviation (RAD)* refers to an axis of +100° or more positive. In other words, *left axis deviation* is an abnormal extension of the mean QRS axis found in persons with an electrically horizontal heart; *right axis deviation* is an abnormal extension of the mean QRS axis found in persons with an electrically vertical heart.

The mean QRS axis is determined by two major factors: (1) the anatomic position of the heart and (2) the direction of ventricular depolarization (the direction in which the stimulus spreads through the ventricles).

The influence of *cardiac anatomic position* on the electrical axis can be illustrated by the effects of respiration. With inspiration, the diaphragm descends and the heart becomes more vertical in the chest cavity. This change in cardiac position generally shifts the electrical axis vertically (to the right). (Patients with emphysema and chronically hyperinflated lungs also have anatomically vertical hearts and electrically vertical QRS axes.) Conversely, with complete expiration, the diaphragm ascends and the heart assumes a more transverse or horizontal position in the chest. With expiration, the electrical axis generally shifts horizontally (to the left).

The second major determinant, the *direction of depolarization through the ventricles,* can be illustrated by left anterior hemiblock (Chapter 7), where there is a delay in the spread of stimuli through the left ventricle and the mean QRS axis is shifted to the left. On the other hand, right ventricular hypertrophy shifts the QRS axis to the right.

Recognition of right and left axis deviations is easy.

RAD, as stated before, is defined as a QRS axis more positive than +100°. Recall that if leads II and III show tall R waves of equal height then the axis must be +90°. As an approximate rule, *if leads II and III show tall R waves and the R wave in lead III exceeds that in lead II, then right axis deviation is present.* In addition, lead I will show an RS pattern, with an S wave that is deeper than the R wave is tall (Figs. 5-8 and 5-10).

The cutoff for LAD is −30°. Fig. 5-4 shows a QRS with an axis of exactly −30°. Notice that lead II shows a biphasic complex (RS complex). Remember that the location of lead II is at +60° (Fig. 5-2) and a biphasic complex indicates that the electrical axis must be at right angles to lead II or at −30° (or at +150°). Thus, with an axis of −30°, lead II will show an RS complex where the R wave equals the S wave in amplitude. *If the electrical axis is more negative than −30° (left axis deviation) then lead II will show an RS complex where the S wave is deeper than the R wave is tall* (Figs. 5-9 and 5-11).

The rules for recognition of axis deviation are summarized as follows:

1. *Right axis deviation* is present if the R wave in lead III is taller than the R wave in lead II. Notice that with right axis deviation lead I shows an RS-type complex, with the S wave deeper than the R wave is tall (Figs. 5-8 and 5-10).
2. *Left axis deviation* is present if lead I shows a tall R wave, lead III shows a deep S wave, and lead II shows a biphasic rS complex (with the amplitude of the S wave exceeding the height of the r wave) (Figs. 5-9 and 5-11) or a QS complex. Leads I and aV$_L$ will both show tall R waves.

RIGHT AXIS DEVIATION

I   II   III

LEFT AXIS DEVIATION

I   II   III

Fig. 5-8. Right axis deviation (RAD)—mean QRS axis more positive than +100°—can be determined by simple inspection of leads I, II, and III. Note that lead III shows an R wave taller than the R wave in lead II.

Fig. 5-9. Left axis deviation (LAD)—mean QRS axis more negative than −30°—can also be determined by simple inspection of leads I, II, and III. Note that lead II shows an rS complex (with the S wave of greater amplitude than the r wave).

RIGHT AXIS DEVIATION

I   II   III   aV_R   aV_L   aV_F

Fig. 5-10. Note the R waves in leads II and III, with the one in lead III greater than the one in lead II, from a patient with RAD.

LEFT AXIS DEVIATION

I   II   III   aV_R   aV_L   aV_F

Fig. 5-11. Note the rS complex in lead II from a patient with LAD.

In Chapter 3 we introduced the terms "electrically vertical" and "electrically horizontal" heart positions (mean QRS axis). Now in this chapter we have added the terms "left axis deviation" and "right axis deviation." What is the difference between these terms? As mentioned, the terms "electrically vertical" and "electrically horizontal" heart positions are qualitative. With an electrically vertical mean QRS axis, leads II, III, and aV_F will show tall R waves. With an electrically horizontal mean QRS axis, leads I and aV_L will show tall R waves. With an electrically vertical heart, the actual mean QRS axis may be normal (for example, $+80°$) or abnormally rightward (for example, $+120°$). Similarly, with an electrically horizontal heart, the actual axis may be normal (for example, $0°$) or abnormally leftward (for example, $-50°$).

RAD, therefore, is simply an extreme form of a vertical mean QRS axis (Fig. 5-12). LAD, similarly, is an extreme form of a horizontal mean QRS axis (Fig. 5-13). Saying that the patient has an electrically vertical or horizontal mean QRS axis does not tell whether actual axis deviation is present or not.

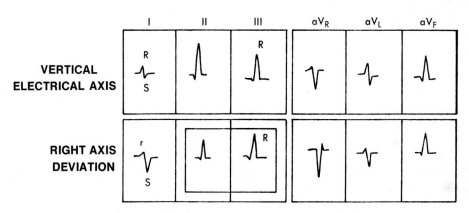

Fig. 5-12. Comparison of a normal vertical axis with actual RAD. See text.

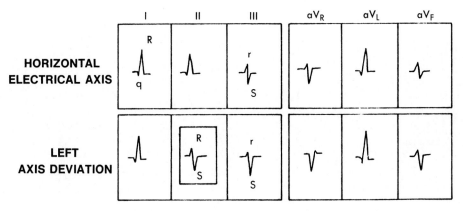

Fig. 5-13. Comparison of a normal horizontal axis with actual LAD. See text.

Clinical Significance

Right axis deviation (RAD, mean QRS axis more positive than $+100°$) may be seen in a variety of settings. It may sometimes be seen in normal persons. Right ventricular hypertrophy (Chapter 6) is an important cause of RAD. Another common cause is myocardial infarction of the lateral wall of the left ventri-cle. Loss of the normal leftward depolarization forces in this setting may lead "by default" to a rightward axis (Fig. 8-11). Left posterior hemiblock (Chapter 7) is a much rarer cause of RAD. Patients with chronic lung disease (emphysema or chronic bronchi-tis) often have electrocardiograms showing RAD. Finally, a sudden shift in the mean

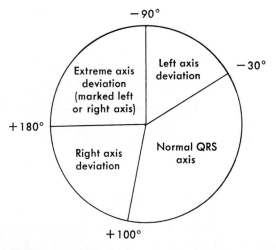

Fig. 5-14. Normal QRS axis and axis deviation. Most electrocardiograms will show either a normal axis or a left or right axis deviation. (Occasionally the QRS axis will be between $-90°$ and $180°$. Such an extreme shift may be caused by marked left or marked right axis deviation.)

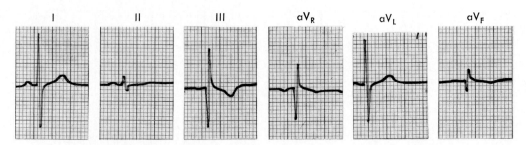

Fig. 5-15. Indeterminate axis. Note the biphasic complexes (RS or QR) in all six frontal plane leads.

QRS axis to the right (not necessarily causing actual RAD) may occur with acute pulmonary embolism (Chapter 10).

Left axis deviation (LAD, mean axis more negative than $-30°$) may also be seen in several settings. Patients with left ventricular hypertrophy (Chapter 6) sometimes, but not always, show LAD. Left anterior hemiblock (Chapter 7) is a fairly common cause of marked LAD (axis more negative than $-45°$). It is also often seen in association with left bundle branch block (Chapter 7). LAD may even be seen in the absence of apparent cardiac disease.

We would like to emphasize that axis deviation, right or left, does not necessarily imply any significant underlying heart disease. However, recognition of axis deviation (Fig. 5-14) often provides helpful, supportive evidence of abnormalities such as left or right ventricular hypertrophy, ventricular conduction disturbances (left anterior or posterior hemiblock), and so on.

Finally, you should realize that the limits for left and right axis deviation ($-30°$ to $+100°$) used in this book are necessarily arbitrary. Some authors use different criteria (for example, $0°$ to $+90°$). These apparent discrepancies reflect the important consideration that there are no absolute criteria in clinical electrocardiography. The best we can do is apply general criteria. The same problems will be found in the next chapter, on left and right ventricular hypertrophy, where different voltage criteria have been described by different authors.

On rare occasions, all six extremity leads will show biphasic (QR or RS) complexes, making it impossible to calculate the mean frontal plane QRS axis. In such cases, the term "indeterminate axis" is used (Fig. 5-15). Indeterminate QRS axis may occur as a normal variant or may be seen in a variety of pathologic settings.

MEAN ELECTRICAL AXIS OF THE P WAVE AND T WAVE

Up to now, we have described only the mean electrical axis of the QRS complex in the frontal plane. Using the same principles, we can also discuss the mean electrical axes of the P wave and T wave in the frontal plane.

For example, when sinus rhythm is present, the normal P wave is always negative in lead aV_R and positive in lead II. Therefore, normally, the P wave is generally directed toward lead II (Fig. 4-3), making the normal mean P wave axis about $+60°$. On the other hand, if the AV junction (and not the sinus node) is pacing the heart, then the atria will be stimulated in a retrograde way. When AV junctional rhythm is present, atrial depolarization spreads upward, toward lead aV_R and away from lead II (Fig. 4-5). In such patients, lead aV_R may show a positive P wave and lead II a negative P wave, and the mean P wave axis may be about $-150°$.

Using the same principles, we can also calculate the mean electrical axis of the T wave in the frontal plane. As a general rule the mean T wave axis and the mean QRS axis normally point in the same general (but not identical) direction. In other words, when the electrical position of the heart is horizontal, the T waves are normally positive in leads I and aV_L, in association with tall R waves in these leads. When the electrical position of the heart is vertical, the T waves will normally be positive in leads II, III, and aV_F, in association with tall R waves in these leads. (However, the T wave is often negative in lead III normally, regardless of the electrical position of the heart.)

To summarize, the concept of mean electrical axis can be applied to the QRS complex, P wave, or T wave. In each case the mean electrical axis describes the general or overall direction in which depolarization or repolarization is directed in the frontal plane.

REVIEW OF CHAPTER 5

The term *"mean QRS axis"* describes the general direction toward which the QRS axis is directed in the frontal plane of the body. Therefore the mean QRS axis is measured in reference to the six extremity (frontal plane) leads. These leads can be arranged in the form of a hexaxial (six axes) diagram (Fig. 5-1, *C*).

The approximate mean QRS axis can be determined by using one of the following rules:

1. The mean QRS axis will be pointed midway between any two leads that show tall R waves of equal height.
2. The mean QRS axis will be pointed at right angles (perpendicular) to any lead showing a biphasic complex and toward other leads showing tall R waves.

The normal mean QRS axis lies between −30° and +100°. An axis more negative than −30° is defined as *left axis deviation* (LAD). An axis more positive than +100° is defined as *right axis deviation* (RAD). LAD is an extreme form of a "horizontal" electrical axis. RAD is an extreme form of a "vertical" electrical axis.

LAD can be readily recognized if *lead II* shows an RS complex in which the S wave is deeper than the R wave is tall. In addition, *lead I* will show a tall R wave and *lead III* a deep S wave. LAD can be seen in cases of left ventricular hypertrophy, left anterior hemiblock, and other pathologic conditions and is sometimes seen in normal people.

RAD is present if the R wave in *lead III* is taller than the R wave in *lead II*. In addition, *lead I* will show an rS complex. RAD can be seen in several conditions, including right ventricular hypertrophy, lateral wall myocardial infarction, chronic lung disease, and left posterior hemiblock, and sometimes in normal people.

In rarer cases the QRS will be biphasic in all six extremity leads, making the mean electrical axis *indeterminate*.

The mean electrical axis of the P wave and T wave can also be estimated in the same manner as the mean QRS axis. With normal sinus rhythm the normal P wave will be about +60° (positive P wave in lead II). Normally the T wave axis in the frontal plane will be similar to the QRS axis, so the T waves will normally be positive in leads with a predominantly positive QRS complex.

Review Questions—Chapter 5

1. The six extremity leads (I, II, III, aV_R, aV_L, and aV_F) from a patient are shown. The standardization mark *(St)* in lead I is 10 mm, indicating proper standardization. What is the mean QRS axis?

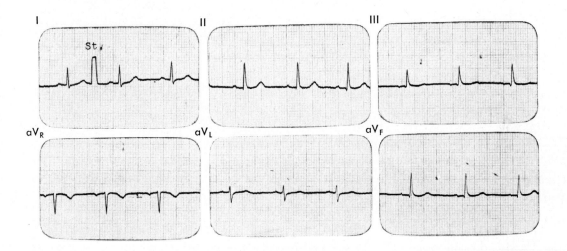

2. *A, B,* and *C* are, in mixed order, leads I, II, and III from a patient with a mean QRS axis of $-30°$. This information should allow you to sort out which lead is which.

3. Examine the following ECG:
   a. Is sinus rhythm present?
   b. What is the mean QRS axis?

4. Examine Fig. 6-5, p. 76. What is the approximate mean QRS axis?

Answers

1. The QRS axis is about +60°. Note that the QRS complex in lead aV$_L$ is biphasic. Therefore the mean QRS axis must point at right angles to −30°. In this case, the axis is obviously +60° since leads II, III, and aV$_F$ are positive. You could also calculate the axis here by noting that leads I and III show R waves of approximately equal amplitude. Therefore the axis must be directed between lead I (0°) and lead III (+120°), or at +60°. (You may have tried to calculate the axis by noting that the R waves in leads II and aV$_F$ were about equal, which would make the axis +75°. However, recall that leads aV$_R$, aV$_L$, and aV$_F$ are *augmented* leads and are not on the same scale as leads I, II, and III. Therefore, in calculating the electrical axis, it is more accurate to compare QRS voltages in leads aV$_R$, aV$_L$, and aV$_F$ *or* in leads I, II, and III.)

2. *A*, lead II; *B*, lead I; *C*, lead III.
   Explanation: You are told that the mean QRS axis is −30°. Therefore, you know that the QRS axis is pointed toward lead I (which is at 0°) and away from lead III (which is at +120°). Obviously lead I must be *B* and lead III must be *C*. Lead II is *A*, which is biphasic. Lead II is at +60° on the hexaxial diagram; and if the mean QRS axis is −30°, then lead II will have to show a biphasic complex since the mean QRS axis is at right angles to that lead.

3. a. Yes, sinus rhythm is present. Note that the P waves are negative in lead aV$_R$ and positive in lead II.

   b. The mean QRS axis is about 0°. Note that the QRS complex is biphasic in lead aV$_F$. In this case, since the QRS axis in lead I is positive, the QRS axis is oriented at right angles to lead aV$_F$, toward lead I or at 0°.

4. +90°. There are R waves of approximately equal magnitude in leads II and III, and lead I shows a biphasic RS complex.

6 Atrial and Ventricular Enlargement

The basics of the normal ECG have been described in the first five chapters. From this point on, we will be concerned primarily with abnormal ECG patterns, beginning in this chapter with a consideration of the effects on the ECG of enlargement of the four cardiac chambers.

Several basic terms must first be defined. "Cardiac enlargement" refers to either *dilation* of a heart chamber or *hypertrophy* of the heart muscle. In dilation of a chamber the heart muscle is *stretched* and the chamber becomes enlarged. For example, with acute congestive heart failure, dilation of the cardiac chambers occurs and is shown by an increase in the size of the cardiac x-ray silhouette. In cardiac hypertrophy the heart muscle fibers actually *increase in size*, with resulting enlargement of the chamber. For example, aortic stenosis, which obstructs the outflow of blood from the left ventricle, leads to hypertrophy of the left ventricular muscle. The atria and the right ventricle can also become hypertrophied in other situations (described later in this chapter). When cardiac hypertrophy occurs, the total number of heart muscle fibers does not increase; rather, each individual fiber becomes larger. One obvious ECG effect of cardiac hypertrophy will be an increase in voltage of the P wave or QRS complex. Not uncommonly hypertrophy and dilation occur together.

Both dilation and hypertrophy usually result from some type of chronic pressure or volume load on the heart muscle. We will proceed with a discussion of the ECG patterns seen with enlargement of each of the four cardiac chambers, beginning with the right atrium.

RIGHT ATRIAL ENLARGEMENT (RAE)

Enlargement of the right atrium (either dilation or actual hypertrophy) may increase the voltage of the P wave. To recognize a large P wave, you must know the dimensions of the normal P wave.

When the P wave is positive (upward), its amplitude is measured in millimeters from the upper level of the baseline, where the P wave begins, to the peak of the P wave. A negative (downward) P wave is measured from the lower level of the baseline to the lowest point of the P wave (Fig. 6-1). Measurement of the width of the P wave is also shown in Fig. 6-1.

Normally the P wave in every lead is less than or equal to 2.5 mm (0.25 mV) in amplitude and less than 0.12 second (three small boxes) in width. A P wave exceeding either of these dimensions in any lead is abnormal.

Enlargement of the right atrium may produce an abnormally tall P wave (greater than 2.5 mm). However, because pure RAE does not generally increase the total duration of atrial depolarization, the width of the P wave will be normal (less than 0.12 sec) (Fig. 6-2). The abnormal P wave in RAE is sometimes referred to as *P pulmonale* because the atrial enlargment is often seen with severe pulmonary disease. Fig. 6-3 shows an actual example of RAE with a P pulmonale pattern.

Fig. 6-1. The normal P wave does not exceed 2.5 mm in height and is less than 0.12 second in width.

P pulmonale

Fig. 6-2. Tall narrow P waves indicate right atrial enlargement (P pulmonale pattern).

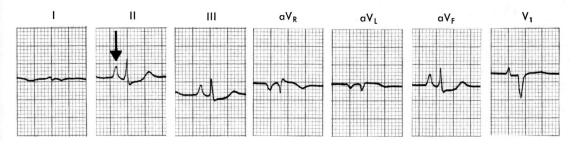

Fig. 6-3. Note the tall P waves, best seen in leads II, III, aV_F, and V_1, from a patient with chronic lung disease. This is the P pulmonale pattern.

The tall narrow P waves characteristic of RAE can usually best be seen in leads II, III, aV_F, and sometimes V_1. The ECG diagnosis of P pulmonale can be made by finding a P wave exceeding 2.5 mm in any of these leads. Recent echocardiographic evidence, however, suggests that the finding of a tall peaked P wave does not always correlate with RAE. On the other hand, patients may have RAE and not tall P waves.

RAE can be seen in a variety of clinical settings. Usually it is associated with right ventricular enlargement. Two of the most common clinical causes of RAE are pulmonary disease and congenital heart disease. The pul-monary disease may be either acute (for example, bronchial asthma, pulmonary embolism) or chronic (for example, emphysema, bronchitis). Congenital heart lesions producing RAE include pulmonic valve stenosis, atrial septal defects, and tetralogy of Fallot.

LEFT ATRIAL ENLARGEMENT (LAE); LEFT ATRIAL ABNORMALITY (LAA)

Enlargement of the left atrium (either by dilation or by actual hypertrophy) also produces distinct changes in the P wave. Normally the left atrium depolarizes after the right atrium. Therefore, enlargement of the left atrium should prolong the total duration

LEFT ATRIAL ENLARGEMENT (ABNORMALITY)

Fig. 6-4. Left atrial enlargement may produce, **A,** wide humped P waves in one or more extremity leads (P mitrale pattern) and/or, **B,** wide biphasic P waves in lead V₁.

Fig. 6-5. Broad humped P waves from a patient with left atrial enlargement (P mitrale pattern).

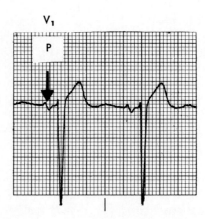

Fig. 6-6. Wide biphasic (initially positive, then negative) P waves from a patient with left atrial enlargement.

of atrial depolarization, indicated by an abnormally wide P wave. LAE characteristically produces a wide P wave of 0.12 second (three small boxes) or more duration. The amplitude (height) of the P wave in LAE may be either normal or increased.

Fig. 6-4 illustrates the characteristic P wave changes seen in LAE. Sometimes, as shown, the P wave will have a distinctive "humped" or "notched" appearance (Fig. 6-4, *A*). The second hump corresponds to the delayed depolarization of the left atrium. These humped P waves are usually best seen in one or more of the extremity leads (Fig. 6-5). The term *"P mitrale"* is sometimes used to describe these wide P waves seen with LAE because they were first described in patients with rheumatic mitral valve disease.

In cases of LAE, lead V_1 sometimes shows a distinctive biphasic P wave (Figs. 6-4, *B*, and 6-6). This biphasic P wave has a small initial positive deflection and a prominent wide negative deflection. The negative component will be of >0.04 second duration or ≥ 1 mm depth. The prominent negative deflection corresponds to the delayed stimulation of the enlarged left atrium. Remember that, anatomically, the left atrium is situated posteriorly, up against the esophagus, while the right atrium lies anteriorly, against the sternum. The initial positive deflection of the P wave in lead V_1, therefore, indicates right atrial depolarization while the deep negative deflection is a result of left atrial depolarization voltages directed posteriorly (away from lead V_1).

In some cases of LAE you will see both the broad often humped P waves in leads I and II and the biphasic P wave in lead V_1. In other cases only the broad humped P waves will be seen. Sometimes a biphasic P wave in lead V_1 will be the only ECG evidence of left atrial enlargment.

Clinically LAE may occur in a variety of settings.

1. Dilation of the left ventricle and left atrium associated with congestive heart failure of multiple causes (ischemic heart disease, cardiomyopathy)
2. Valvular heart disease, particularly aortic stenosis, aortic regurgitation, mitral regurgitation, and mitral stenosis (With mitral stenosis there is valvular obstruction to the emptying of the left atrium into the left ventricle. This will eventually result in a backup of pressure through the pulmonary vessels to the right ventricle. Therefore, with advanced mitral stenosis, the ECG may show a combination of LAE with signs of right ventricular hypertrophy, described below.)
3. Hypertensive heart disease, which causes left ventricular enlargement and eventually LAE

Some patients, particularly those with coronary artery disease, may show broad P waves without actual LAE. The abnormal P waves in these cases probably represent an atrial conduction delay. Therefore, the more general term *"left atrial abnormality"* is used by some authors in preference to left atrial "enlargement" to describe abnormally broad P waves.

RIGHT VENTRICULAR HYPERTROPHY (RVH)

Although atrial enlargement (dilation or hypertrophy) produces characteristic changes in the P wave, the QRS complex will be modified primarily by ventricular *hypertrophy*. The ECG changes that will be described indicate actual hypertrophy of the ventricular muscle and not simply ventricular dilation.

The ECG changes produced by both right and left ventricular hypertrophy can be predicted on the basis of what you already know about the normal QRS patterns. Normally (as described in Chapter 4) the left and right ventricles depolarize simultaneously and the left ventricle is electrically predominant because it is normally the larger chamber. As a result, leads placed over the right side of the chest, such as lead V_1, record rS-type complexes $\left(\begin{array}{c} r \\ \bigvee \\ S \end{array} \right)$, in which the deep negative S wave indicates the spread of depolarization voltages away from the right side and toward the left side. Conversely, a lead placed over the left chest, such as V_5 or V_6, records a qR-type complex $\left(\begin{array}{c} R \\ \bigwedge \\ q \end{array} \right)$, in which the tall positive R wave indicates the predominant depolarization voltages that point to the left generated by the left ventricle.

Now, if the right ventricle becomes sufficiently hypertrophied, this normal electrical predominance of the left ventricle can be overcome. In such cases of RVH, what type of QRS complex might you expect to see in the right chest leads? With RVH, the right chest leads will show tall R waves, indicating the spread of positive voltages from the hypertrophied right ventricle toward the right. Figs. 6-7 and 6-8 show actual examples of RVH. Instead of the rS complex normally seen in lead V_1, we now see a tall positive (R) wave, indicating marked hypertrophy of the right ventricle.

How tall an R wave in lead V_1 do you have to see to make a diagnosis of RVH? As a general rule, the normal R wave in lead V_1 in adults is usually smaller than the S wave in that lead. An R wave exceeding the S wave

RIGHT VENTRICULAR HYPERTROPHY

Fig. 6-7. Note the tall R wave in lead V_1 (with an inverted T wave caused by right ventricular strain). There is also right axis deviation (R wave in lead III taller than that in lead II). This patient had tetralogy of Fallot.

in lead V_1 is suggestive, but not diagnostic, of RVH. Sometimes, as shown in Fig. 6-8, a small q wave precedes the tall R wave in lead V_1 in cases of RVH.

Along with tall right chest R waves, RVH also often produces two additional ECG signs: right axis deviation and right ventricular strain T wave inversions.

As noted in Chapter 5, the normal mean QRS axis in adults lies approximately between $-30°$ and $+100°$. A mean QRS axis of $+100°$ or more is called *right axis deviation*. One of the most common causes of

right axis deviation is RVH. Therefore, whenever you see an ECG with right axis deviation, you should search carefully for other confirmatory evidence of RVH (Figs. 6-7 and 6-8). (Remember the simple rule of thumb that *right axis deviation is present if the R wave of lead III is taller than the R wave of lead II.*)

RVH (and left ventricular hypertrophy, to be discussed next) not only produces depolarization (QRS) changes but also affects repolarization (the ST-T complex). For reasons not fully understood, hypertrophy of the

RIGHT VENTRICULAR HYPERTROPHY

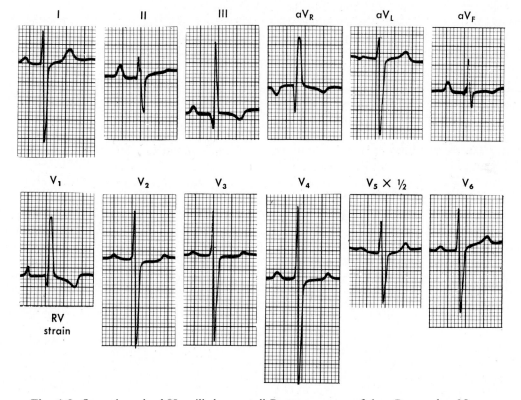

Fig. 6-8. Sometimes lead V_1 will show a tall R wave as part of the qR complex. Note the peaked P waves (leads II, III, and V_1) because of right atrial enlargement. T wave inversion in V_1 and ST depressions in V_2 and V_3 are due to right ventricular strain. There is also a prolonged PR interval (0.24 sec), indicating first-degree AV block.

heart muscle alters the normal sequence of repolarization. In RVH the characteristic repolarization change is the appearance of inverted T waves in the right and middle chest leads, as shown in Figs. 6-7 and 6-8. These right chest T wave inversions are referred to as a right ventricular *strain* pattern. (Strain is a descriptive term. The exact mechanism for the strain pattern is not understood.)

To summarize, with RVH, the ECG may show tall R waves in the right chest leads, with the R wave greater than the S wave in lead V_1.* Right axis deviation and right ventricular strain T wave inversions are also often present. Some cases of RVH are more subtle, and the ECG may show only one of the above patterns. The appearance of all three patterns (tall right precordial R waves, right axis deviation, and right ventricular strain) firmly establishes the diagnosis of RVH. However, the absence of these patterns does not necessarily exclude RVH.

RVH may occur in a variety of clinical settings. Probably the most common cause is congenital heart disease (for example, pulmonic stenosis, atrial septal defects,† tetralogy of Fallot, Eisenmenger syndrome, and so on). Patients with long-standing severe pulmonary disease may develop pulmonary artery hypertension and RVH. Mitral stenosis, as mentioned previously, may produce a combination of LAE and RVH. Right ventricular strain T wave inversions (in V_1 to V_3) may also occur without other ECG signs of RVH, as in acute pulmonary embolism (pp. 149 to 151).

---

*With RVH the chest leads to the left of the leads showing tall R waves may show a variable pattern. Sometimes the middle left chest leads show poor R wave progression, with rS or RS complexes all the way to lead V_6 (Fig. 6-8). In other cases normal R wave progression will be present and the left chest leads will also show R waves (Fig. 6-7).

†Patients with right ventricular enlargement from atrial septal defect often show a right bundle branch block pattern (RSR′) in lead V_1 with a vertical or rightward QRS axis.

In patients with RVH associated with emphysema the ECG may not show any of the patterns described above. Instead of tall R waves in the right precordial leads, the ECG generally shows very poor R wave progression. Right axis deviation is commonly present (discussed on p. 65). (See Fig. 10-14.)

LEFT VENTRICULAR HYPERTROPHY (LVH)

The ECG changes produced by LVH, like those from RVH, are predictable. Normally, as noted, the left ventricle is electrically predominant over the right ventricle and produces prominent S waves in the right chest leads and tall R waves in the left chest leads. When LVH is present, the balance of electrical forces is tipped even further to the left. Thus, when LVH is present, the chest leads will show abnormally tall R waves (left chest leads) and abnormally deep S waves (right chest leads).

The following criteria and guidelines have been established to help in the ECG diagnosis of LVH:

1. If the depth of the S wave in lead V_1 (S_{V_1}) added to the height of the R wave in either lead V_5 or V_6 (R_{V_5} or R_{V_6}) exceeds 35 mm (3.5 mV), then suspect LVH (Fig. 6-9).

2. You should also realize that high voltage in the chest leads is commonly seen as a normal finding, particularly in young adults with thin chest walls. Consequently, high voltage in the chest leads (S_{V_1} + R_{V_5} or R_{V_6} > 35 mm) is not a *specific* indicator of LVH (Fig. 6-10).

3. In some cases LVH will produce tall R waves in lead aV_L. An R wave of 13 mm or more in lead aV_L (Fig 6-8) is another sign of LVH.* Occasionally a

---

*Occasionally LVH will develop with an electrically vertical axis. In such cases a qR pattern with a tall R wave (exceeding 20 mm) may appear in lead aV_F.

LEFT VENTRICULAR HYPERTROPHY

Fig. 6-9. This patient had severe hypertension. Note the pattern of left ventricular hypertrophy: tall voltage in the chest leads and aV$_L$ (R = 16 mm) with strain pattern in these leads. In addition, there is the pattern of left atrial enlargement, including a biphasic P wave in lead V$_1$ and a broad notched P wave in lead II.

Fig. 6-10. Tall voltage in chest leads (R_{V_1} + S_{V_5} = 36 mm) in a 20-year-old man. This is a normal variant caused by the patient's thin chest wall. The ST-T complexes are normal, without evidence of left ventricular strain. What is the heart rate? (Answer: about 60 beats/min.)

LEFT VENTRICULAR STRAIN PATTERN

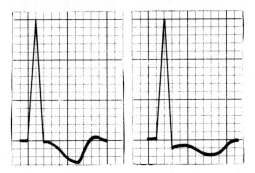

Fig. 6-11. Note the characteristic wavy ST-T pattern with T wave inversion in leads showing tall R waves.

tall R wave in lead aV_L may be the only ECG sign of LVH and the voltage in chest leads may be normal. In other cases the chest voltages may be abnormally high, with a normal R wave in lead aV_L.

4. Furthermore, just as RVH is associated with a right ventricular strain pattern, so left ventricular strain ST-T changes are often seen in LVH. Fig. 6-11 illustrates the characteristic shape of the ST-T complex with left ventricular strain. Notice that the ST-T complex has a distinctive asymmetric appearance, with slight ST segment depression followed by a broadly inverted T wave. In some cases these left ventricular strain T wave inversions may be very deep. The left ventricular strain pattern is seen in leads with tall R waves (Fig. 6-9).

5. With LVH the electrical axis is usually horizontal. Actual left axis deviation (axis $-30°$ or more negative) may also be seen. In addition, the QRS complex may become wider. Not uncommonly patients with LVH will eventually develop complete left bundle branch block. (See Chapter 7.)

6. Finally, ECG signs of LAE (broad notched P waves in the extremity leads or wide biphasic P waves in lead V_1) are often seen in patients with ECG evidence of LVH. Most conditions that lead to LVH ultimately produce LAE as well.

A variety of clinical conditions are associated with LVH. In adults, three of the most common are (1) valvular heart disease, such as aortic stenosis, aortic regurgitation, or mitral regurgitation, (2) hypertension, and (3) cardiomyopathies (p. 152).

To summarize, the diagnosis of LVH can be made with reasonable certainty from the ECG if you find high QRS voltages with a left ventricular strain pattern. As mentioned, high voltage in the chest or extremity leads can sometimes be seen in normal subjects so the diagnosis of LVH should not be made on this finding alone.* T wave inversion resulting from left ventricular strain can also occur without other evidence of LVH.

---

*The voltage criteria used here for diagnosing LVH in the chest and extremity leads are by no means absolute numbers. Some authors use somewhat different voltage criteria.

• • •

We have described the patterns of RVH with right ventricular strain and LVH with left ventricular strain. However, the subject is somewhat more complicated than this because the ST-T changes of ventricular strain can also occur in the absence of actual ventricular hypertrophy.

For example, you can see right ventricular strain (T wave inversions in the right to middle chest leads) without actual RVH. Acute right ventricular strain, for example, is sometimes seen with massive pulmonary embolism (Fig. 10-13), where there is a sudden severe stress on the right side of the heart.

Left ventricular strain can also occur without actual LVH. In such cases the ECG will show the characteristic ST-T changes of Fig. 6-11 *without* high QRS voltages. Acute left ventricular strain may occur, for example, with sudden increases in systemic blood pressure.

ECG IN CARDIAC ENLARGEMENT: A PERSPECTIVE

The ECG findings associated with enlargement of each of the four cardiac chambers have been presented. In some cases combined patterns will be seen in the same tracing; for example, LAE and RVH in cases of mitral stenosis or LAE and LVH with hypertension. You may be wondering what the ECG shows if both left and right ventricles become hypertrophied (biventricular hypertrophy). In such cases the ECG usually shows mainly evidence of LVH.

Finally, always remember that in the assessment of cardiac size the ECG is only an indirect laboratory test and not an absolute measurement. A person may have underlying cardiac enlargment that does not show up on the ECG. Conversely, as we have mentioned, high voltage may be present in normal persons without cardiac enlargement. In cases where the degree of cardiac chamber enlargement must be determined with more precision, an *echocardiogram* should be obtained.

REVIEW OF CHAPTER 6

Cardiac *dilation* refers to stretching of muscle fibers, with enlargement of one or more of the cardiac chambers. Cardiac *hypertrophy* refers to an abnormal increase in the actual size of the heart muscle fibers. The ECG can indicate either right or left atrial dilation or hypertrophy, but generally only indicates right or left ventricular hypertrophy.

Right atrial enlargement shows the following: Tall peaked P waves (*P pulmonale pattern*), greater than 2.5 mm in height, are usually best seen in leads II, III, aV$_F$, and sometimes V$_1$.

Left atrial enlargement (abnormality) shows the following: Wide sometimes humped P waves (*P mitrale pattern*), of 0.12 second or more duration, are seen in one or more of the extremity leads. Lead V$_1$ sometimes shows a biphasic P wave with a prominent, wide, negative deflection.

Right ventricular hypertrophy may show the following:
1. Tall R wave in lead V$_1$, where the R wave is equal to or larger than the S wave in that lead, is seen.
2. RAD is often present.
3. Right ventricular strain pattern (T wave inversions in the right to middle chest leads) is often present.

Left ventricular hypertrophy may show the following:
1. The voltage of the S wave in lead V$_1$ plus the voltage of the R wave in lead V$_5$ or V$_6$ exceeds 35 mm (S$_{V_1}$ + R$_{V_5}$ or R$_{V_6}$ > 35 mm).
2. High-voltage R wave in lead aV$_L$ (13 mm or more) may be present when the heart is electrically horizontal. When the axis is vertical, lead aV$_F$ may show a tall R wave (>20 mm) as part of a qR complex.
3. Left ventricular strain pattern (inverted T waves in leads with a qR pattern) may be present.

The diagnosis of LVH should *not* be made solely on the basis of high voltage in the chest leads, since this may occur normally, particularly in young adults and thin-chested people.

T wave inversions in both left ventricular strain and right ventricular strain may also occur without LVH or RVH.

Review Questions—Chapter 6

1. Answer these questions about the following ECG:
   a. What is the approximate heart rate?
   b. Is sinus rhythm present?
   c. Where is the transition zone in the chest leads?
   d. Mention three signs of LVH.

2. In the following ECG
   a. What is the heart rate?
   b. Name two abnormal findings.

Answers

1. a. About 100 beats/min.
   b. No. Notice the retrograde P waves, positive in lead aV_R and negative in lead II, owing to an AV junctional (or ectopic atrial) rhythm.
   c. Around lead V_4.
   d. Tall voltage in chest leads (S_{V_1} + R_{V_6} > 35 mm); tall voltage in lead aV_L (R wave > 13 mm); left ventricular strain pattern in leads I, aV_L, and V_5 and V_6.

2. a. About 75 beats/min.
   b. The PR interval is prolonged (about 0.22 sec) because of first-degree AV block (Chapter 15). Also, the P wave in lead II is abnormally wide and notched (notice the two humps) as a result of left atrial enlargement.

7 Ventricular Conduction Disturbances

Bundle Branch Blocks

The normal process of ventricular stimulation was outlined in Chapter 4. The electrical stimulus reaches the ventricles from the atria by way of the AV junction. As mentioned, the first part of the ventricles normally stimulated (depolarized) is the left side of the ventricular septum. Soon after, the depolarization spreads to the main mass of the left and right ventricles by way of the left and right bundle branches. Normally the entire process of ventricular depolarization is completed within 0.1 second. Therefore, the normal width of the QRS complex is less than or equal to 0.1 second (two and a half small boxes on the ECG graph paper). Any process that interferes with the normal stimulation of the ventricles may prolong the QRS width. In this chapter we will be concerned primarily with the effects of blocks within the bundle branch system on the QRS complex.

RIGHT BUNDLE BRANCH BLOCK (RBBB)

Consider, first, the effect of cutting the right bundle branch. Obviously this will delay right ventricular stimulation and widen the QRS complex. Furthermore, the shape of the QRS complex with a right bundle branch block (RBBB) can be predicted on the basis of some familiar principles.

Normally, as noted above, the first part of the ventricles to be depolarized is the interventricular septum (Fig. 4-6, *A*). The left side of the interventricular septum is stimulated first (by a branch of the left bundle). This septal depolarization produces the small septal r wave in lead V_1 and the small septal q wave in lead V_6 seen on the normal ECG (Fig. 7-1, *A*). Clearly, RBBB should not affect this first septal phase of ventricular stimulation, since the septum is stimulated by a part of the left bundle.

The second phase of ventricular stimulation is the simultaneous depolarization of the left and right ventricles (Fig. 4-6, *B*). RBBB should not affect this phase either, since the left ventricle is normally electrically predominant, producing deep S waves in the right chest leads and tall R waves in the left chest leads (Fig. 7-1, *B*).

The change in the QRS complex produced by RBBB is a result of the delay in the total time needed for stimulation of the right ventricle. This means that following the completion of left ventricular depolarization, the right ventricle continues to depolarize. This delayed right ventricular depolarization produces a third phase of ventricular stimulation. The electrical voltages in the third phase are directed to the right, reflecting the delayed depolarization and slow spread of the depolarization wave outward through the right ventricle. Therefore a lead placed over the right side of the chest (for example, lead V_1) will record this third phase of ventricular stimulation as a positive wide deflection (R′

RIGHT BUNDLE BRANCH BLOCK

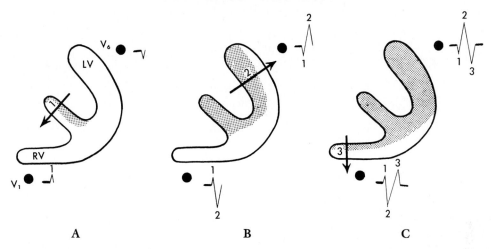

Fig. 7-1. Step-by-step sequence of ventricular depolarization in RBBB. See text.

wave). The same delayed and slow right ventricular depolarization voltages spreading to the right will produce a wide negative (S wave) deflection in the left chest leads (for example, lead V_6) (Fig. 7-1, C).

Putting together what we have just explained in a step-by-step fashion, we can now derive the pattern seen in the chest leads with RBBB. Lead V_1 will show an rSR' complex with a broad R' wave. Lead V_6 will show a qRS-type complex with a broad S wave. The tall wide R wave in the right chest leads and the deep terminal S wave in the left chest leads represent the same event viewed from opposite sides of the chest—the slow spread of delayed depolarization voltages through the right ventricle.

To make the diagnosis of RBBB, forget about the extremity leads. You need look only at the chest leads, and at leads V_1 and V_6 in particular. The characteristic appearance of the QRS complex in these leads makes the diagnosis of RBBB simple.

Fig. 7-1 shows how the delay in ventricular depolarization with RBBB produces the characteristic ECG patterns we have been describing.

To summarize, in RBBB the ventricular stimulation process can be divided into three phases. The first two phases consist of the normal septal and ventricular depolarization. The third phase is the delayed stimulation of the right ventricle. These three phases of ventricular stimulation with RBBB are represented on the ECG by the triphasic complexes seen in the chest leads—lead V_1 showing an rSR' complex with a wide R' wave, lead V_6 showing a qRS pattern with a wide S wave.

We have said that with an RBBB the QRS complex in lead V_1 generally shows an rSR' pattern. Occasionally (as shown in Fig. 7-3) the S wave never quite makes its way below the baseline, giving the complex in lead V_1 the appearance of a large notched R wave.

Figs. 7-2 and 7-3 show some typical examples of RBBB. Do you notice anything abnormal about the ST-T complexes in these tracings? If you look carefully, you will notice

RIGHT BUNDLE BRANCH BLOCK

Fig. 7-2. Note the wide rSR′ complex in lead V_1 and the qRS complex in lead V_6. Inverted T waves in the right precordial leads (V_1 to V_3 in this case) are common with RBBB and are called secondary T wave inversions.

that the T waves in the right chest leads are inverted (negative). T wave inversions in the right chest leads are a characteristic finding in RBBB. These T wave inversions are referred to as *secondary changes* because they are related to the abnormal process of ventricular stimulation. In contrast, *primary T wave abnormalities* reflect some actual change in repolarization, independent of any QRS change. For example, T wave inversions resulting from ischemia (p. 132), hypokalemia (p. 143), or digitalis (p. 140) are all examples of primary T wave abnormalities.

Some ECGs will show both primary and secondary ST-T changes. For example, in Fig. 7-3 the T wave inversions in V_1 to V_3, II, III, and V_F can be explained solely on the basis of the RBBB since they occur in leads with an rSR′-type complex. However, T

wave inversions or ST segment depressions in other leads (V_4 and V_5) represent a primary change resulting perhaps from ischemia or a drug effect.

Complete vs Incomplete RBBB

RBBB can be further divided into complete and incomplete forms depending on the width of the QRS complex. Complete RBBB is defined by a QRS complex (rSR′ in lead V_1 and qRS in lead V_6) of 0.12 second or more width. Incomplete RBBB shows the QRS shape described in the preceding section but the QRS duration is between 0.1 and 0.12 second.

Clinical Significance

RBBB may be caused by a number of factors. First, some normal people will show an

RIGHT BUNDLE BRANCH BLOCK

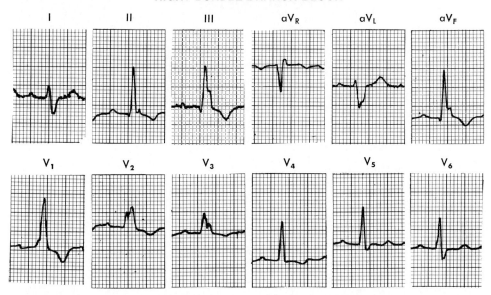

Fig. 7-3. Sometimes, with RBBB, instead of the classic rSR′ pattern, the right precordial leads will show a wide notched R wave (seen here in leads V_1 to V_3). Note the secondary T wave inversions in leads V_1 to V_3, II, III, and aV_F, all of which show rSR′-type complexes. However, the abnormal ST changes in V_4 and V_5 are primary since they are present in leads without an R′ wave.

RBBB pattern without any underlying heart disease; therefore, RBBB per se is not necessarily abnormal. In many persons, however, RBBB is associated with organic heart disease. RBBB may be caused by any conditions that affect the right side of the heart (for example, atrial septal defect with left-to-right shunting of blood, chronic pulmonary disease with pulmonary artery hypertension, and valvular lesions such as pulmonic stenosis). In some cases, individuals (particularly older people) develop RBBB because of chronic degenerative changes in the conduction system. RBBB may also occur with myocardial ischemia and infarction. Pulmonary embolism, which produces acute right-sided heart strain, may also produce RBBB.

The conduction disturbance does not, in itself, require any specific treatment.

LEFT BUNDLE BRANCH BLOCK (LBBB)

Left bundle branch block (LBBB) also produces a pattern with a widened QRS complex. However, the shape of the QRS complex with LBBB is very different from that with RBBB. The reason for this difference is that RBBB affects mainly the terminal phase of ventricular activation. LBBB, on the other hand, affects the early phase of ventricular depolarization as well.

Recall that the first phase of ventricular stimulation—depolarization of the left side of the septum—is started by a part of the left bundle branch. LBBB, therefore, will block this normal pattern of septal depolarization. When LBBB is present, the septum depolarizes from right to left and not from left to right. Thus the first major change on the

LEFT BUNDLE BRANCH BLOCK

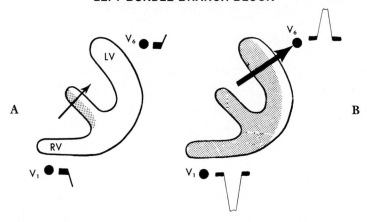

Fig. 7-4. The sequence of ventricular depolarization in LBBB produces a wide QS complex in lead V_1 and a wide R wave in lead V_6.

ECG produced by LBBB will be a loss of the normal septal r wave in lead V_1 and the normal septal q wave in lead V_6 (Fig. 7-4, *A*). Furthermore, the total time for left ventricular depolarization will be prolonged with LBBB, resulting in an abnormally wide QRS complex. Lead V_6 will show a wide entirely positive (R) wave (Fig. 7-4, *B*). The right chest leads (such as V_1) record a negative QRS (QS) complex because the left ventricle is still electrically predominant with LBBB and produces greater voltages than the right ventricle. The major change is that the total time for completion of left ventricular depolarization is delayed. Therefore, with LBBB, the entire process of ventricular stimulation is oriented toward the left chest leads—the septum depolarizing from right to left, with stimulation of the electrically predominant left ventricle prolonged. Fig. 7-4 illustrates the sequence of ventricular activation in LBBB.*

---

*A variation of this pattern that sometimes occurs is for lead V_1 to show an rS complex with a very small r wave and a wide S wave. This superficially suggests that the septum is being stimulated normally from left to right. However, lead V_6 in such cases will show an abnormally wide and notched R wave *without* an initial q wave.

Sometimes the QS wave in lead V_1 with LBBB will show a small notching at its point, giving it a characteristic **W** shape. Similarly the R wave in lead V_6 may show a notching at its peak, giving it a distinctive **M** shape. An actual example of an LBBB pattern is shown in Fig. 7-5.

Just as there are secondary T wave inversions with RBBB, so there are also secondary T wave inversions with LBBB. As you can see from the example in Fig. 7-5, the T wave in the leads with tall R waves is inverted (negative). This T wave inversion (for example, in the left precordial leads) is characteristic of LBBB. However, T wave inversions in the right precordial leads cannot be explained solely on the basis of LBBB and, if present, reflect some primary abnormality, such as ischemia (Fig. 8-21).

To summarize, the diagnosis of LBBB can be made simply by inspection of leads V_1 and V_6. Lead V_1 usually shows a wide, entirely negative, QS complex (rarely a wide rS complex) while lead V_6 will show a wide tall R wave without a q wave. You should have no problem differentiating left and right bundle branch block patterns. Fig. 7-6 compares the complexes seen with RBBB and LBBB. Oc-

LEFT BUNDLE BRANCH BLOCK

Fig. 7-5. Note the characteristic wide QS complex in lead V_1 and the wide R wave in lead V_6 with slight notching at the peak. The inverted T waves in leads V_5 and V_6 are also characteristic of LBBB (secondary T wave inversions).

Fig. 7-6. Comparison of leads V_1 and V_6, with normal conduction, right bundle branch block, and left bundle branch block. Normally lead V_1 shows an rS complex and lead V_6 a qR complex. With RBBB, lead V_1 shows a wide rSR' complex and lead V_6 a qRS complex. With LBBB, lead V_1 shows a wide QS complex and lead V_6 a wide R wave.

casionally an ECG will show wide QRS complexes that are not typical of an RBBB or LBBB pattern. In such cases, the general term *intraventricular delay* is used (Fig. 7-7).

Complete vs Incomplete LBBB

As with RBBB, there are complete and incomplete forms of LBBB. With complete LBBB, the QRS complex has the characteristic appearance described previously, and the QRS complex is 0.12 second or wider. With incomplete LBBB, the QRS complex is between 0.1 and 0.12 second.

Clinical Significance

Unlike RBBB, which is occasionally seen in normal people, LBBB is usually a sign of organic heart disease. LBBB is often seen in elderly patients with chronic degenerative changes in their myocardial conduction system. LBBB may develop in patients with long-standing hypertensive heart disease, with valvular lesions (such as aortic stenosis or aortic regurgitation), or with different types of cardiomyopathy (p. 152). LBBB is also seen in patients with coronary artery disease. Most patients with LBBB have under-

Fig. 7-7. Intraventricular conduction delay. The QRS here is abnormally wide (0.11 sec). However, such a pattern is not typical of LBBB or RBBB. In this case it was caused by a lateral infarction. (See Chapter 8.)

lying left ventricular hypertrophy (p. 80). As described in Chapter 9, when LBBB occurs with an acute myocardial infarction it is often a forerunner of complete heart block. In rare instances some otherwise normal individuals will show an LBBB pattern.

If you find LBBB in a patient, it usually does not require any specific treatment. The major exception is patients with acute myocardial infarction who develop a *new* LBBB pattern on the ECG. Since there is danger that complete heart block may occur, the cardiologist may insert a temporary pacemaker in such a patient (see p. 221).

In patients who have LBBB *without* acute infarction, the risk of developing complete heart block is very small. However, if a patient with LBBB complains of dizziness or fainting, a Holter monitor study should be performed to exclude intermittent AV block.

Finally, in some cases the presence of LBBB may be an important clue to previously undiagnosed but clinically important abnormalities—in particular, coronary artery disease, valvular disease, cardiomyopathy, or hypertensive heart disease.

PACEMAKER PATTERNS

Pacemakers are battery-operated devices that are capable of electrically stimulating the heart. They are used primarily in cases where the patient's own heart rate is not adequate; for example, in complete heart block. In most cases, the pacemaker electrode is inserted into the right ventricle. Therefore, the ECG will show an LBBB pattern, reflecting delayed activation of the left ventricle. Fig. 7-8 gives an example of a pacemaker tracing. The vertical spike preceding each QRS complex is the pacemaker spike, followed by a wide QRS complex with an LBBB morphology (QS complex in lead V_1 and wide R wave in lead V_6). Pacemakers are discussed in greater detail in Chapter 20.

Up to this point, we have mentioned three major causes of a wide QRS complex: RBBB, LBBB, and pacemaker patterns. Later (p. 155) we will complete the list of the differential diagnosis of a wide QRS complex, including a number of other patterns, such as hyperkalemia, the Wolff-Parkinson-White preexcitation syndrome, and toxicity due to certain drugs (for example, quinidine or procainamide).

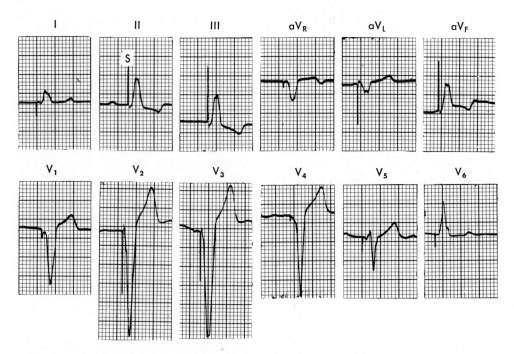

Fig. 7-8. A pacemaker inserted into the right ventricle generally produces a pattern resembling LBBB, with a wide QS complex in lead V_1 and a wide R wave in lead V_6, caused by delayed depolarization of the left ventricle. Note the pacemaker spike in each lead preceding the QRS complex. In some leads (such as lead II) the spike *(S)* is positive; in others (V_1 to V_6) it is negative.

HEMIBLOCKS

We will conclude this chapter on ventricular conduction disturbances by introducing a slightly more complex but important topic, the hemiblocks. Up to now we have discussed the left bundle branch system as if it were a single pathway. Actually it has been known for many years that the left bundle subdivides into major two branches, or *fascicles* (*fasciculus*, Latin, small bundle). The left bundle subdivides into an anterior fascicle and a posterior fascicle. The right bundle branch, on the other hand, is a single pathway and consists of just one main fascicle or bundle.

This revised concept of the bundle branch system as a trifascicular highway (one right fascicle, two left fascicles) is illustrated in Fig. 7-9.

To summarize, the bundle of His divides into a right bundle branch and a left main bundle branch. The left main bundle branch then subdivides into an anterior and a posterior fascicle.

It makes sense to suppose that a block can occur at any single point (or at multiple points) in this trifascicular system. We have already described the ECG pattern seen with a block in the right bundle branch. The pattern of LBBB can obviously occur in one of two ways: by a block at the left main bundle before it divides or by blocks in both subdivisions (anterior and posterior fascicles).

The next question is, what happens if a block occurs in just the anterior or just the posterior fascicle of the left bundle? A block in either fascicle of the left bundle branch system is called a *hemiblock*. Recognition of hemiblocks on the ECG is intimately related to the subject of axis deviation, presented in Chapter 5. Somewhat surprisingly, a hemiblock (unlike a full left or right bundle branch block) does not widen the QRS complex markedly. It has been found experimentally that the main effect of cutting these fascicles is to markedly change the QRS axis. Specifically, *left anterior* hemiblock results in a marked left axis deviation ($-45°$ or more);

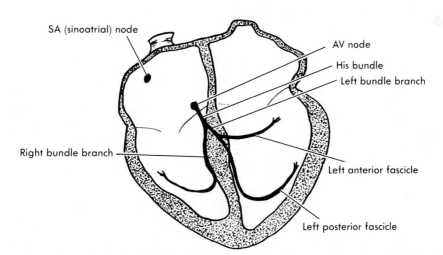

Fig. 7-9. Trifascicular conduction system. Note that the left bundle branch subdivides into a left anterior fascicle and a left posterior fascicle. This diagram is a revision of the original drawing of the conduction system in Fig. 1-1.

left posterior hemiblock produces a right axis deviation (+120° or more).

Discussion of the exact manner in which hemiblocks produce a shift in the QRS axis lies beyond the scope of this book.

To summarize, hemiblocks are partial blocks in the left bundle branch system and involve either the anterior or the posterior fascicle. The diagnosis of a hemiblock is made from the mean QRS axis in the extremity (frontal plane) leads. This is in contrast to the diagnosis of complete (or incomplete) right or left bundle branch block, which is made primarily from the QRS patterns in the chest (horizontal plane) leads.

Left anterior hemiblock. Left anterior hemiblock is diagnosed by finding a mean QRS axis of −45° or more and a QRS width of less than 0.12 second. A mean QRS axis of −45° or more negative can be easily recognized because left axis deviation is present and the S wave in lead aV$_F$ equals or exceeds the R wave in lead I (Fig. 7-10).

Left posterior hemiblock. Left posterior hemiblock (Fig. 9-8, *B*) is diagnosed by finding a mean QRS axis of +120° or more, with a QRS width of less than 0.12 second. *However, the diagnosis of left posterior hemiblock can be considered only if other, more common, causes of right axis deviation* (right ventricular hypertrophy, normal variant, emphysema, lateral wall infarction [Fig. 8-11], and pulmonary embolism) *are first excluded.*

Left anterior hemiblock is relatively common, while isolated left posterior hemiblock is rare.

We will discuss the clinical importance of the hemiblocks and bifascicular and trifascicular blocks further in the section on complete heart block (Chapter 15). In general, the finding of *isolated* left anterior or left posterior hemiblock is not of much clinical significance.

DIAGNOSIS OF HYPERTROPHY IN THE PRESENCE OF BUNDLE BRANCH BLOCKS

The ECG diagnosis of hypertrophy (Chapter 6) in the presence of bundle branch blocks may pose special problems. Therefore, a few general guidelines will be given.

When right ventricular hypertrophy (RVH) occurs with RBBB, right axis deviation is often present. A tall peaked P wave (P

Fig. 7-10. Left anterior hemiblock. Note the marked left axis deviation, without significant widening of the QRS duration.

pulmonale, p. 74) with RBBB should also suggest underlying RVH.

The usual voltage criteria for left ventricular hypertrophy can be used in the presence of RBBB. Unfortunately, RBBB often masks these typical voltage increases. However, if you see evidence of left atrial abnormality (LAA, p. 75) with RBBB, suspect underlying LVH.

The finding of LBBB, regardless of the QRS voltage, is highly suggestive of underlying LVH. Finding LBBB with prominent QRS voltages (p. 80) and evidence of LAA virtually assures the diagnosis of LVH.

Finally, it should be emphasized that the *echocardiogram* is more accurate than the ECG in the diagnosis of cardiac enlargement (see p. 84).

DIAGNOSIS OF MYOCARDIAL INFARCTION IN THE PRESENCE OF BUNDLE BRANCH BLOCKS

The ECG diagnosis of myocardial infarction in the presence of bundle branch blocks is discussed in Chapter 8.

REVIEW OF CHAPTER 7

RBBB shows the following characteristic patterns in the chest leads: an rSR' pattern with a prominent wide final R' wave in V_1 and a qRS pattern with a wide final S wave in V_6. The QRS width is 0.12 second (three small time boxes) or more.

Incomplete RBBB shows the same chest lead patterns as RBBB, but the QRS width is between 0.1 and 0.12 second.

LBBB shows the following characteristic patterns in the chest leads: a deep wide QS pattern (occasionally an rS pattern with a wide S wave) in V_1 and a prominent, often notched, R wave *without* a preceding q wave in V_6. The QRS width is 0.12 second or more.

Incomplete LBBB shows the same chest lead patterns as LBBB, but the QRS width is between 0.1 and 0.12 second.

Pacemaker patterns produced by an electrode in the right ventricle generally resemble LBBB but have a pacemaker spike before each QRS complex.

Hemiblocks can occur because the left bundle divides into two smaller fascicles (bundles): the left anterior fascicle and the left posterior fascicle. Conduction through either or both of these fascicles can be blocked.

Left anterior hemiblock is characterized by a mean QRS axis of $-45°$ or more. (When the mean QRS axis is $-45°$, left axis deviation is present and the height of R_I is equal to the depth of S_{aV_F}. When the mean QRS axis is more negative than $-45°$, S_{aV_F} becomes larger than R_I.)

Left posterior hemiblock is characterized by right axis deviation. However, in making the diagnosis of left posterior hemiblock the other more common causes of right axis deviation (such as right ventricular hypertrophy, lateral wall infarction, chronic lung disease, or normal variants) must first be excluded.

Review Questions—Chapter 7

1. Draw the shape of the QRS complexes you would expect to see in leads V_1 and V_6 with RBBB and LBBB.
2. Examine the following set of chest leads:
   a. What is the approximate QRS width?
   b. What conduction disturbance is present?
   c. Why are the T waves in leads V_1 and V_3 inverted (negative)?

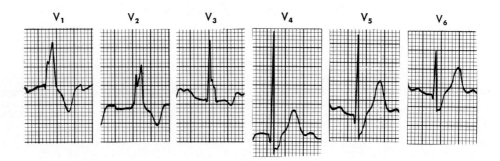

3. Answer these questions about the following ECG:
   a. What is the QRS width?
   b. What type of axis deviation is present?
   c. What ventricular conduction disturbance is present?
   d. What evidence is there of left ventricular hypertrophy?

True or false (4 to 6):

4. Left anterior hemiblock does not markedly widen the QRS complex.
5. LBBB is generally seen in patients with organic heart disease.
6. Bundle branch blocks may occur transiently.

Answers

1. See p. 94.
2. a. 0.12 second.
   b. RBBB.
   c. Secondary T wave inversions may be seen in the right chest leads with RBBB (see p. 90).

3. a. 0.08 second (normal).
   b. Left axis deviation (see p. 65).
   c. Left anterior hemiblock (see p. 98).
   d. Tall R wave in lead aV_L (18 mm) with strain pattern in that lead (see p. 80).
4. True.
5. True.
6. True.

8 Myocardial Ischemia and Infarction—I

Transmural Infarct Patterns

In this chapter and the next, we will discuss one of the most important topics of clinical electrocardiography—the diagnosis of myocardial ischemia and infarction (ischemic heart disease). We will begin with a discussion of certain basic terms.

MYOCARDIAL ISCHEMIA

Myocardial cells require oxygen and other nutrients to function. Oxygenated blood is supplied by the coronary arteries. If blood flow becomes inadequate due to severe narrowing or complete blockage of a coronary artery, ischemia of the heart muscle will develop. The term *"ischemia"* means literally "to hold back blood." Myocardial ischemia may occur transiently. For example, patients who experience angina pectoris with exercise are having transient myocardial ischemia. If the ischemia is more severe, actual necrosis (death) of a portion of heart muscle may occur. The term *"myocardial infarction"* (MI) refers to myocardial necrosis caused by severe ischemia.

In this discussion we will be referring primarily to ischemia and infarction of the left ventricle, the predominant chamber of the heart. Right ventricular infarction will be discussed briefly.

TRANSMURAL AND SUBENDOCARDIAL ISCHEMIA

Fig. 8-1 shows a cross section of the left ventricle. The left ventricle can be subdivided into an outer layer, the *epicardium,* and an inner layer, the *subendocardium.* This distinction is important because myocardial ischemia or infarction is sometimes limited to just the inner layer (subendocardial ischemia and infarction) and sometimes affects the entire thickness of the ventricular wall (transmural ischemia and infarction).

MYOCARDIAL BLOOD SUPPLY

It is also important to understand certain basic facts about the blood supply to the left

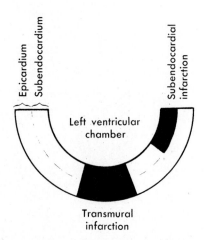

Fig. 8-1. Cross section of the left ventricle showing the difference between a *subendocardial* infarct, which involves the inner half of the ventricular wall, and a *transmural* infarct, which involves the full thickness of the wall.

ventricle. The cardiac blood supply is delivered by the three main coronary arteries (Fig. 8-2). The right coronary artery supplies the inferior (diaphragmatic) portion of the heart. The left anterior descending coronary artery generally supplies the ventricular septum and part of the left ventricular wall. The left circumflex coronary artery supplies the lateral wall of the left ventricle. This circulation pattern may be variable. For example, in some cases the circumflex artery also supplies the inferior portion of the left ventricle. MIs tend to be *localized* to the portion (anterior or inferior) of the left ventricle supplied by one of these arteries.

TRANSMURAL MI

We will begin by describing the effect of a transmural MI on the ECG. In the next chapter we will consider the ECG patterns of subendocardial ischemia and infarction.

Transmural infarction, as mentioned, is characterized by ischemia and, ultimately, by necrosis of a portion of the entire thickness of the left ventricular wall. Not surprisingly, transmural infarction produces changes in both myocardial depolarization (QRS complex) and myocardial repolarization (ST-T complex).

The earliest changes seen with an acute transmural infarction occur in the ST-T complex. There are two sequential phases to these ST-T changes seen with MI: the *acute* phase and the *evolving* phase. The acute phase is marked by the appearance of ST segment elevations and sometimes tall positive (hyperacute) T waves in certain leads. The evolving phase (occurring after hours or days) is characterized by the appearance of deep T wave inversions in those leads that previously showed ST elevations.

Transmural MI can also be described in terms of the location of the infarct: *anterior* means involving the anterior and/or lateral wall of the left ventricle; *inferior* means involving the inferior (diaphragmatic) wall of

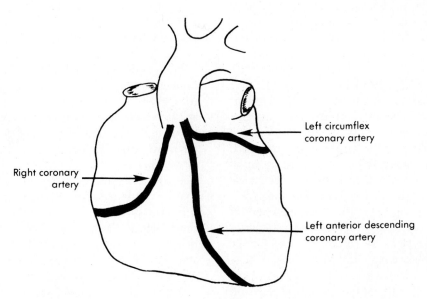

Right coronary
artery

Left circumflex
coronary artery

Left anterior descending
coronary artery

Fig. 8-2. Three major coronary arteries that supply blood to the heart.

Fig. 8-3. Myocardial infarcts are generally localized to either the anterior, **A,** or the inferior (diaphragmatic), **B,** portions of the left ventricle.

the left ventricle (Fig. 8-3). The anatomic location of the infarct determines the leads in which the typical ECG patterns appear. For example, with an acute anterior wall MI the ST segment elevations and tall hyperacute T waves appear in one or more of the anterior leads (chest leads V_1 to V_6, limb leads I and aV_L) (Fig. 8-4). With an inferior wall MI the ST segment elevations and tall hyperacute T waves are seen in inferior leads II, III, and aV_F (Fig. 8-5).

One of the most important characteristics of the ST-T changes seen in MI is their *reciprocity*. The anterior and inferior leads tend to show inverse patterns. Thus, in an anterior infarction with ST segment elevations in leads V_1 to V_6, I, and aV_L, leads II, III, and aV_F will characteristically show ST segment depression. Conversely, in an acute inferior wall infarction, leads II, III, and aV_F will show ST segment elevation, with reciprocal ST segment depressions in one or more of leads V_1 to V_6, I, and aV_L. (These reciprocal changes are illustrated in Figs. 8-4 and 8-5.)

The ST segment elevation seen in acute MI is called a "current of injury" and indicates the acute injury to the epicardial layer of the heart, which occurs with transmural infarction. The exact reason why acute MI produces ST segment elevation is complex and not fully understood. Normally, the ST seg-

ment is isoelectric (neither positive nor negative) because there is no net current flow at this time. Myocardial infarction produces an abnormal electrical charge on the myocardial cell membranes. As a result there is abnormal current flow (current of injury) that produces the ST segment deviations.

The ST segment elevation seen with acute MI may have a variable appearance. The different shapes and appearances of these ST segment elevations are shown in Fig. 8-6. In some cases, as shown, the ST segment is plateau shaped; in other cases it is dome shaped, and sometimes it is obliquely elevated.

The ST segment elevations (and reciprocal ST depressions) are the *earliest* ECG signs of infarction and are generally seen within minutes of the infarct. As mentioned previously, tall positive (hyperacute) T waves may also be seen at this time (Figs. 8-7 and 8-8) and have the same significance as the ST elevations. In some cases hyperacute T waves actually precede the appearance of ST elevation.

After a variable time lag of hours to days, the ST segment elevations start to return to the baseline. At the same time the T waves begin to be inverted in leads that previously showed ST segment elevations. This phase of T wave inversions is called the evolving phase of the infarct. Thus, with an anterior wall infarction the T waves become inverted in one

ECG SEQUENCE WITH ANTERIOR WALL INFARCTION

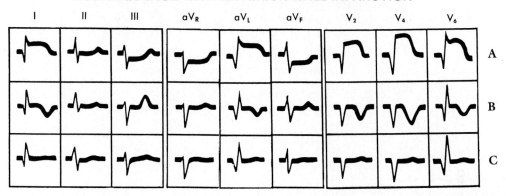

Fig. 8-4. Note the reciprocal ST-T changes in the inferior leads (II, III, and aV$_F$). **A,** Acute phase: ST elevations and new Q waves. **B,** Evolving phase: deep T wave inversions. **C,** Resolving phase: partial or complete regression of ST-T changes (and sometimes of Q waves).

ECG SEQUENCE WITH INFERIOR WALL INFARCTION

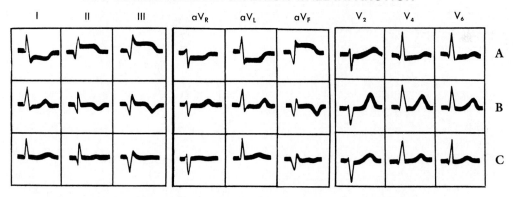

Fig. 8-5. Note the reciprocal ST-T changes in the anterior leads (I, aV$_L$, V$_2$, V$_4$). **A,** Acute phase: ST elevations and new Q waves. **B,** Evolving phase: deep T wave inversions. **C,** Resolving phase: partial or complete regression of ST-T changes (and sometimes of Q waves).

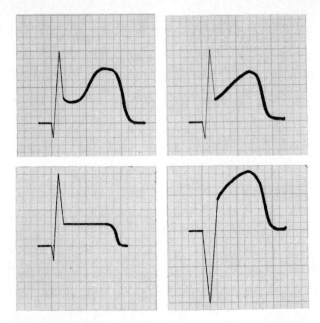

Fig. 8-6. ST segment elevations seen with acute infarction may have variable shapes.

Fig. 8-7. Chest leads from a patient with acute anterior wall infarction. **A,** Note the tall positive (hyperacute) T waves in leads V_2 to V_5 in the earliest phase of the infarction. **B,** Recorded several hours later. There is marked ST segment elevation in the same leads (current of injury pattern) with abnormal Q waves in leads V_1 and V_2.

Fig. 8-8. Hyperacute T waves with anterior wall infarction. This patient was complaining of severe chest pain. Note the very tall (hyperacute) T waves in the chest leads. There are also slight ST segment elevations in lead aV_L with reciprocal ST depressions in leads II, III, and aV_F. In lead V_4, note the premature atrial contraction *(PAC)*.

or more of the anterior leads (V_1 to V_6, I, aV_L). With an inferior wall infarction the T waves become inverted in one or more of the inferior leads (II, III, aV_F). These T wave inversions are illustrated in Figs. 8-4 and 8-5.

QRS Changes: Q Waves of Transmural Infarction

Transmural infarction also produces distinctive changes in the QRS (depolarization) complex. The characteristic sign of a transmural infarct is the appearance of new Q waves.

Why do transmural MIs lead to Q waves? Recall that a Q wave is simply an initial negative deflection of the QRS complex. If the entire QRS complex is negative $\left(\bigvee\right)$, we call it a *QS complex*. A Q wave (negative deflection) in any lead simply indicates that the electrical voltages are directed away from that particular lead. When transmural infarction occurs, there is necrosis of heart muscle in a localized area of the ventricle; therefore the electrical voltages produced by this portion of the myocardium will disappear. Instead of positive (R) waves over the infarcted area, Q waves will be recorded (either a QR or a QS complex).

To summarize, abnormal Q waves are the characteristic markers of transmural infarction.* Q waves signify the loss of positive electrical voltages caused by the death of heart muscle.

---

*As discussed in the next chapter, the equation of pathologic Q waves with transmural necrosis is an oversimplification. Not all transmural infarcts lead to Q waves, and not all Q wave infarcts correlate with transmural necrosis.

The new Q waves of an MI generally appear within the first day or so of the infarct. With an anterior wall infarction, the Q waves will be seen in one or more of leads V_1 to V_6, I, and aV_L (Fig. 8-4). With an inferior wall MI, the new Q waves will appear in leads II, III, and aV_F (Fig. 8-5).

LOCALIZATION OF INFARCTS

As mentioned, MIs are generally localized to a specific portion of the left ventricle, affecting either the anterior or the inferior wall. Anterior infarcts (Figs. 8-9 to 8-11) are sometimes considered as anteroseptal, strictly anterior, or anterolateral depending on the leads that show signs of the infarct.

Anterior Wall Infarcts

The characteristic feature of anterior wall infarcts is a *loss of the normal R wave progression in the chest leads*. Normally (as described in

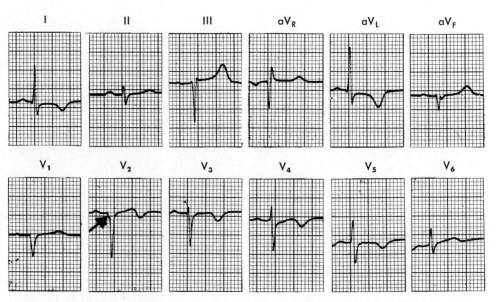

Fig. 8-9. Anterior wall infarction. Note the QS complexes in leads V_1 and V_2, indicating anteroseptal infarction. There is also a characteristic notching (*arrow, V_2*) of the QS complex, often seen with infarcts. In addition, note the diffuse ischemic T wave inversions in leads I, aV_L, and V_2 to V_5, indicating generalized anterior wall ischemia.

Chapter 4) there is a progressive increase in the height of the R wave as you move from the right to the left chest leads. An anterior infarct interrupts this normal R wave progression, resulting in pathologic Q waves in one or more of the chest leads.

Anteroseptal infarcts. Normally, as mentioned earlier, the ventricular septum is depolarized from left to right, so leads V_1 and V_2 show small positive r waves (septal r waves). Consider the effect of damaging the septum. Clearly, you would expect to see a loss of septal depolarization voltages; thus, in leads V_1 and V_2 the normal septal r waves will be lost and an entirely negative QS complex will appear.

The septum is supplied with blood by the left anterior descending coronary artery, and septal infarction generally suggests that there has been an occlusion of this artery or one of its branches.

Fig. 8-10. Evolving anterior wall infarction. The patient sustained the infarct 1 week earlier. Note the abnormal Q waves (leads I, aV_L, and V_2 to V_5) with slight ST segment elevations and deep T wave inversions. Left axis deviation resulting from left anterior hemiblock is present as well. (See Chapter 7.)

Strictly anterior infarcts. Normally leads V_3 and V_4 show RS- or Rs-type complexes. If the anterior wall of the left ventricle is infarcted, then the positive R waves that reflect the voltages produced by this muscle area will be lost. Instead, Q waves, as part of QS or QR complexes, will be seen in leads V_3 and V_4. Strictly anterior infarcts generally also result from oc-clusion of the left anterior descending coronary artery.

Anterolateral infarcts. Infarction of the lateral wall of the left ventricle produces changes in the more laterally situated chest leads, for example, leads V_5 and V_6. With lateral wall infarction, abnormal Q waves, as part of QS or QR complexes, appear in leads V_5 and V_6 (Fig.

Fig. 8-11. Evolving anterior wall infarction. The infarct occurred 1 week earlier. Note the poor R wave progression in leads V_1 to V_5 with Q waves in leads I and aV_L. T waves are slightly inverted in these leads. Right axis deviation in this case is the result of loss of lateral wall forces, with Q waves in I and aV_L.

7-7). Lateral wall infarction is often caused by an occlusion of the left circumflex coronary artery but may also result from occlusion of the left anterior descending coronary artery or a branch of the right coronary artery.

Differentiating anterior wall infarctions. The above classification of anterior infarcts—as anteroseptal, strictly anterior, and anterolateral—is not absolute. Often there is overlap. You can simply describe MIs by calling any infarct that shows ECG changes in one or more of leads I, aV_L, and V_1 to V_6 as "anterior" and then specifying which leads show Q waves and ST-T changes.

Inferior Wall Infarcts

Infarction of the inferior (diaphragmatic) portion of the left ventricle is indicated by changes in leads II, III, and aV_F (Figs. 8-12 to 8-14). These three leads, as shown in the frontal plane axis diagram, are oriented downward or inferiorly (Fig. 5-1). Thus these leads will record voltages from the inferior portion of the ventricle. An inferior wall infarct will produce abnormal Q waves in leads II, III, and aV_F.

Inferior wall infarction is generally caused by occlusion of the right coronary artery and, less commonly, by a left circumflex coronary obstruction.

"Posterior" Infarcts

The posterior (back) surface of the left ventricle can also be infarcted. This may be difficult to diagnose because characteristic abnormal ST elevations may not appear in any of the 12 conventional leads. Instead, a tall R wave and ST segment depression may occur in chest leads V_1 and V_2 (reciprocal to the Q wave and ST segment elevations that would be recorded at the back of the heart). During the evolving phase of such infarcts, when deep T wave inversions appear in the posterior leads, the anterior chest leads will show reciprocally tall positive T waves (Fig. 8-15).

In most cases of posterior MI the infarct extends either to the lateral wall of the left ventricle, producing characteristic changes in

Fig. 8-12. Acute inferior wall infarction. Note the ST elevations in leads II, III, and aV_F with reciprocal ST depressions in leads I and aV_L. Abnormal Q waves are also present in leads II, III, and aV_F.

Fig. 8-13. Inferior wall infarct. This patient sustained a myocardial infarction 1 month previously. Note the abnormal Q waves and symmetric T wave inversions in leads II, III, and aV$_F$. There is also T wave flattening in lead V$_6$. Q waves and ST-T changes after infarction may persist indefinitely or may resolve partially or completely.

lead V$_6$, or to the inferior wall of the left ventricle, producing characteristic changes in leads II, III, and aV$_F$ (Fig. 8-15). Because of the overlap between *inferior* and *posterior* infarcts the more general term "inferoposterior" can be used when the ECG shows changes consistent with either inferior or posterior infarction.

Right Ventricular (RV) Infarcts

A related topic is right ventricular (RV) infarction. Recent studies show that a high per-

centage of patients with an inferoposterior infarct have associated RV involvement. In one autopsy study RV infarction was noted in about one of four cases of inferoposterior MI but not in cases of anterior MI. Clinically patients with an RV infarct may have elevated central venous pressure (distended neck veins) because of the abnormally high diastolic filling pressures in the right side of the heart. If the RV damage is severe, hypotension and even cardiogenic shock may result. AV conduction disturbances are not uncom-

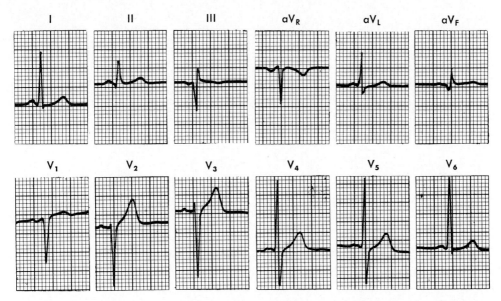

Fig. 8-14. Old inferior wall infarct. Note the prominent Q waves in leads II, III, and aV_F from a patient who sustained an MI 1 year previously. The ST-T changes have essentially reverted to normal.

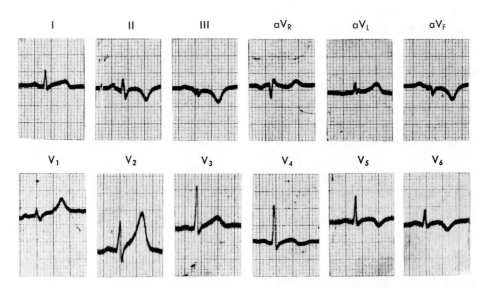

Fig. 8-15. Posterior infarction. Note the tall R waves in V_1 and V_2. In addition, there is evidence of a prior inferior infarction (Q waves in II, III, aV_F) and probably a lateral infarction as well (T wave inversions in V_4 to V_6) Note also the reciprocally tall positive T waves in anterior precordial leads V_1 and V_2. (From Goldberger, A.L.: Myocardial infarction: electrocardiographic differential diagnosis, ed. 3, St. Louis, 1984, The C.V. Mosby Co.)

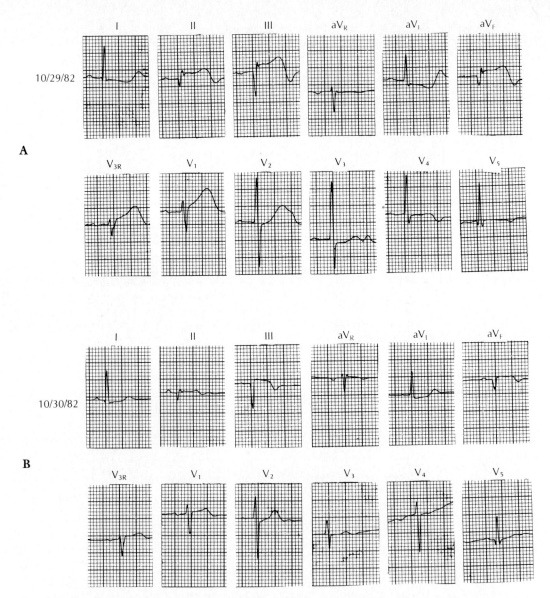

Fig. 8-16. Acute right ventricular infarction with inferior wall infarction. **A,** Q waves and ST segment elevations in leads II, III, and aV$_F$ are accompanied by ST elevations in the right precordial leads (V$_{3R}$ and V$_1$). ST-T changes in V$_5$ and V$_6$ are consistent with lateral wall ischemia. ST depression in I and aV$_L$ is probably reciprocal to an inferior wall injury current. **B,** Follow-up tracing showing diminution of acute ST changes. The patient was hypotensive, and right-sided heart catheterization showed elevated right-sided heart filling pressures but relatively low pulmonary capillary wedge pressure. The patient responded favorably to volume expansion. (From Goldberger, A.: Myocardial infarction, ed. 3, St. Louis, 1984, The C.V. Mosby Co.)

mon in this setting. The presence of jugular venous distension in a patient with an acute inferoposterior MI should always suggest this diagnosis. In addition, many of these patients will show ST segment elevations in leads reflecting the right ventricle, such as V_1 to V_3 and V_{3R} to V_{5R} (p. 31, footnote), as shown in Fig. 8-16.

Recognition of RV infarction is of major clinical importance. Volume expansion may be critical in patients who are hypotensive and have a low or normal pulmonary capillary wedge pressure despite elevated systemic venous pressure. Patients with an acute RV infarct may also be at increased risk for the development of ventricular fibrillation during placement of a temporary pacemaker.

SEQUENCE OF Q WAVES AND ST-T CHANGES WITH TRANSMURAL INFARCTS

Up to now we have discussed separately the ventricular depolarization (QRS) and repolarization (ST-T) changes produced by a transmural MI. As shown in the examples in Figs. 8-4 and 8-5, these changes occur simultaneously.

Ordinarily the earliest sign of transmural infarction is ST segment elevations (with reciprocal ST depressions). The ST elevations (current of injury pattern) usually persist for hours to days. During this same period Q waves will begin to appear in leads showing ST elevations. Following these changes, the ST segments start to return to the baseline; and the T waves become inverted during the evolving phase.

In the weeks or months following an infarct, what should you expect to happen to the Q waves and the ST-T changes described above? The answer is that you cannot make any certain predictions. In most cases the abnormal Q waves will persist for months, and even years, after the acute infarction. However, the Q waves may occasionally diminish in size and even disappear entirely. In some cases abnormal T wave inversions will persist

indefinitely. In others there will be improvement in the ECG but minor nonspecific ST-T abnormalities (such as slight T wave flattening) may persist (Figs. 8-4 and 8-5).

NORMAL AND ABNORMAL Q WAVES

One of the diagnostic problems frequently faced is deciding whether or not Q waves are abnormal. Not all Q waves are indicators of MI. For example, we normally expect to see a Q wave in lead aV_R. Furthermore, small "septal" q waves are normally seen in the left chest leads (V_4 to V_6) and in one or more of leads I, aV_L, II, III, and aV_F. Recall from Chapter 4 the significance of these septal q waves. The ventricular septum depolarizes from left to right. Left chest leads record this spread of voltages toward the right as a small negative deflection (q wave) as part of a qR complex, where the R wave represents the spread of left ventricular voltages toward the lead. When the electrical axis is horizontal, such qR complexes will be seen in leads I and aV_L. When the electrical axis is vertical, qR complexes will appear in leads II, III, and aV_F.

These normal septal q waves must be differentiated from the pathologic Q waves of infarction. Normal septal q waves are characteristically narrow and of low amplitude. As a rule septal q waves are less than 0.04 second in duration. (The width of a q wave or a Q wave is measured on the upper level of the baseline from the point where it begins to the point where it returns to the baseline.) A Q wave of 0.04 second or more in lead I, in all three inferior leads (II, III, aV_F), or in leads V_3 to V_6 is generally abnormal.

What about a Q wave of 0.04 second or more width in leads V_1 and V_2? A large QS complex can be seen as a normal variant in lead V_1 and rarely in leads V_1 and V_2. However, QS waves in these leads may be the only evidence of an anteroseptal MI. An abnormal QS complex resulting from infarction will sometimes show a notch as it descends or it will be slurred instead of descending and rising abruptly (Fig. 8-9). Further criteria for differentiating normal from abnormal Q waves in these leads lie beyond the scope of this book.

What about a wide Q wave in lead aV_L or Q waves in leads III and aV_F, which can also occur normally? Here again, the precise criteria to differentiate normal from abnormal Q waves in these leads lie beyond the scope of this book. However, the following can be taken as general rules:

1. An inferior wall MI should be diagnosed with certainty only when abnormal Q waves are seen in leads II, III, and aV_F. If you see Q waves just in leads III and aV_F, then the likelihood of MI is increased by the presence of abnormal ST-T changes in all three inferior limb leads.

2. An anterior wall infarction should not be diagnosed from lead aV_L alone. Look for abnormal Q waves and ST-T changes in the other anterior leads (I and V_1 to V_6).

Furthermore, just as not all Q waves are abnormal, so not all abnormal Q waves are a result of MI. For example, poor R wave progression in the chest leads, sometimes with actual QS complexes in the right to middle chest leads (for example, V_1 to V_3), may occur with left bundle branch block, left ventricular hypertrophy, and chronic lung disease in the absence of MI. Prominent noninfarctional Q waves are often a characteristic feature of the ECG in idiopathic hypertrophic subaortic stenosis (IHSS) (Fig. 8-17). Noninfarction Q waves also occur in dilated cardiomyopathy (Fig. 10-15). As mentioned before, nor-

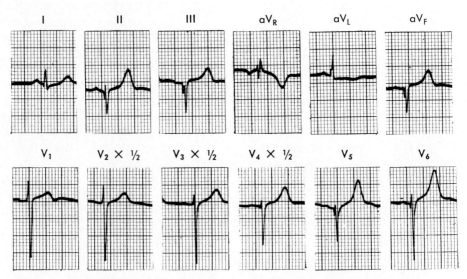

Fig. 8-17. Idiopathic hypertrophic subaortic stenosis (IHSS). Note the prominent pseudoinfarctional Q waves, which are the result of septal hypertrophy. (From Goldberger, A.L.: Myocardial infarction: electrocardiographic differential diagnosis, ed. 3, St. Louis, 1984, The C.V. Mosby Co.)

mal people may sometimes have a QS wave in lead V_1 and rarely in leads V_1 and V_2. Q waves in the absence of MI are sometimes referred to as *pseudoinfarct patterns.**

---

*See Goldberger, A.L.: Myocardial infarction: electrocardiographic differential diagnosis, ed. 3, St. Louis, 1984, The C.V. Mosby Co.

VENTRICULAR ANEURYSM

Following a large MI, some patients will develop a ventricular aneurysm. An aneurysm is a portion of infarcted ventricular myocardium that does not contract normally. Instead, during ventricular contraction (systole) the aneurysmic portion bulges outward while the rest of the ventricle is contracting. Ventricular aneurysms may occur on the anterior

Fig. 8-18. Anterior wall aneurysm. The patient sustained an infarct several months prior to this ECG. Note the prominent Q waves in leads V_1 to V_3 and aV_L with persistent ST elevations in these leads and with reciprocal ST depressions in the inferior leads (II, III, and aV_F). Persistent ST elevations more than 2 weeks after an infarct suggest possible aneurysm.

or inferior surface of the heart. The ECG may be helpful in making the diagnosis of ventricular aneurysm following an MI. Patients with ventricular aneurysms frequently show persistent ST segment elevations following the infarct. As mentioned earlier, the ST segment elevations seen with acute infarction generally resolve within several days. The persistence of ST segment elevations for 2 weeks or more is suggestive of a ventricular aneurysm (Fig. 8-18). On the other hand, the absence of persisting ST segment elevations does not rule out the possibility of an aneurysm.

Ventricular aneurysms are of clinical importance for several major reasons. The aneurysm may lead to congestive heart failure, or it may be associated with serious ventricular arrhythmias in some patients. In addition, a thrombus may form in an aneurysm and break off, resulting in stroke or some other embolic complication.

MULTIPLE INFARCTIONS

Up to this point we have discussed localized single infarcts. Not infrequently patients may have two or more MIs at different times. For example, a patient with a previous inferior wall infarction may develop a new anterior wall infarct. In such cases the ECG will initially show abnormal Q waves in leads II, III, and aV$_F$. During the anterior infarct new Q waves and ST-T changes will develop in the anterior leads. Fig. 8-19 shows the ECG of a patient with multiple infarcts (anterior and inferior).

SILENT MI

Most patients with acute MI have symptoms. They may experience the classic syndrome of crushing substernal chest pain. In other cases the pain may be atypical (for example, indigestion, high back pain, jaw pain). However, in some cases of infarction the patient may experience few if any symptoms. Therefore, it

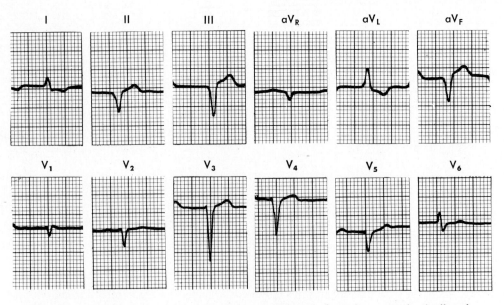

Fig. 8-19. Multiple infarcts. This ECG shows evidence of previous anterior wall and inferior wall MIs. Note the poor R wave progression and QS complexes in chest leads V$_1$ to V$_5$, as well as the QS waves in leads II, III, and aV$_F$.

Fig. 8-20. Acute anterior wall infarction and the RBBB pattern. Note the wide QRS complexes with an rSR′ wave in lead V_1 and a qRS pattern in V_5, indicating RBBB. There is, furthermore, a pattern of acute anterior wall infarction (Q waves and ST elevations in leads I and aV_L plus marked reciprocal ST depressions in II, III, and aV_F). Finally, note the left axis deviations caused by the left anterior hemiblock. This combination (left anterior hemiblock and RBBB) is an example of bifascicular block and may herald complete heart block in patients with an acute anterior infarction.

is not unusual to see abnormal Q waves on a patient's ECG that suggest a previous infarct, without any clinical history of a definite MI. Such "silent infarcts" are particularly common in the elderly.

DIAGNOSIS OF MI IN THE PRESENCE OF BUNDLE BRANCH BLOCK

Up to now we have described the effects of an MI on the normal ECG. In some cases the diagnosis of infarction is made more difficult because the patient's baseline ECG may show a bundle branch block pattern or because the patient may develop a bundle branch block as a complication of the infarct. In such cases the ECG picture becomes more complex.

Right Bundle Branch Block with MI

The diagnosis of an MI can be made relatively easily in the presence of right bundle branch block (RBBB). Remember that RBBB affects primarily the terminal phase of ventricular depolarization, producing a wide R' wave in the right chest leads and a wide S wave in the left chest leads. MI affects the initial phase of ventricular depolarization, producing abnormal Q waves. When RBBB and an infarct occur together, you will see a combination of both patterns. The QRS complex will be abnormally wide (0.12 sec or more) as a result of the bundle branch block, lead V_1 will show a terminal positive deflection, and lead V_6 will show a wide S wave. If the infarction is anterior, there will be a loss of R wave progression with abnormal Q waves in the anterior leads and characteristic ST-T changes. If the infarct is inferior, pathologic Q waves and ST-T changes will be seen in leads II, III, and aV_F. Fig. 8-20 shows RBBB and acute MI. (See also p. 342.)

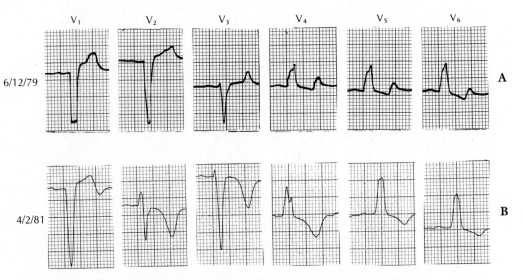

Fig. 8-21. A, Typical left bundle branch block pattern. Note the poor R wave progression in the right precordial leads and the dicordance of QRS and ST-T vectors reflected by ST elevations in the right precordial and ST depressions with T wave inversions in the left precordial leads. **B,** Subsequently the ECG from this patient showed development of primary T wave inversions in leads V_1 to V_3 caused by anterior ischemia and probable infarction. (From Goldberger, A.L.: Myocardial infarction: electrocardiographic differential diagnosis, ed. 3, St. Louis, 1984, The C.V. Mosby Co.)

Left Bundle Branch Block with MI

The diagnosis of left bundle branch block (LBBB) in the presence of MI is considerably more complicated and confusing than that of RBBB. The reason is that LBBB interrupts both the early and the late phases of ventricular stimulation (Chapter 7). It also produces secondary ST-T changes. As a general rule LBBB will hide the diagnosis of an infarct. *Thus a patient with a chronic LBBB pattern who then develops an acute MI may not show the characteristic changes of infarction described in this chapter.* Occasionally patients with LBBB will develop primary ST-T changes indicative of ischemia or actual infarction. As discussed in Chapter 7, the secondary T wave inversions of uncomplicated LBBB are seen in the left chest leads (V_4 to V_6) (with prominent R waves). The appearance of T wave inversions in the right chest leads (with prominent S waves) is a primary abnormality that cannot be ascribed to the LBBB itself (Fig. 8-21).

The problem of diagnosing infarction with LBBB is further complicated by the fact that the LBBB pattern, in and of itself, has several features that resemble those seen with infarction. An LBBB pattern, therefore, can mimic an infarct pattern. As you recall from Chapter 7, LBBB patterns typically show poor R wave progression in the chest leads because of the reversal in the way the ventricular septum is activated. With LBBB the ventricular septum is depolarized from right to left, the reverse of what happens normally. Consequently, with LBBB, there is a loss of the normal septal R waves in the right chest leads. This loss of normal R wave progression simulates the pattern seen in an anterior wall infarct.

Fig. 7-5 shows an example of LBBB with

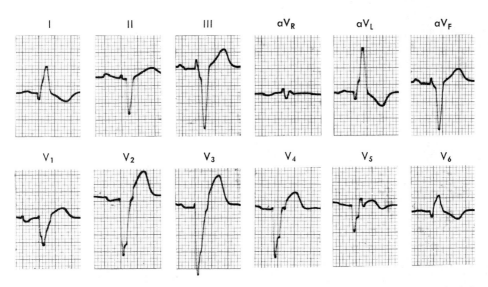

Fig. 8-22. Anterior wall infarction with LBBB. Note the prominent Q waves in the left chest leads as part of QR complexes. See text. (From Goldberger, A.L.: Myocardial infarction: electrocardiographic differential diagnosis, ed. 3, St. Louis, 1984, The C.V. Mosby Co.)

poor R wave progression. Anterior wall infarction was not present. Notice that the ST segments in the right chest leads are elevated, resembling the pattern seen during the hyperacute or acute phase of an infarction. This pattern of ST segment elevation in the right chest leads is also commonly seen with LBBB in the absence of infarction.

As a general rule a patient with an LBBB pattern should not be diagnosed as having had a myocardial infarction simply on the basis of poor R wave progression in the right chest leads or ST elevations in these leads.

However, the presence of Q waves as part of QR complexes in the left chest leads (V_5 and V_6) with LBBB generally indicates underlying MI (Fig. 8-22). In addition, the appearance of ST elevations in the left chest leads or in leads with prominent R waves from a patient with LBBB also suggests ischemia (Fig. 8-22, lead V_5).

In the next chapter, we will continue this discussion of the ECG with ischemia and infarction, focusing on the ECG patterns seen with *subendocardial* ischemia.

REVIEW OF CHAPTER 8

Myocardial ischemia occurs when the blood supply to the myocardium is not adequate. *Myocardial infarction* (MI) refers to necrosis of the myocardium caused by severe ischemia.

Myocardial ischemia or infarction can affect the entire thickness of the ventricular muscle (*transmural* injury), or it may be localized to just the inner layer of the ventricle (*subendocardial* ischemia or infarction). Transmural MI produces a typical sequence of ST-T changes and abnormal Q waves. The ST-T changes can be divided into two phases: (1) an acute phase, marked by ST segment elevations (current of injury pattern) and sometimes tall positive T waves (hyperacute T waves), and (2) an evolving phase, characterized by the appearance of deeply inverted T waves in leads that showed the hyperacute T waves and ST elevations. These ST-T changes occur during a period of hours or days and usually slowly resolve over a period of weeks or months. Usually during the first day or so after transmural infarction, new abnormal Q waves will appear in one or more leads.

When ST segment elevations persist for more than 2 or 3 weeks after an acute MI, this may be a sign that a ventricular aneurysm has developed. The abnormal Q waves tend to persist but may become smaller with time and, rarely, may even disappear.

Transmural MI can also be described in terms of the location of the infarct. With *anterior* infarction, ST segment elevations and abnormal Q waves occur in one or more of leads V_1 to V_6, I, and aV_L. (Reciprocal ST depressions may be seen in leads II, III, and aV_F.) With *inferior* infarction, ST elevations and Q waves will appear in leads II, III, and aV_F and there may be reciprocal ST depressions in one or more of the anterior leads.

Right ventricular MI is a common complication of inferoposterior infarcts. In acute cases the ECG may also show elevated ST segments in the right chest leads.

The pathologic Q waves of infarction must be distinguished from normal Q waves. For example, small normal "septal" q waves as part of qR complexes may be seen in the left chest leads (V_4 to V_6), in leads II, III, and aV_F (with a vertical electrical axis), and in leads I and aV_L (with a horizontal axis). These septal q waves are normally less than 0.04 sec in width.

A QS wave may be seen normally in lead V_1 and occasionally in leads V_1 and V_2. Q waves may also be seen as normal variants in leads aV_F, III, and aV_L.

Multiple MIs may occur and the ECG will show old Q waves from the preceding infarct as well as new Q waves with ST-T changes from the current infarct.

When *right bundle branch block* complicates acute MI, the diagnosis of both conditions is possible. The RBBB prolongs the QRS width, and lead V_1 shows a tall positive final deflection. In addition, abnormal Q waves and ST segment elevations resulting from the acute MI will be present in the chest leads (with an anterior MI) and in leads II, III, and aV_F (in inferior MI).

When *left bundle branch block* complicates acute MI, it is often difficult to diagnose the MI because the LBBB may mask both the abnormal Q waves of the MI and the ST segment elevations and T wave inversions of the ischemia. In addition, LBBB may produce a QS wave in the right chest leads with ST segment elevation and poor R wave progression across the chest *without* MI. The presence of QR complexes in the left chest leads with LBBB is suggestive of underlying MI. T wave inversion in the right chest leads or ST segment elevation in the left chest leads or in leads with prominent R waves suggests ischemia with underlying LBBB.

Review Questions—Chapter 8

See the end of Chapter 9.

9 Myocardial Ischemia and Infarction—II
Subendocardial Ischemia and Infarct Patterns

Transmural myocardial infarction (MI) may be associated with abnormal Q waves and the typical progression of ST-T changes described in Chapter 8. In other cases (described in this chapter), however, myocardial ischemia with or without actual infarction may be limited to the *subendocardial* layer of the ventricle.

SUBENDOCARDIAL ISCHEMIA

How can subendocardial ischemia occur without transmural ischemia or infarction? The subendocardium is most distant from the coronary blood supply and closest to the high pressure of the ventricular cavity and therefore is particularly vulnerable to ischemia. It can become ischemic while the outer layer of the ventricle (epicardium) remains normally perfused with blood.

The most common ECG change with subendocardial ischemia is ST segment depression (shown in Fig. 9-1). The ST segment depression caused by subendocardial ischemia may be limited to the anterior leads (I, aV_L, and V_1 to V_6) or to the inferior leads (II, III, and aV_F), or may be seen more diffusely in both groups of leads. As shown in Fig. 9-1, the ST segment depression seen with subendocardial ischemia has a characteristic squared-off shape. (ST segment elevations may be seen in lead aV_R.)

Recall from the previous chapter that acute transmural infarction produces ST segment elevation, a current of injury pattern. This ST segment elevation results from epicardial injury. With pure subendocardial ischemia just the opposite pattern occurs—ST segment depression (except in lead aV_R, which often shows ST elevation).

To summarize, myocardial ischemia involving just the subendocardium produces ST segment depression while acute ischemia involving the epicardium produces ST elevation. This difference in the direction of the injury current vector in epicardial versus subendocardial ischemia is depicted in Fig. 9-2.

ECG Changes with Angina Pectoris

The term "angina pectoris" refers to transient attacks of chest pain caused by myocardial ischemia. Angina is a symptom of coronary artery disease. The classic attack of angina is experienced as a dull, burning, or boring sub-

Fig. 9-1. Subendocardial ischemia may produce ST depressions.

sternal pressure or pain. Angina is typically precipitated by exertion, stress, exposure to cold, and so on, and is relieved by rest and nitroglycerin.

Many patients with classic angina will show an ECG pattern of subendocardial ischemia, with ST segment depressions during an attack. When the pain disappears, the ST depressions generally return to the baseline.

Fig. 9-3 shows an example of ST depressions during a spontaneous episode of angina. Not all patients with angina will show ST depressions during chest pain. The presence of a normal ECG does not rule out underlying coronary artery disease. However, the appearance of transient ST segment depression with chest pain is a strong indicator of myocardial ischemia.

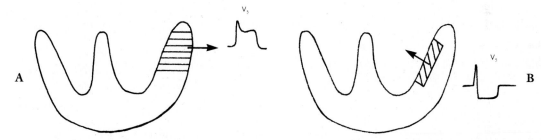

Fig. 9-2. Epicardial versus subendocardial injury currents. **A,** Acute epicardial ischemia as seen in a case of transmural MI. Electrical forces *(arrow)* responsible for the ST segment are deviated toward the outer layer of the heart, causing ST elevations in the overlying lead. **B,** Acute subendocardial ischemia. The electrical forces *(arrow)* responsible for the ST segment are deviated toward the inner layer of the heart, causing ST depressions in lead V_5, which faces the outer surface of the heart.

Fig. 9-3. This patient complained of chest pain while being examined. **A,** Note the marked ST depressions in lead V_4. **B,** Five minutes later, after nitroglycerin, the ST segments have reverted to normal, with relief of the angina.

Exercise Testing

Many patients with coronary artery disease will have a normal ECG while at rest; however, during exercise, ischemic changes may appear on their ECGs because of the extra oxygen requirements imposed on their heart muscle by exertion. To assist in diagnosing coronary artery disease, the ECG can be recorded while the patient is being exercised under controlled conditions. Such *stress elec-*

trocardiography can be performed while the patient walks on a treadmill or pedals a bicycle. The test is stopped when the patient develops angina, fatigue, or diagnostic ST changes or when the heart rate reaches 85% to 90% of a maximum predetermined rate, predicted from the patient's age. (This is known as *submaximal testing.*)

Fig. 9-4, *A,* shows the normal resting ECG of a patient. Fig. 9-4, *B,* shows marked ST

Fig. 9-4. Positive exercise test. **A,** Baseline rhythm strip from a patient with coronary artery disease. **B,** Note the marked ST depressions with increased heart rate. (From Goldberger, A.L.: Myocardial infarction: electrocardiograhic differential diagnosis, ed. 3, St. Louis, 1984, The C.V. Mosby Co.)

Fig. 9-5. Physiologic ST segment depression with exercise. Note the J junction depression *(arrow)* with upsloping of the ST segments. (From Goldberger, A.L.: Myocardial infarction: electrocardiographic differential diagnosis, ed. 3, St. Louis, 1984, The C.V. Mosby Co.)

segment depressions recorded while the patient was exercising. The appearance of ST segment depressions constitutes a positive (abnormal) result. Most cardiologists accept horizontal or downward ST depression of at least 1 mm or more, lasting at least 0.08 second, as a positive (abnormal) test result (Fig. 9-4, *B*). ST depression less than 1 mm, or depression of only the J point, with a rapid upward sloping of the ST segment, is considered a negative (normal) test response (Fig. 9-5).

Exercise electrocardiography is often helpful in diagnosing coronary artery disease. However, like all tests, it may give both false-positive and false-negative results. For example, about 10% of normal men and an even higher percentage of normal women will have false-positive exercise tests. False-positive tests also can be seen in patients taking digitalis and in those with hypokalemia, left ventricular hypertrophy, ventricular conduction disturbances, or Wolff-Parkinson-White syndrome (p. 152). False-negative tests also can occur despite the presence of significant underlying coronary artery disease.

The likelihood that an exercise test will be abnormal is, in part, a reflection of the extent of the coronary obstructions. Thus only about 40% of subjects with stenosis of a single coronary vessel will have a positive test while over 60% of those with two-vessel disease and over 80% with three-vessel disease will have positive test results. Therefore, a normal exercise test does not exclude coronary artery disease.

To summarize, subendocardial ischemia, such as occurs with typical angina pectoris (and as may sometimes be elicited with stress testing), often produces ST segment depressions in one or more leads.

SUBENDOCARDIAL INFARCTION

If the ischemia to the subendocardial region is severe enough, actual subendocardial infarction may occur. In such cases the ECG may show persistent ST segment depression instead of the transient ST depressions seen with reversible subendocardial ischemia.

Fig. 9-6 shows an example of subendocardial infarction. Do Q waves appear with pure subendocardial infarction? The answer is that if only the subendocardium is infarcted abnormal Q waves usually do not appear. As a rule Q waves are seen only with transmural infarction. Subendocardial infarction generally affects ventricular repolarization (ST-T complex) and not depolarization (QRS complex). However, exceptions may occur (see p. 134).

Another pattern sometimes seen in cases of *nontransmural* (non–Q wave) infarctions is T wave inversion with or without ST segment depressions. Fig. 9-7 shows a subendocardial infarction pattern with deep T wave inversions. (T wave inversions may also be seen in some cases of noninfarctional ischemia.)

To summarize, subendocardial infarction can produce either (1) persistent ST segment depressions without Q waves or (2) T wave inversions without Q waves.

VARIETY OF ECG CHANGES SEEN WITH MYOCARDIAL ISCHEMIA

It should be apparent by now that myocardial ischemia can produce a wide variety of ECG changes. For example, transmural infarction (discussed earlier) causes abnormal Q waves as well as ST segment elevations followed by T wave inversions. Ventricular aneurysm may be associated with persistent ST segment elevations. Subendocardial ischemia (seen, for example, during anginal attacks or during a stress test) may produce transient ST segment depressions. Actual subendocardial infarction may lead to persistent ST depressions or to T wave inversions without Q waves.

ECG Changes Associated with Noninfarctional Ischemia

The foregoing list does not include all the possible ECG patterns seen in myocardial

Fig. 9-6. Subendocardial infarction. This patient complained of severe chest pain. Subsequently cardiac enzymes were elevated. Note the marked ST depressions, best seen in chest leads V_2 to V_5, consistent with subendocardial infarction. There is also a premature ventricular contraction *(PVC)* in lead I. Slight ST elevations are seen in lead aV_R and lead III.

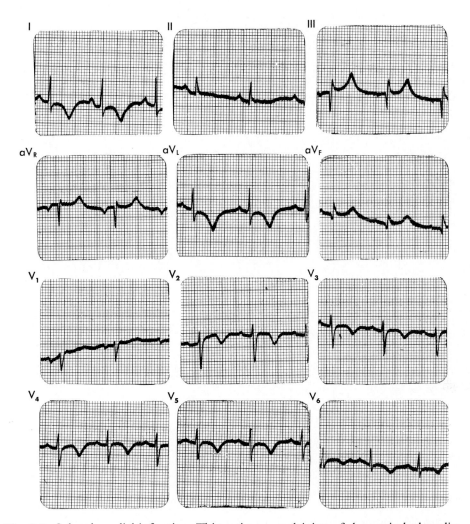

Fig. 9-7. Subendocardial infarction. This patient complaining of chest pain had cardiac enzyme elevations. Note the deep T wave inversions in leads I, aV$_L$, and V$_2$ to V$_6$. (Prominent Q waves in leads III and aV$_F$ may represent an old inferior wall infarction.) Patients with subendocardial infarcts may have deep ST segment depressions or T wave inversions.

ischemia. We will mention two other ECG patterns and then summarize the entire range of ECG abnormalities associated with ischemic heart disease.

As has already been mentioned, not every ischemic episode leads to an actual MI. The typical anginal attack is caused by transient subendocardial ischemia and often produces ST segment depressions. Similarly, in other cases, myocardial ischemia without infarction may occur involving various portions of the ventricle. Depending on the degree of ischemia, a number of different ECG patterns may be seen. In some cases, myocardial ischemia may produce only subtle changes in the ST-T complex. For example, you may see only slight T wave flattening or minimal T wave inversions. These changes are referred to as *nonspecific ST-T changes* (see also Chapter 10).

Nonspecific ST-T changes are abnormal but are *not* definite indicators of ischemia.

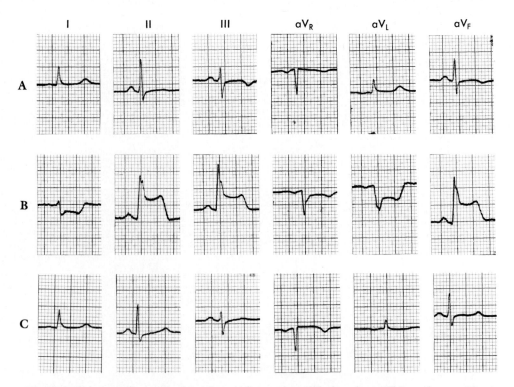

Fig. 9-8. Prinzmetal's (variant) angina with transient ST elevations. This patient, a 30-year-old man, had a history of exertional as well as rest angina. **A,** The baseline resting ECG shows nonspecific inferior lead ST-T changes. **B,** With chest pain, marked ST segment elevation occurs in leads II, III, and aV_F and there is reciprocal ST depression in leads I and aV_L. The rightward shift and slight widening of the QRS axis are consistent with left posterior hemiblock. **C,** Return of the ST segments to baseline after nitroglycerin administration. Cardiac catheterization in this case showed a 99% right coronary obstruction with intermittent spasm producing total occlusion and transient ST elevations. (From Goldberger, A.L.: Myocardial infarction: electrocardiographic differential diagnosis, ed. 3, St. Louis, 1984, The C.V. Mosby Co.)

They may be a sign of ischemic heart disease. However, they may also be caused by many other conditions, such as drug effects, hyperventilation, electrolyte abnormalities, and so on. Therefore, you should *not* make a definite diagnosis of myocardial ischemia solely on the basis of nonspecific ST-T changes.

To complete our discussion of noninfarctional ischemia, we will mention one other pattern, *Prinzmetal's angina*. Recall that the ECG with classic or typical angina may show the pattern of subendocardial ischemia with ST segment depressions. There is a small but important group of patients who have an atypical form of angina first reported by Dr. Myron Prinzmetal. Their angina is atypical because during episodes of chest pain they have ST segment elevations, a pattern we described previously with acute transmural infarction. However, in these patients with Prinzmetal's angina the ST segment elevations are transient. Following the episode of chest pain, the ST segments return to the baseline, without the characteristic evolving pattern of Q waves and T wave inversions seen in acute transmural MI. Thus Prinzmetal's angina is atypical because the ECG shows ST elevations rather than the ST depressions seen in typical angina.

Patients with Prinzmetal's angina are also atypical because their chest pain often occurs at rest or at night (in contrast to classic angina pectoris, which usually occurs with exertion or emotional stress). Prinzmetal's angina pattern is significant because it is a marker of coronary artery *spasm,* causing transient transmural ischemia. These episodes of spasm may occur in patients with otherwise normal coronary arteries. In other cases, spasm is associated with high-grade coronary obstruction (Fig. 9-8).

At this point we can summarize the diversity of ECG changes seen with ischemic heart disease (Fig. 9-9).

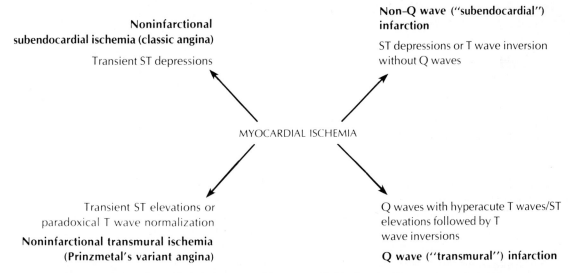

Fig. 9-9. Diversity of ECG changes with myocardial ischemia. T wave inversions may also occur with noninfarctional ischemia, and the ECG either be normal or show only nonspecific ST-T changes. (From Goldberger, A.L.: Myocardial infarction: electrocardiographic differential diagnosis, ed. 3, St. Louis, 1984, The C.V. Mosby Co.)

DIFFERENTIAL DIAGNOSIS OF ST ELEVATIONS AND ST DEPRESSIONS

ST elevations (current of injury pattern) are the earliest sign of acute transmural MI. Transient ST elevations, as mentioned, are also seen with Prinzmetal's angina. ST elevations persisting for 2 or more weeks after an acute MI may be a sign of a ventricular aneurysm.

However, not all ST segment elevations are indicators of ischemia. For example, acute pericarditis (p. 145) is also associated with ST elevations. (The ECG changes with acute pericarditis are described in Chapter 10.) In other cases ST elevation may occur as a normal variant (Fig. 10-10). Many young adults have ST elevations, usually most prominent in the chest leads. This pattern of benign ST segment elevation is called the "early repolarization variant" (also described in Chapter 10). Finally, chronic ST elevations are often seen in leads V_1 and V_2 associated with the patterns of left ventricular hypertrophy and left bundle branch block.

Subendocardial ischemia with or without actual infarction is characterized by ST segment depression. However, not all the ST depressions you will see are indicative of subendocardial ischemia. We have already mentioned some other causes of ST depressions. For example, in Chapter 6 we described the left ventricular "strain" pattern often seen with left ventricular hypertrophy. As shown in Fig. 6-11, the ST segment may also be slightly depressed with the left ventricular strain pattern. Another cause of ST depressions is the reciprocal ST depression seen during an acute transmural infarct. Remember that acute anterior wall infarction may be associated with reciprocal ST depression in one or more of leads II, III, and aV_F. Conversely, acute inferior wall infarction may be associated with reciprocal ST segment depressions in one or more of the anterior leads (I, aV_L, V_1 to V_6). Therefore, whenever you see ST depressions, it is important to look at all the leads and to evaluate these changes in context. As in the case of the *reciprocal* ST depressions seen with acute transmural infarcts, not all ST segment depressions are indicative of subendocardial ischemia.

The ST segment may also be depressed by two other important factors (both described in Chapter 10). The first is *digitalis effect*. As shown in Fig. 10-1, digitalis may produce scooping of the ST-T complex with slight ST segment depression. The second factor that can produce ST segment depression is *hypokalemia*. As shown in Fig. 10-7, with a low serum potassium the ST segment may be slightly depressed. Prominent U waves may also appear. In some cases it may be difficult to sort out which of these two factors is responsible for the ST depressions you are seeing. For example, a patient with left ventricular hypertrophy and strain may be taking digitalis and may also be having subendocardial ischemia.

DIFFERENTIAL DIAGNOSIS OF DEEP T WAVE INVERSIONS

Deep T wave inversions, as described previously, are seen during the evolving phase of transmural MI (Fig. 8-4, *B*) and also sometimes in nontransmural (subendocardial) MI (Fig. 9-7). These T wave inversions are the result of a delay in regional repolarization produced by the ischemic injury. However, just as not all ST segment elevations reflect ischemia, so not all deep T wave inversions are abnormal. For example, T wave inversions may be seen normally in leads with a negative QRS complex (such as aV_R). The T wave may be normally inverted in lead V_1 and sometimes in lead V_2 in adults. Furthermore, as mentioned earlier (p. 51, footnote), some adults show a persistent *juvenile T wave inversion pattern* with inverted T waves in the right and middle chest leads (V_1 to V_3).

Furthermore, not all abnormal T wave inversions are caused by myocardial infarction.

Fig. 9-10. Acute subarachnoid hemorrhage with giant T wave inversions. Subarachnoid hemorrhage may cause deeply inverted T waves, usually with markedly prolonged QT intervals, simulating the pattern seen in MI. (From Goldberger, A.L.: Myocardial infarction: electrocardiographic differential diagnosis, ed. 3, St. Louis, 1984, The C.V. Mosby Co.)

T wave inversions in the right chest leads may be caused by right ventricular strain (Fig. 10-13) and in the left chest leads by left ventricular strain (Fig. 6-9). Diffusely inverted T waves are seen during the evolving phase of pericarditis. Very deep widely splayed T wave inversions (with a long QT interval and sometimes prominent U waves) have been described in some patients with cerebrovascular accidents, particularly subarachnoid hemorrhage ("CVA T wave pattern") (Fig. 9-10). The cause of these marked repolarization changes with some types of cerebrovascular injury is not certain, but it probably reflects changes in the autonomic nervous system and not primary myocardial damage. As described in Chapter 7, secondary T wave inversions (resulting from abnormal depolarization) are seen in the right chest leads with RBBB and in the left chest leads with LBBB. Deep T wave inversions have also been reported following bouts of tachycardia (posttachycardia T wave syndrome) and after electronic ventricular pacing (postpacemaker T wave pattern). Patients with the mitral valve prolapse syndrome may have inverted T waves in the inferolateral leads (II, III, aV$_F$, V$_5$, and V$_6$).

This list of noninfarctional factors causing deep T wave inversions is by no means complete, but it should convey the point that *T wave inversions are not always indicative of myocardial ischemia.* For a more complete discussion of the differential diagnosis of the ST-T changes of myocardial infarction, readers are referred to the Bibliography.

COMPLICATIONS OF MI

Up to now we have outlined the diagnosis of MI from the ECG and also the differential diagnosis of these patterns. We will conclude this section with a brief review of the major complications of MI.

The complications of MI can be divided into two groups: (1) mechanical and (2) electrical. The *mechanical* complications include heart failure, cardiogenic shock, left ventricular aneurysms, rupture of the heart, pericarditis, papillary muscle dysfunction, and emboli. (Diagnosis of these problems lies outside the scope of this book.) The *electrical* complications include the arrhythmias and conduction disturbances seen as a consequence of myocardial ischemia. MI can lead to virtually any arrhythmia. (The whole subject of arrhythmias is discussed in Part II of this book.) The conduction disturbances include AV block (heart block) and intraventricular block (bundle branch block). (The conduction disturbances are discussed in Chapters 7 and 15.)

THE ECG IN MI: A CLINICAL PERSPECTIVE

One final note of caution should be made. The ECG is a reasonably sensitive, but hardly perfect, indicator of acute MI. Most patients with an acute MI will show the ECG changes described in Chapters 8 and 9. However, particularly during the early minutes or hours after an infarct, the ECG may be relatively nondiagnostic or even normal. Furthermore,

as mentioned, an LBBB pattern may completely mask the changes of an acute infarct. Therefore the ECG must always be considered in clinical perspective and the diagnosis of infarction not be dismissed simply because the ECG does not show the classic changes.

It should also be emphasized that the distinction between transmural and subendocardial (nontransmural) MIs on the basis of the ECG findings is an oversimplification. In some cases extensive infarction may occur without Q waves while in others nontransmural injury may occur with Q waves. Furthermore, recent evidence suggests that "subendocardial" infarction may have as ominous a long-term prognosis as "transmural" infarction. For these reasons a number of authorities have suggested that electrocardiographers abandon the terms "transmural" and "subendocardial" and instead use "Q wave" and "non–Q wave" when describing an infarction.

REVIEW OF CHAPTER 9

Subendocardial ischemia generally produces ST segment depressions, which may appear only in the anterior leads (I, aV_L, and V_1 to V_6) or only in the inferior leads (II, III, and aV_F) or may appear diffusely in both groups of leads. (Lead aV_R often shows ST segment elevation.)

These ischemic ST segment depressions may be seen during attacks of typical angina pectoris. Similar ST segment depressions may develop during exercise (with or without chest pain) in people with ischemic heart disease. Recording the ECG during exercise (stress electrocardiography) is a method of determining the presence of ischemic heart disease. ST segment depression of 1 mm or more, lasting 0.08 second or more, is generally considered a *positive* (abnormal) response. However, *false-negative* (normal) results can occur in patients with ischemic heart disease and *false-positive* results can occur in normal people.

With *subendocardial infarction* the ECG may show persistent ST segment depressions. Another pattern sometimes seen with subendocardial (nontransmural) infarction is deep T wave inversions with or without ST segment depressions. Abnormal Q waves *do not* usually occur with subendocardial infarction.

Prinzmetal's angina occurs in patients who develop transient ST segment elevations, suggestive of epicardial or transmural ischemia, during attacks of angina. These patients often have atypical chest pain, which occurs at rest or at night, in contrast to classic angina, which is typically exertional and is associated with ST segment depressions. Prinzmetal's (variant) angina pattern is generally a marker of coronary artery spasm with or without underlying coronary obstructions.

The ST segment elevations of acute transmural MI can be simulated by the ST segment elevations of Prinzmetal's angina as well as by the normal variant ST segment elevations seen in some healthy people ("early repolarization pattern") and by the ST segment elevations of acute pericarditis.

The abnormal ST segment depressions of subendocardial ischemia or infarction can be simulated by the pattern of left ventricular strain, digitalis effect (Chapter 10), or hypokalemia (Chapter 10).

T wave inversions may be a sign of ischemia or infarction but may also occur in a variety of other settings, including normal variants, ventricular strain, pericarditis, subarachnoid hemorrhage, secondary ST-T changes due to bundle branch block, and so on.

Review Questions—Chapters 8 and 9

1. Answer the following questions about the ECG below:
   a. What is approximate heart rate?
   b. Are there any ST segment elevations?
   c. Are there any abnormal Q waves?
   d. What is the diagnosis?

2. Answer these questions about the ECG below:
   a. Is sinus rhythm present?
   b. What is the approximate mean QRS axis?
   c. Is the R wave progression in the chest leads normal?
   d. Are the T waves normal?
   e. What is the diagnosis?

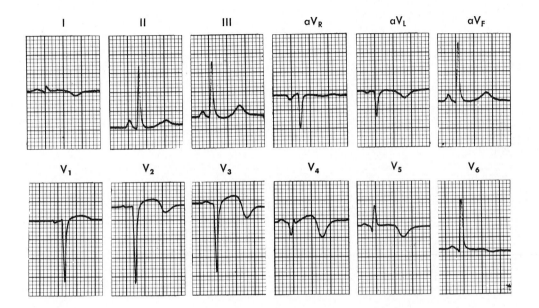

3. With an acute anterior wall infarction, the ST segments in leads II, III, and aV_F are likely to be _____.

4. Persistent ST elevations several weeks or more after an infarct may be a sign of _____ _____.

5. A patient with severe chest pain has persistent diffuse ST segment depressions with abnormal elevations of cardiac enzymes. The most likely diagnosis is
   a. Prinzmetal's angina
   b. Subendocardial infarction
   c. Hyperacute infarction
   d. Angina pectoris

6. What ECG abnormality is shown and of what symptom might this patient have been complaining?

7. Does this ECG tracing show evidence of a previous MI?

Answers

1. a. 100 beats/min.
   b. Yes. Leads II, III, and aV$_F$ (with reciprocal ST depressions in leads V$_2$ to V$_4$, I, and aV$_L$).
   c. Yes. Best seen in leads III and aV$_F$.
   d. Acute inferior wall infarction.
2. a. Yes. Positive P wave in leads II, negative in lead aV$_R$.
   b. About +90°. (Between 80° and 90° is acceptable.)
   c. No.
   d. No. Note the inverted T waves in leads V$_2$ to V$_6$, I, and aV$_L$.
   e. (Evolving) anterior wall infarction.
3. Reciprocally depressed.

4. Ventricular aneurysm.
5. b.
6. Marked ST segment depressions. This patient had severe ischemic chest pain with a subendocardial infarct.
7. Yes. There is evidence of anterior wall infarction, with loss of R wave progression in the chest leads. There is also evidence of inferior wall infarction, with large Q waves in leads III and aV$_F$. In addition, note the tall R wave in lead aV$_L$ (14 mm) with a strain pattern in leads I and aV$_L$. This patient had a history of hypertension, producing left ventricular hypertrophy.

10 Miscellaneous ECG Patterns

This chapter presents an electrocardiographic potpourri—a discussion of several ECG patterns that have not been covered in detail up to this point. We will briefly discuss drug effects, electrolyte disturbances, pericardial disease, early repolarization, pulmonary embolism, Wolff-Parkinson-White syndrome, and several other miscellaneous ECG patterns.

DRUG EFFECTS

Numerous drugs can affect the ECG. Generally the changes produced are slight and nonspecific. However, several commonly used drugs produce distinct ECG changes. We will describe the ECG patterns seen with digitalis, quinidine, and related agents.

Digitalis is used to treat heart failure and certain arrhythmias and is one of the most frequently employed drugs. One of the effects of digitalis is to shorten repolarization time in the ventricles. This effect shortens the QT interval. Digitalis also often produces a characteristic scooping of the ST-T complex, as shown in Figs. 10-1 and 10-2. This scooping of the ST-T complex is called *digitalis effect*. Notice that when digitalis effect occurs the ST segment and T wave are fused together and it is impossible to tell where one ends and the other begins. Digitalis effect can be seen in any patient taking therapeutic or toxic doses of any of the digitalis preparations (for example digoxin, digitoxin). Digitalis *effect* must be distinguished from digitalis *toxicity* (Chapter 16), which involves arrhythmias, conduction disturbances, and systemic side effects produced by excessive amounts of digitalis.

Quinidine, procainamide (Pronestyl, Procan SR), and disopyramide (Norpace) are antiarrhythmic drugs with similar properties. They may be useful in the therapy of ventricular or atrial arrhythmias. In contrast to digitalis, they prolong ventricular repolarization. Therefore, they may prolong the QT interval and flatten the T wave. In toxic doses they may also prolong ventricular depolarization, leading to a widening of the QRS complexes. Occasionally these agents will produce prominent U waves with a pattern resembling that seen in hypokalemia (p. 143).

Quinidine, a drug used to treat ventricular arrhythmias, may in selected cases actually

DIGITALIS EFFECT

Fig. 10-1. Note the characteristic scooping of the ST-T complex produced by digitalis. Not all patients taking digitalis exhibit these changes, however.

DIGITALIS EFFECT

Fig. 10-2. Note the characteristic scooping of the ST-T complex, best seen in leads V_5 and V_6. Low voltage is also present, with a total QRS amplitude of 5 mm or less in all six extremity leads.

QUINIDINE EFFECTS

Fig. 10-3. Lead V_6. Quinidine blood level 2.9 µg/ml (therapeutic range). Note the prolonged repolarization with prominent U waves, similar to the pattern of hypokalemia. Some patients in whom repolarization is markedly prolonged, with large U waves caused by quinidine, may be at increased risk of ventricular tachycardia (torsades de pointes, p. 209) or ventricular fibrillation (quinidine syncope). A similar syndrome has been reported with disopyramide (Norpace) and procainamide (Pronestyl, Procan SR). (From Goldberger, E.: Textbook of clinical cardiology, St. Louis, 1981, The C.V. Mosby Co.)

cause fainting or even sudden death as a result of ventricular tachycardia *(quinidine syncope)*.* This paradoxical effect is most likely to occur in patients who develop very long QT intervals and prominent U waves (Fig. 10-3). The dispersion of repolarization in such cases may allow for "reentrant" (p. 155) ventricular arrhythmias, in particular, "torsades de pointes," a potentially lethal complication that can occur in patients taking therapeutic doses. (See also pp. 209 and 210.)

ELECTROLYTE DISTURBANCES

Abnormal serum concentrations of potassium and calcium can produce marked effects on the ECG. Hyperkalemia can, in fact, be lethal because of its cardiac toxicity.

Hyperkalemia

Hyperkalemia produces a distinct sequence of ECG changes affecting both depolarization

---

*The same toxicity may occur with procainamide and disopyramide.

(QRS) and repolarization (ST-T). The normal serum potassium concentration is between 3.5 and 5.0 mEq/L. The first change seen with abnormal elevation of the serum potassium concentration is narrowing and peaking of the T wave. As shown in Figs. 10-4 and 10-5, the T wave with hyperkalemia has a characteristic "tented" shape and may become quite tall. With further elevation of the serum potassium concentration, the PR interval becomes prolonged, and the P waves become smaller and may disappear entirely. Further elevations in the serum potassium concentration produce an intraventricular conduction delay, with widening of the QRS complex (Fig. 10-6). As serum potassium concentration rises further, the QRS complex continues to widen, leading to a large undulating ("sine-wave") pattern and eventual asystole. The sequence of ECG changes seen with progressive hyperkalemia is outlined in Fig. 10-4. Because hyperkalemia may be fatal, recognition of the earliest ECG signs of T wave peaking may prove life saving (Fig. 10-

EFFECTS OF HYPERKALEMIA

Fig. 10-4. The earliest change with hyperkalemia is peaking ("tenting") of the T wave. With progressive increases in serum potassium, the QRS complexes widen, P waves disappear, and, finally, ventricular fibrillation develops. These changes do not necessarily occur with a specific serum K^+ level. For example, some patients can have a normal ECG with a K^+ of 7 mEq/L whereas others will have ventricular fibrillation at 9 mEq/L or less.

5). Hyperkalemia may be seen in several clinical settings. The most common is kidney failure, where there is reduced excretion of potassium.

Hypokalemia

Hypokalemia also produces distinct changes in the ST-T complex. The most common pattern seen in hypokalemia is ST segment depression with prominent U waves and prolonged repolarization* (Figs. 10-7 and 10-8).

---

*Technically the QT interval with hypokalemia may remain normal while repolarization is prolonged (as shown by the prominent U waves). However, the T wave and U wave often merge, so the QT interval cannot always be accurately measured.

Recall from Chapter 2 that a U wave is a small deflection following the T wave. In hypokalemia the U wave typically becomes enlarged and may even exceed the height of the T wave. Hypokalemia may be caused by several factors. The most common clinical causes are (1) urinary potassium losses resulting from diuretic therapy and (2) potassium losses associated with metabolic alkalosis from vomiting or gastric suction.

Hypercalcemia and Hypocalcemia

Hypercalcemia shortens ventricular repolarization. Hypocalcemia lengthens ventricular repolarization.

Hypercalcemia causes shortening of the

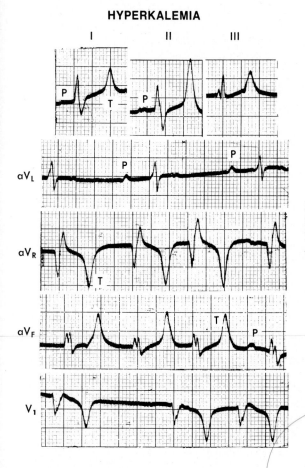

HYPERKALEMIA

Fig. 10-5. Note the peaked T waves, widened QRS complexes, and prolonged PR intervals. Intermittently a junctional rhythm is present with no P waves.

Fig. 10-6. In this patient the K$^+$ concentration was 8.5 mEq/L. Note the absence of P waves and the bizarre wide QRS complexes.

HYPOKALEMIA

Fig. 10-7. Variable ECG patterns may be seen with hypokalemia, ranging from slight T wave flattening to the appearance of prominent U waves, sometimes with ST depressions or T wave inversions. These patterns are not directly related to the specific level of serum potassium.

QT interval. It may be life threatening at high levels and may lead to coma and death. A short QT interval in a comatose patient may be the first clue to the diagnosis of hypercalcemia. Hypercalcemia may be caused by numerous factors, including malignant tumors (especially breast and lung), multiple myeloma, hyperparathyroidism, excessive amounts of vitamin D, and so on.

Hypocalcemia causes lengthening or prolongation of the QT interval. Common causes include intestinal malabsorption, pancreatitis, kidney failure (azotemia, uremia), and hypoparathyroidism.

PERICARDITIS AND PERICARDIAL EFFUSION

Pericarditis is an inflammation of the pericardium (the sac that surrounds the heart). It may be caused by a number of factors—including viral or bacterial infection, metastatic tumors, collagen vascular diseases, myocardial infarction, uremia, and others.

As mentioned in Chapter 8, the ECG patterns in pericarditis resemble those seen in acute myocardial infarction. The early phase of acute pericarditis is characterized by ST segment elevations. This is a current of injury pattern resulting from the epicardial inflam-

HYPOKALEMIA

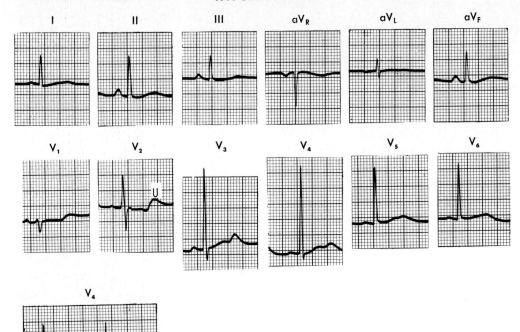

Fig. 10-8. The serum K^+ was 2.2 mEq/L. Notice the prominent U waves.

ACUTE PERICARDITIS

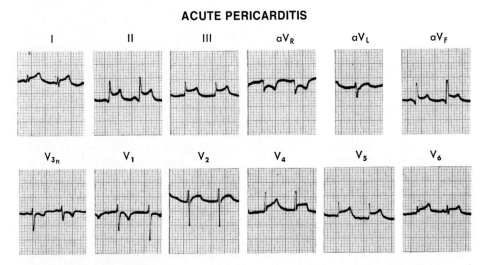

Fig. 10-9. Note the diffuse ST elevations in leads I, II, aV_F, and V_4 to V_6. Reciprocal ST depressions are seen in lead aV_R.

mation that occurs along with inflammation of the pericardium. Fig. 10-9 shows an example of the ST segment elevations seen in acute pericarditis. The major difference between the ST segment elevations of pericarditis and myocardial infarction is the distribution of these changes. The ST segment elevations of acute myocardial infarction are characteristically limited to either the anterior leads or the inferior leads because of the localized area of infarction. The pericardium envelops the heart, and the ST-T changes seen with pericarditis are therefore more generalized. The ST segment elevations in pericarditis are usually seen in both the anterior and the inferior leads. For example, in Fig. 10-9, the ST segment elevations are seen in leads I, II, aV_L, aV_F, and V_2 to V_6.

Not only does acute pericarditis affect ventricular repolarization (ST segment), it also affects the repolarization of the atria, which starts during the PR segment (end of the P wave to beginning of the QRS). In particu-

lar, pericardial inflammation often causes an atrial current of injury, reflected by elevation of the PR segment in lead aV_R and depression of the PR segment in other limb leads and the left chest leads (V_5 and V_6). Thus in acute pericarditis the PR and ST segments typically point in opposite directions—the PR segment being elevated (often by only 1 mm or so) in aV_R while the ST segment is usually slightly depressed in that lead. Other leads may show PR depression and ST elevation.

Fig. 10-10 illustrates these subtle but often helpful repolarization changes in acute pericarditis. The presence of PR segment changes may be a useful clue in the differential diagnosis of ST segment elevation, suggesting acute pericarditis as the cause.

The ST segment elevations seen in acute pericarditis are followed (after a variable time) by T wave inversions (Fig. 10-11). This sequence of ST elevations followed by inversion of the T wave is the same as that described with myocardial infarction. In

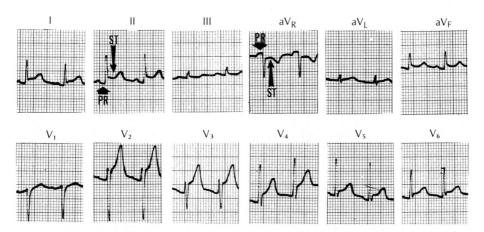

Fig. 10-10. Acute pericarditis causing diffuse ST segment elevations in leads I, II, aV_F, and V_2 to V_6, with reciprocal ST depression in aV_R. In contrast, an atrial of current injury causes PR segment elevation in lead aV_R with reciprocal PR depression in the left chest leads and lead II. (From Goldberger, A.L.: Myocardial infarction: electrocardiographic differential diagnosis, ed. 3, St. Louis, 1984, The C.V. Mosby Co.)

PERICARDITIS, EVOLVING PATTERN

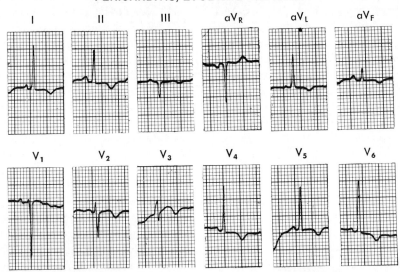

Fig. 10-11. Note the diffuse T wave inversions in leads I, II, III, aV_L, aV_F, and V_2 to V_6.

some cases the T wave inversions caused by pericarditis will resolve completely with time and the ECG will return to normal. In other cases the T wave inversions may persist for long periods.

We have commented on the similarity between the ECG patterns of acute pericarditis and acute myocardial infarction because both produce ST segment elevations followed by T wave inversions. However, the ST-T changes due to pericarditis, as noted, tend to be more diffuse than the localized changes of myocardial infarction. Another major difference is that pericarditis does not produce abnormal Q waves, such as those seen in transmural infarction. With transmural myocardial infarction, abnormal Q waves occur because of the death of heart muscle and consequent loss of positive depolarization voltages (see Chapter 8). Pericarditis, on the other hand, generally causes only a superficial inflammation and does not produce transmural myocardial necrosis. Thus Q waves never result from pericarditis alone.

Pericardial effusion refers to an abnormal accumulation of fluid in the pericardial sac. In most cases, this fluid accumulates as the result of pericarditis. In some cases, however, such as myxedema (hypothyroidism) or rupture of the heart, pericardial effusion may occur in the absence of pericarditis. The major clinical significance of pericardial effusion is the danger of pericardial tamponade, where the fluid actually "chokes off" the heart, leading to a drop in blood pressure and sometimes to cardiac arrest (see Chapter 17).

The most common ECG sign of pericardial effusion (with or without actual tamponade) is low voltage of the QRS complexes. In such cases the low voltage is probably due to short-circuiting of cardiac voltages by the fluid surrounding the heart.

In our discussion of hypertrophy patterns (Chapter 6), we mentioned the criteria for high voltage. *Low voltage* is said to be present when the total amplitude of the QRS complexes in each of the six extremity leads is 5 mm or less. Fig. 10-2 shows an example of low voltage. Separate criteria have been established for diagnosing low voltage in the precordial leads. However, for general clinical purposes, only the six extremity leads need be examined.

The following is a list of the major factors that can lead to low voltage complexes:

1. Pericardial effusion
2. Obesity
3. Emphysema
4. Diffuse myocardial injury (for example, extensive myocardial infarction or myocardial fibrosis)
5. Normal variant
6. Infiltration of the heart muscle (for example, amyloidosis)

Obesity can cause low voltage because of the fat tissue that lies between the heart and the chest wall. In emphysema there is increased inflation of the lungs. This extra air acts to insulate the heart. Of the causes of low voltage listed above, obesity and emphysema are by far the most common. However, when you see low voltage, pericardial effusion should always be first on your list because it can lead to fatal tamponade (p. 238).

Myxedema (hypothyroidism), as noted, may cause a pericardial effusion without actual pericarditis. Hypothyroidism also generally causes sinus bradycardia (Chapter 11). Therefore, the combination of low voltage and sinus bradycardia should suggest the possible diagnosis of myxedema.

To summarize, pericarditis causes a diffuse current of injury pattern with ST segment elevations in the anterior and inferior leads, followed by T wave inversions in these leads. Abnormal Q waves, however, are not seen with pericarditis alone. Pericardial effusion is one of the causes of low voltage on the ECG.

EARLY REPOLARIZATION VARIANT

In Chapter 4 we described the normal ST segment as usually being isoelectric, riding along the baseline and gradually rising into the T wave, as shown in Fig. 2-10. Slight ST segment deviations (usually less than 1 mm)

from the baseline may be seen normally. We have already described ST segment elevations in several abnormal conditions: acute myocardial infarction, Prinzmetal's angina, ventricular aneurysm, and pericarditis.

Fig. 10-12 shows an example of marked ST segment elevations in a *normal* young adult. In this case the ST elevations represent a common, benign, normal variant referred to as the *early repolarization* pattern. With the early repolarization pattern, benign ST elevations up to 3 mm above the baseline may be seen in the chest leads (Fig. 10-12). As noted, this pattern of normal variant ST elevations is most common in young adults but may occur in older persons as well, simulating the pattern of acute pericarditis or myocardial infarction. The ST elevations seen with early repolarization are stable over time and do not undergo the evolving sequence of ST-T changes observed in acute pericarditis and MI. Furthermore, ST elevations seen in early repolarization are not associated with reciprocal ST depression (except in lead aV_R), in contrast to those in acute MI.

PULMONARY EMBOLISM

The ECG is not a sensitive test for pulmonary embolism. In some cases the obstruction of the pulmonary artery system produced by the embolism can lead to ECG changes. However, there is no single ECG pattern diagnostic of pulmonary embolism. The following patterns may all be seen (Fig. 10-13):

1. As mentioned earlier, the appearance of a *new RBBB pattern* (wide rSR' in lead V_1) should suggest the possibility of pulmonary embolism, particularly in a patient with shortness of breath.
2. Right ventricular strain (Chapter 6) is characterized by inverted T waves in the right chest leads (V_1 to V_4). Acute pulmonary embolism may cause *right ventricular dilation and strain* (Fig. 10-13) with T wave inversions in these leads.
3. Occasionally acute pulmonary embolism may produce a distinctive ECG

Fig. 10-12. ST segment elevation, usually most marked in the chest leads, is sometimes seen as a normal variant. This pattern may be confused with ST segment elevations of acute myocardial infarction or pericarditis.

ACUTE PULMONARY EMBOLISM

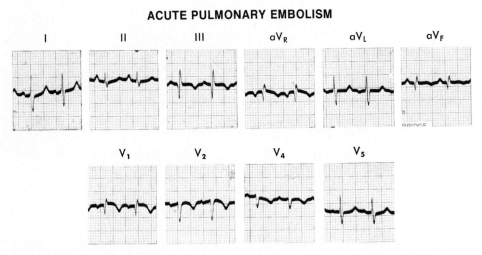

Fig. 10-13. Several features occasionally seen with pulmonary embolism are sinus tachycardia, S waves in lead I with Q waves and T wave inversions in lead III ($S_I Q_{III} T_{III}$ pattern), and poor R wave progression with T wave inversions in chest leads V_1 to V_4 resulting from acute right ventricular strain.

pattern with an S wave in lead I and a new Q wave in lead III with slight T wave inversions in that lead. This $S_I Q_{III} T_{III}$ *pattern* (Fig. 10-13) superficially resembles the pattern seen with inferior wall myocardial infarction, which produces Q waves and T wave inversions in leads II, III, and aV_F. The $S_I Q_{III} T_{III}$ pattern is probably caused by acute right ventricular dilation.

4. The mean *QRS may be shifted to the right* with acute pulmonary embolism.
5. The ECG pattern may show *subendocardial ischemia with ST segment depressions.*
6. Sinus tachycardia is the most common *arrhythmia* seen with pulmonary embolism. Other *arrhythmias,* such as ventricular ectopy, atrial fibrillation, and atrial flutter, also occur. (These arrhythmias are discussed in Part II.)

The appearance of the above ECG changes, particularly in combination, is suggestive but not diagnostic of pulmonary embolism. Many patients with massive pulmonary emboli may have only minor, relatively nonspecific, changes on their ECG. Thus, both the diagnostic sensitivity and the specificity of the ECG with pulmonary embolism are limited. Fig. 10-13 shows a classic example of the ECG changes in pulmonary embolism.

CHRONIC LUNG DISEASE (EMPHYSEMA)

Patients with chronic lung disease from emphysema often have a relatively characteristic combination of ECG findings (Fig. 10-14), including (1) low voltage, (2) poor R wave progression in the chest leads, and (3) a vertical or rightward QRS axis in the frontal plane. Excessive pulmonary air trapping

CHRONIC LUNG DISEASE

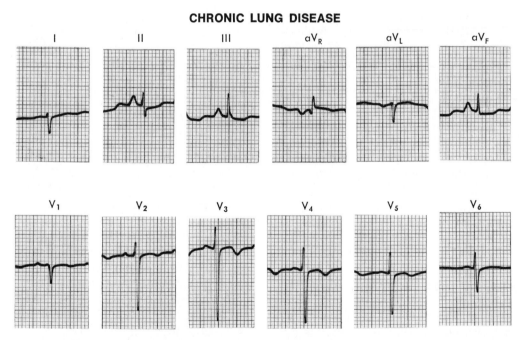

Fig. 10-14. Note the characteristic relatively low voltages in the limb leads, right axis deviation, P pulmonale, and poor R wave progression. T wave inversions (V_1 to V_5) are due to right ventricular strain.

causes the low voltage. The poor R wave progression results in part from the downward displacement of the diaphragm, so the chest leads are actually placed *relatively* higher than usual. In addition, right ventricular dilation may contribute to the delayed chest lead transition zone. Finally, the anatomically vertical position of the heart in the chest of a patient with emphysema, and sometimes right ventricular enlargement, causes the mean QRS axis to be vertical or even rightward (greater than + 100°).

CONGESTIVE HEART FAILURE (CHF)

Congestive heart failure (CHF) is a complex syndrome that may result from multiple causes, including ischemic heart disease, systemic hypertension, valvular heart disease, and chronic lung disease. The ECG may provide helpful clues to a specific diagnosis in some of these patients. For example, prominent Q waves and typical ST-T changes suggest underlying ischemic heart disease. Left ventricular hypertrophy patterns (p. 80) may be seen with hypertensive heart disease, aortic valve disease (stenosis or regurgitation), or mitral regurgitation. The combination of left atrial enlargement (or atrial fibrillation) and signs of right ventricular hypertrophy should suggest mitral stenosis. Left bundle branch block (p. 91) may be seen with congestive heart failure due to ischemic heart disease, valvular abnormalities, hypertension, or cardiomyopathy.

In some patients marked enlargement and decreased function of the left (and often the right) ventricle occur without severe ischemic disease, hypertension, or significant valvular lesions. The term *"dilated (congestive) cardiomyopathy"* is applied in such cases. Dilated cardiomyopathy can occur in the absence of any apparent cause (idiopathic) or may be associated with excessive chronic alcohol ingestion (alcoholic cardiomyopathy), viral infection, and a variety of other etiologies.

Patients with dilated cardiomyopathy from any cause may show a distinctive ECG pattern (the *ECG-CHF* triad), which is characterized by

1. Relatively low limb lead voltage (such that the QRS in each of the six limb leads ≤ 8 mm in amplitude)
2. Relatively prominent precordial lead QRS voltages (such that the sum of the S wave in either lead V_1 or lead V_2 plus the R wave in V_5 or $V_6 \geqslant 35$ mm)
3. Poor R wave progression, defined by a QS- or rS-type complex in leads V_1 to V_4

When this triad is present (Fig. 10-15), it strongly suggests underlying cardiomyopathy but does not indicate a specific etiology. It may occur not only in primary dilated cardiomyopathy but also in heart disease associated with previous infarcts or significant valvular dysfunction. Furthermore, it is of only modest sensitivity; that is, its absence does not exclude underlying cardiomyopathy.

WOLFF-PARKINSON-WHITE SYNDROME

The Wolff-Parkinson-White (WPW) syndrome is an unusual and distinctive ECG abnormality caused by preexcitation of the ventricles. Normally the electrical stimulus passes to the ventricles from the atria via the AV junction. The physiologic lag of conduction through the AV junction results in the normal PR interval of 0.12 to 0.2 second. Imagine the consequences of having an accessory conduction pathway between the atria and ventricles that would bypass the AV junction and preexcite the ventricles. This is exactly what occurs in the WPW syndrome: an accessory conduction fiber (the bundle of Kent) connects the atria and ventricles, bypassing the AV junction (Fig. 10-16).

Preexcitation of the ventricles in the WPW syndrome produces the following three characteristic changes on the ECG:

1. The PR interval is shortened (often but not always <0.12 sec) because of ventricular preexcitation.

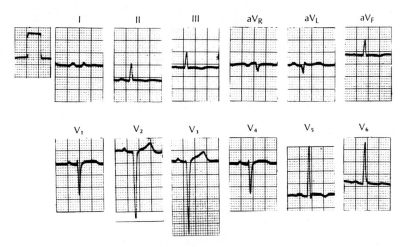

Fig. 10-15. Severe idiopathic dilated cardiomyopathy in a 29-year-old man. Poor precordial R wave progression simulates anterior wall infarction. The triad of relatively low limb lead QRS voltages, prominent precordial QRS voltages, and poor R wave progression in the chest leads is highly specific for dilated cardiomyopathy. (From Goldberger, A.L.: Myocardial infarction: electrocardiographic differential diagnosis, ed. 3, St. Louis, 1984, the C.V. Mosby Co.)

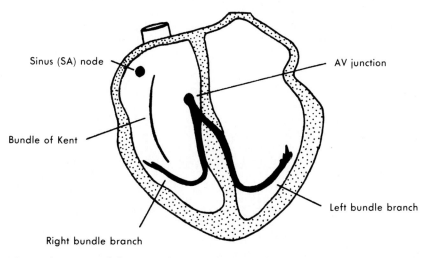

Fig. 10-16. Anatomy of the preexcitation syndrome (Wolff-Parkinson-White) pattern. In a small percentage of the population an accessory fiber (bundle of Kent) connects the atria and ventricles. The consequences of this extra conduction path are discussed in the text.

2. The QRS complex is widened, giving the superficial appearance of a bundle branch block pattern. The wide QRS in the WPW syndrome is caused not by a delay in ventricular depolarization but by early stimulation of the ventricles. The QRS complex will be widened to the degree that the PR interval is shortened.

3. There is slurring, or notching, of the upstroke of the QRS complex. This is called a *delta* wave (Fig. 10-17).

Fig. 10-17 shows an example of the WPW pattern, with the classic triad of a short PR interval, widened QRS complex, and delta wave. The WPW syndrome, as noted, superficially resembles a bundle branch block pattern because of the widened QRS complex. Depending on whether the left or right ventricle is preexcited first, the ECG in the WPW syndrome will show a pattern resembling either a right bundle branch block with tall R waves in right chest leads (type A pattern) or a left bundle branch block with a negative QS complex in lead V_1 (type B pattern).

The significance of the WPW syndrome is twofold. First, patients with this pattern are prone to atrial arrhythmias, especially paroxysmal atrial tachycardia and atrial fibrillation. Second, the ECG of these patients is often mistaken as indicating a bundle branch block or myocardial infarction (Fig. 10-17).

The WPW syndrome predisposes to parox-

WOLFF-PARKINSON-WHITE PATTERN

Fig. 10-17. Note the characteristic triad of the WPW (type B) pattern: wide QRS complexes, short PR intervals, and delta wave (*arrow* in lead V_1). The Q waves in leads II, III, and aV_F result from abnormal ventricular conduction rather than from inferior myocardial infarction.

ysmal atrial tachycardia in particular because of the accessory conduction pathway. For example, an impulse traveling down the AV junction may recycle up the bundle of Kent and then back down the AV junction, and so on.* This type of reentry mechanism *(circus movement)* may also account for other types of tachycardias.

Another type of preexcitation variant, the Lown-Ganong-Levine (LGL) pattern, is caused by a bypass tract (James fiber) that connects the atria and AV junction. Bypassing the AV node results in a short PR interval (less than 0.12 sec). However, the QRS width will not be prolonged because ventricular activation occurs normally. Therefore, the LGL pattern (Fig. 10-18) consists of a short PR interval with a normal-width QRS and no delta wave; the WPW syndrome consists of a short PR interval with a wide QRS and a delta wave. Patients with the LGL pattern may also have "reentrant" paroxysmal atrial tachycardia (PAT).

---

*When a patient with the WPW syndrome develops paroxysmal atrial tachycardia, the QRS complex generally becomes narrow. The wide QRS complex seen in WPW syndrome with normal sinus rhythm occurs because the stimulus travels concomitantly down the bundle of Kent and down the AV junction, resulting in a *fusion* beat. When atrial tachycardia occurs, the impulse usually travels down the AV junction and back up the bundle of Kent in retrograde fashion resulting in loss of the delta wave.

DIFFERENTIAL DIAGNOSIS OF WIDE QRS COMPLEXES

Discussion of the WPW syndrome allows us now to review all the major ECG patterns that produce a widened QRS complex. This list includes four major categories:

1. Bundle branch block, including the classic RBBB or LBBB patterns
2. "Toxic" conduction delays caused by some extrinsic factor, such as hyperkalemia or drugs (quinidine and related antiarrhythmics, phenothiazines, tricyclic antidepressants)
3. Beats arising in the ventricles, which may be premature ventricular contractions (PVCs, p. 198), ventricular escape beats (p. 237), or pacemaker beats (p. 96)
4. Wolff-Parkinson-White type preexcitation

Differentiation among these possibilities is usually easy. Right and left bundle branch blocks were described earlier. Hyperkalemia produces widening of the QRS complex often with loss of P waves. Widening of the QRS complex in any patient taking quinidine or procainamide (Pronestyl) should always suggest possible drug toxicity. Pacemakers generally produce an LBBB pattern with a pacemaker spike before each QRS complex. The WPW syndrome is recognized by the combination of a short PR interval and a wide QRS complex, usually with a delta wave.

Fig. 10-18. Possible Lown-Ganong-Levine (LGL) type of preexcitation with short PR intervals (0.12). In addition, note the single premature atrial contraction.

ST-T CHANGES: SPECIFIC AND NONSPECIFIC

The concluding topic of Part I of this book is a review of the major factors causing ST-T (repolarization) changes. The term *"nonspecific ST-T change,"* defined earlier (Chapter 9), is commonly used in clinical electrocardiography. Many factors, such as drugs, ischemia, electrolyte imbalances, infections, pulmonary disease, and so on, can affect the ECG. As mentioned earlier, the repolarization phase (ST-T complex) is particularly sensitive to such effects. The ST-T complex can show a variety of nonspecific changes as a result of multiple factors (Figs. 10-19 and 10-20). Nonspecific ST-T changes include slight ST depressions, T wave flattening, or slight T wave inversions, diagrammed in Fig. 10-19.

In contrast to these nonspecific ST-T changes, we have described certain fairly specific ST-T changes associated with particular conditions, such as the tall tented T waves of hyperkalemia. Some of these relatively specific ST-T changes are shown in Fig. 10-21. However, even such apparently specific ST changes can be misleading. For example, ST elevation is characteristic of acute transmural myocardial infarction yet ST elevations are also seen in Prinzmetal's angina and ventricular aneurysms as well as in pericarditis and benign (normal) early repolarization. Similarly, deep T wave inversions are most characteristic of ischemia but may occur in other conditions as well (p. 132).

To summarize, we can group repolarization abnormalities (ST-T changes) into two general categories: *First* are the nonspecific ST-T changes, which include slight ST segment deviation or flattening or inversion of the T wave. These changes are not diagnostic of any particular condition but must always be interpreted in clinical context. *Second* are the relatively specific ST-T changes that are more strongly, but not always definitively, di-

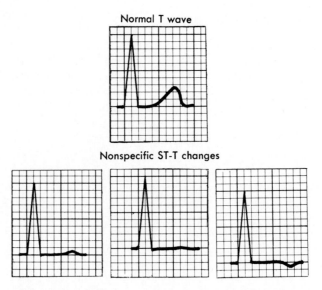

Normal T wave

Nonspecific ST-T changes

Fig. 10-19. Flattening of the T wave *(left* and *middle)* or slight T wave inversion *(right)* is an abnormal but relatively nonspecific change that may be caused by numerous factors.

Fig. 10-20. Nonspecific ST-T changes. Note the diffuse T wave flattening.

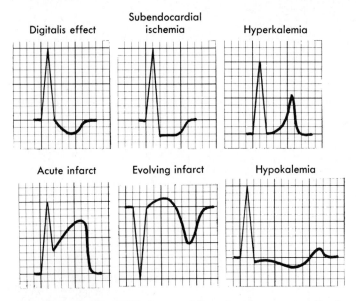

Fig. 10-21. Relatively specific ST-T changes. Note that they are not absolutely specific for the abnormalities shown.

agnostic of some particular underlying cause (for example, hyperkalemia, myocardial ischemia).

PEDIATRIC ELECTROCARDIOGRAPHY

The normal ECG patterns seen in children differ considerably from those seen in adults (Chapter 4). The topic of pediatric electrocardiography falls outside the scope of this book, but a few critical points of difference between pediatric and adult ECGs will be mentioned briefly. The normal ECG of the newborn and infant resembles the pattern seen in right ventricular hypertrophy, with tall R waves in the right chest leads and right axis deviation. During the first decade of life the T waves in the right to middle chest leads are normally inverted. This pattern sometimes persists into adolescence and adulthood and is called the *juvenile* T wave variant. As mentioned in Chapter 6, children and young adults may also show tall voltage in the chest leads as a normal variant.

REVIEW OF CHAPTER 10

The ECG can be influenced by numerous factors.

Many *drugs* can affect the ECG. *Digitalis effect* refers to the characteristic scooped-out depression of the ST segment produced by therapeutic doses of digitalis. (*Digitalis toxicity* refers to the arrhythmias and conduction disturbances produced by excessive doses of digitalis.) *Quinidine* and *procainamide* can prolong the QT interval and, in toxic doses, can also widen the QRS complex. *Quinidine syncope* results from ventricular tachycardia, paradoxically caused by this antiarrhythmic drug. Patients likely to develop this complication often show prolonged QT intervals and large U waves.

Electrolyte disturbances can also affect the ECG.

Hyperkalemia produces a sequence of changes. First, there is narrowing and peaking (tenting) of the T wave. Further elevation of the serum potassium concentration leads to PR prolongation and then to loss of P waves and QRS widening, followed by eventual ventricular fibrillation and asystole.

Hypokalemia may produce ST segment depressions and prominent U waves. The QT interval becomes prolonged. (In some cases you are actually measuring the QU interval and not the QT interval because it may be impossible to tell where the T wave ends and the U wave begins.)

Hypercalcemia may shorten the QT interval, and *hypocalcemia* may prolong the QT interval.

Pericarditis produces diffuse ST segment elevations, usually in one or more of the chest leads and also in leads I, aV_L, II, and aV_F. PR segment elevation in lead aV_R with PR depression in other leads may also occur due to an atrial current of injury. Abnormal Q waves do not develop. The ST segment elevations are followed by T wave inversions after a variable time.

Pericardial effusion produces *low voltage* of the QRS complex (QRS amplitude of 5 mm or less in all six extremity leads). Low voltage is not specific for pericardial effusion but may also occur with obesity, emphysema, and diffuse myocardial injury or infiltration or as a normal variant.

Normally, the ST segment is isoelectric. However, some normal people, young adult males in particular, may show normal variant ST segment elevations *(early repolarization variant)*. These benign ST elevations are usually best seen in the chest leads (up to 3 mm of elevation). The pattern may simulate acute myocardial infarction or pericarditis but does not show the successive changes that usually occur with myocardial infarcts or pericarditis.

Pulmonary embolism may produce any of the following ECG patterns: (1) acute RBBB, (2) right ventricular strain T wave inversions, (3) $S_I Q_{III} T_{III}$ pattern, (4) right axis shift, (5) ST depressions resulting from subendocardial ischemia, and (6) various arrhythmias.

The *WPW pattern* shows (1) a short PR interval (usually but not always <0.12 sec), (2) a wide QRS complex, and (3) slurring or notching of the initial part of the QRS complex. This slurring is called a *delta* wave. Patients with the WPW pattern are particularly prone to attacks of supraventricular tachycardias (paroxysmal atrial tachycardia or rapid atrial fibrillation). Another form of preexcitation, the Lown-Ganong-Levine pattern, is characterized by a short PR interval and a normal QRS.

The differential diagnosis of ECG patterns with a wide QRS complex includes four major possibilities: (1) right or left bundle branch block, (2) toxic conduction delays caused by hyperkalemia or drugs, (3) beats arising in the ventricles, such as PVCs or pacemaker beats, and (4) WPW pattern of preexcitation.

Review Questions—Chapter 10

1. The following factors may all affect ventricular repolarization (ST-T complex). Put an "L" next to those that may prolong ventricular repolarization (lengthen the QT interval). Put an "S" next to those that may shorten the QT interval.
   Digitalis
   Quinidine
   Procainamide
   Hypokalemia
   Hypocalcemia
   Hypercalcemia
2. Put an "X" next to those factors that can widen the QRS complex.
   Hypokalemia
   Hyperkalemia
   Wolff-Parkinson-White syndrome
   Digitalis effect
   Quinidine toxicity
   Right bundle branch block

3. Which of the following factors can produce ST segment elevations?
   Hypokalemia
   Early repolarization pattern
   Digitalis effect
   Ventricular aneurysm
   Hypocalcemia
   Left ventricular strain
   Pericarditis
4. Match ECGs *A*, *B*, and *C* with the following causes:
   Digitalis effect
   Hyperkalemia
   Hypokalemia

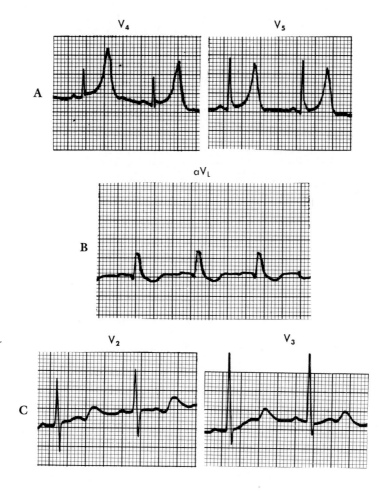

Answers

1. Digitalis (S); quinidine (L); procainamide (L); hypokalemia (L); hypocalcemia (L); hypercalcemia (S).
2. Hyperkalemia (X); Wolff-Parkinson-White syndrome (X); quinidine toxicity (X); right bundle branch block (X).
3. Early repolarization variant; ventricular aneurysm; pericarditis.
4. Digitalis effect, *B*; hyperkalemia, *A*; hypokalemia, *C*.

PART TWO

Cardiac Rhythm Disturbances

11 Sinus Rhythms

NORMAL SINUS RHYTHM (NSR)

The diagnosis of normal, or regular, sinus rhythm (NSR) was already described in Chapter 3. When the sinus (SA) node is pacing the heart, atrial depolarization spreads from right to left and downward toward the AV junction. An arrow representing this atrial depolarization wave will point downward and toward the left. Therefore, as de-

NORMAL SINUS RHYTHM

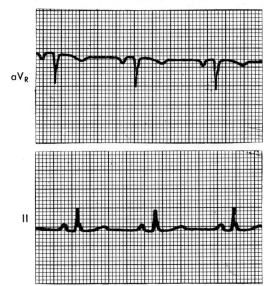

Fig. 11-1. Each QRS complex is preceded by a P wave that is negative in lead aV_R and positive in lead II.

scribed earlier, with NSR, the P wave is negative in lead aV_R and reciprocally positive in lead II (Fig. 4-3).

Do not be confused by the polarity of the P wave in other leads. With NSR the P wave may be upright, negative, or biphasic in one or more of the extremity leads. In diagnosing normal sinus rhythm, pay attention to the polarity of the P wave in lead aV_R and lead II. The diagnosis of NSR requires examining lead aV_R and finding a negative P wave preceding each QRS complex. Each sinus beat will also produce a positive P wave preceding the QRS complex in lead II (Fig. 11-1).

By convention, *NSR* is defined as sinus rhythm with a heart rate between 60 and 100 beats/min. Sinus rhythm with a heart rate of less than 60 beats/min is called *sinus bradycardia;* one with a heart rate greater than 100 beats/min is called *sinus tachycardia.*

REGULATION OF THE HEART RATE

The heart, like the other organs, has a special nerve supply from the autonomic nervous system, which controls involuntary muscle action. The autonomic nerve supply to the heart consists of two opposing groups of nerve fibers: the sympathetic nerves and the parasympathetic nerves. The sympathetic fibers supply the sinus node, the atria, the AV junction, and the ventricles. Sympathetic stimulation produces an increased heart rate and also increases the strength of myocardial contraction. The parasympathetic nervous supply to the heart is from the vagus nerve, which supplies the sinus node, atria, and AV junction. Vagal stimulation produces a slowing of the heart rate as well as a slowing of conduction through the AV junction. In this way, the autonomic nervous system exerts a counterbalancing control of heart rate. The sympathetic nervous system acts as a cardiac accelerator, while the parasympathetic (vagal) fibers produce a braking effect. For example, when you become excited or upset, increased sympathetic stimuli (and diminished parasympathetic tone) result in an increased heart rate and increased contractility, producing the familiar sensation of a pounding heart (palpitations).

SINUS TACHYCARDIA

Sinus tachycardia *is simply sinus rhythm with a heart rate exceeding 100 beats/min.* Generally in adults the heart rate with sinus tachycardia is between 100 and 180 beats/min.

Fig. 11-2 shows an example of sinus tachycardia. Each QRS complex is preceded by a P wave. Note that the P waves are positive in lead II. With sinus tachycardia at very fast rates, the P waves may merge with the preceding T wave and become difficult to distinguish.

Sinus tachycardia is an arrhythmia, but not necessarily an abnormal rhythm. For example, most normal persons develop a sinus tachycardia during exercise or excitement. In general, a sinus tachycardia will be seen with any condition that produces an increase in sympathetic tone or a decrease in vagal tone.

The following conditions are commonly associated with sinus tachycardia:

1. Anxiety, emotion, and exertion
2. Drugs such as epinephrine, ephedrine, and isoproterenol (Isuprel) that increase sympathetic tone
3. Drugs such as atropine that block vagal tone
4. Fever
5. Congestive heart failure (Sinus tachycardia caused by increased sympathetic tone is generally seen with pulmonary edema.)
6. Pulmonary embolism (Sinus tachycardia is the most common arrhythmia seen with acute pulmonary embolism [Chapter 10].)
7. Acute myocardial infarction, which may produce virtually any arrhythmia (Sinus tachycardia persisting after an acute infarct is generally a bad prognostic sign and implies extensive heart damage.)
8. Hyperthyroidism (Sinus tachycardia occurring at rest is a common finding.)
9. Hypotension and shock associated with myocardial infarction, sepsis, or blood loss

Treatment of sinus tachycardia must be directed at the underlying cause (for example, infection, hyperthyroidism, congestive heart failure, and so on). Patients with a sinus tachycardia may complain of palpitations, as mentioned before.

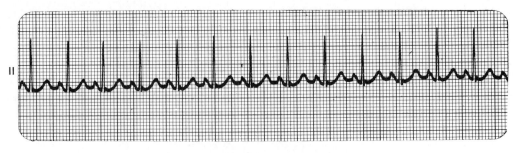

Fig. 11-2. Sinus tachycardia.

Sinus tachycardia is our first example of a supraventricular tachycardia (SVT). A *supraventricular tachycardia* is a tachycardia in which the pacemaker is located in either the atria or AV junction, *above* the ventricles. In subsequent chapters we will describe other types of SVTs, such as paroxysmal atrial tachycardia (PAT), atrial fibrillation, and atrial flutter.

SINUS BRADYCARDIA

With sinus bradycardia, sinus rhythm is present and the heart rate is less than 60 beats/min (Fig. 11-3).

Sinus bradycardia is usually caused by a relative increase in vagal tone or a decrease in sympathetic tone that slows the pacemaker rate of the SA node. Sinus bradycardia commonly occurs in the following conditions:

1. As a normal variant (Many normal people have a resting pulse rate of less than 60 beats/min, and trained athletes may have a pulse rate as low as 35 beats/min.)
2. Drugs that increase vagal tone, such as digitalis or edrophonium (Tensilon), or that decrease sympathetic tone, such as propranolol (Inderal) or reserpine (In addition, calcium channel–blocking drugs such as diltiazem hydrochloride and verapamil may cause marked sinus bradycardia.)
3. Hypothyroidism (This is generally associated with a sinus bradycardia, just

as hyperthyroidism produces a resting sinus tachycardia.)
4. "Sick sinus syndrome" (Some patients, particularly among the elderly, will have marked sinus bradycardia without obvious cause, probably from degenerative disease of the sinus node. This "sick sinus syndrome" is discussed further at the end of this chapter and in Chapter 18. [See also Fig. 11-6.])
5. Sleep apnea syndrome
6. Carotid sinus syndrome

Most people with sinus bradycardia have no symptoms. If the heart rate is very slow (in the 40s), light-headedness and even syncope may occur. In such cases a drug such as atropine, which blocks vagal tone, may be needed acutely to increase the heart rate. In cases of chronic sinus bradycardia causing symptoms (for example, in the sick sinus syndrome) an electronic pacemaker may be needed.

SINUS ARRHYTHMIA

Even in healthy persons the sinus node does not pace the heart at a perfectly regular rate. Actually, there is normally a slight beat-to-beat variation in sinus rate. Sometimes, as shown in Figs. 11-4 and 11-5, when this beat-to-beat variability in sinus rate is more accentuated, the term *"sinus arrhythmia"* is used. Sinus arrhythmia, therefore, is sinus rhythm with an irregular rate.

The most common cause of sinus arrhythmia is respiration. With inspiration the heart

Fig. 11-3. Sinus bradycardia.

Fig. 11-4. Phasic sinus arrhythmia. Normally there is a slight increase in the heart rate with inspiration and a slight decrease with expiration.

Fig. 11-5. Nonphasic sinus arrhythmia. The monitor lead shows a markedly irregular rhythm. Each QRS complex is preceded by a P wave, with a constant PR interval. This arrhythmia resulted from viral myocarditis. (Note that the T waves are biphasic.)

rate normally increases slightly; with expiration it slows slightly. This respiratory, or *phasic,* sinus arrhythmia is caused by slight changes in vagal tone occurring during the different phases of respiration (Fig. 11-4).

Occasionally a *nonphasic* sinus arrhythmia occurs, and the heart rate varies from beat to beat without relation to the respiratory cycle (Fig. 11-5).

Phasic sinus arrhythmia is a normal finding, particularly in children. A nonphasic sinus arrhythmia, while not strictly normal, does not have any special pathologic or therapeutic significance.

SINUS ARREST AND ESCAPE BEATS

Up to this point, we have described normal sinus rhythm, sinus tachycardia with a rapid sinus rate, sinus bradycardia with a slow sinus rate, and sinus arrhythmia where the sinus rate is variable. Suppose for some reason the sinus node fails to function for one or more beats. Such failure of the sinus node to pace is called *sinoatrial block (SA block)*. SA block may occur intermittently, where there is simply a missing beat (no P wave or QRS complex) at occasional intervals, or it may be more extreme. An example of the latter is *sinus pause* or *arrest* (Fig. 11-6), where the sinus node fails to function altogether for a prolonged period. This type of block will lead to cardiac arrest with asystole unless the sinus node regains function or some other pacemaker (escape pacemaker) takes over. Fortunately, as mentioned earlier, other parts of the cardiac conduction system are capable

SINUS PAUSE

Fig. 11-6. Sinus pause in a patient with sick sinus syndrome. The monitor lead shows sinus bradycardia with a long pause.

monitor

JE

Fig. 11-7. Junctional escape beat *(JE)*. The monitor strip shows a sinus pause with each escape beat.

of producing electrical stimuli and functioning as an escape pacemaker in these circumstances. Escape beats may come from the atria, the AV junction, or the ventricles.

Fig. 11-7 shows an example of a junctional escape beat. The characteristics of escape beats are described in Chapter 12.

SA block and sinus arrest can be caused by numerous factors, including hypoxia (decreased oxygen in the tissues), myocardial ischemia (inadequate myocardial blood supply), hyperkalemia, digitalis toxicity, and toxic reactions to other drugs such as the beta-blockers and calcium-channel blockers (diltiazem, verapamil). In elderly people the sinus node may undergo degenerative changes and fail to function effectively. In such cases periods of SA block and even sinus

arrest may occur, leading to light-headedness and syncope at times. The term *"sick sinus syndrome,"* mentioned previously, is used to refer to this type of sinus node dysfunction and is described further in Chapter 18 (Figs. 11-6 and 18-13).

Disturbances of sinus rhythm (in particular sinus bradycardia, sinus arrhythmia, and sinus arrest) are common with inferior wall infarctions. These arrhythmias may be a result of sinus node ischemia or of increased vagal tone, a frequent accompaniment of inferior MI. They are usually transient and self-limited. Occasionally one or more injections of atropine will be necessary if the rate slows excessively, and in rare cases a temporary pacemaker may be required.

In summary, the term *arrhythmia* refers to

any heart rhythm other than strictly normal sinus rhythm. Sinus bradycardia, sinus tachycardia, sinus arrhythmia, and SA block are all examples of arrhythmias. However, arrhythmias such as sinus bradycardia in a resting person, sinus tachycardia with exercise, or phasic sinus arrhythmia with respiratory changes in heart rate may be normal findings.

In other settings, such as hypothyroidism or pulmonary emboli, sinus bradycardia or sinus tachycardia respectively may be important diagnostic clues.

The next few chapters describe other common arrhythmias where the cardiac pacemaker is located *outside* the sinus node—in the atria, AV junction, or ventricles.

REVIEW OF CHAPTER 11

In *NSR* (normal sinus rhythm) each heartbeat originates in the sinus node. The P wave is always negative in lead aV_R and positive in lead II. The rate is between 60 and 100 beats/min.

In *sinus tachycardia* the heart rate is greater than 100 beats/min while in *sinus bradycardia* it is less than 60 beats/min. There are multiple causes of sinus bradycardia and sinus tachycardia, and both arrhythmias may occur normally.

In *sinus arrhythmia* there is variability of the sinus rate from beat to beat, and it may be either phasic with respiration or nonphasic. *SA block* describes failure of the sinus node to function for one or more beats. *Sinus arrest,* leading to fatal asystole, may occur unless NSR resumes or unless *escape beats* from other foci in the atria, AV junction, or ventricles take over. SA block and sinus arrest may be seen particularly in elderly people as a consequence of the *sick sinus syndrome*. Digitalis toxicity or toxic reactions to other drugs (beta-blockers, calcium-channel blockers) must always be excluded in anyone with marked sinus bradycardia, SA block, or sinus arrest.

Review Questions—Chapter 11

1. Is NSR present?

2. Is NSR present?

Answers

1. Yes. The P waves are negative in lead aV_R and positive in lead II. Don't be confused by the unusual QRS complexes (positive in lead aV_R and negative in lead II) produced by the abnormal axis deviation. Diagnosis of NSR depends only on the P waves.

2. No. Each QRS complex is preceded by a P wave. However, notice that the P waves are *negative* in lead II. These retrograde P waves were produced in this case by a junctional (or ectopic atrial) rhythm.

12 Supraventricular Arrhythmias—I

Premature Atrial Contractions, Paroxysmal Atrial Tachycardia, AV Junctional Rhythms

The normal pacemaker of the heart is the sinus (SA) node, and normally it initiates each heartbeat. However, pacemaker stimuli can arise from other parts of the heart—the atria, the AV junction, or the ventricles. The terms "ectopy," "ectopic pacemaker," and "ectopic beat" are used to describe these non-sinus beats. Ectopic beats are often premature; that is, they come before the next sinus beat is due. Thus we may find premature atrial contractions (PACs), premature AV junctional contractions (PJCs), and premature ventricular contractions (PVCs). Ectopic beats can also come after a pause in the normal rhythm, as in the case of AV junctional or ventricular *escape* beats. Ectopic beats originating in the AV junction or atria are referred to as *supraventricular* (that is, coming from *above* the ventricles).

In this chapter and the next we will describe ectopic atrial and AV junctional (supraventricular) rhythms. Chapter 14 deals with ventricular ectopy.

PREMATURE ATRIAL CONTRACTIONS (PACs)

Premature atrial contractions (PACs)* are ectopic beats arising from somewhere in either the left or the right atrium but not in the sinus node. The atria, therefore, are depolarized from an ectopic site. Following atrial stimulation, the stimulus will spread normally through the AV junction into the ventricles. For this reason, ventricular depolarization (QRS) is generally not affected by PACs.

PACs have the following major features (Fig. 12-1):

1. The beat is premature, occurring before the next normal beat is due. This is in contrast to escape beats (p. 169), which come after a pause in the normal rhythm.

2. The PAC is often, but not always, preceded by a visible P wave. This P wave usually has a slightly different shape and/or slightly different PR interval from the P wave seen with the normal sinus beats. The PR interval of the PAC may be either longer or shorter than the PR interval of the normal beats.

3. Following the PAC there is generally a slight pause before the normal sinus beat resumes.

4. Occasionally, no clear P wave will be seen preceding the PAC (Fig. 12-2). In such cases the P wave may be "buried" in the T wave of the preceding beat.

5. The QRS complex of the PAC is usually identical or very similar to the QRS complex of the preceding beats. Re-

---

*The terms "premature atrial contractions," "premature atrial beats," "premature atrial depolarizations," and "atrial extrasystoles" are used synonymously in the current literature.

member that with PACs the atrial pacemaker is in an ectopic location, but the ventricles are depolarized in a normal way. This contrasts with premature ventricular contractions (PVCs), discussed in Chapter 14, where the QRS complex is abnormally wide because of abnormal depolarization of the ventricles. (Occasionally, PACs will result in aberrant ventricular conduction so the QRS is wider than normal. Differentiation of such PACs "with aberration" from pre-

mature ventricular contractions may be difficult.)

Sometimes, when the PAC is very premature, the stimulus will reach the AV junction shortly after it has already been stimulated by the preceding normal beat. Because the AV junction, like all other conduction tissue, requires time to recover its capacity to conduct impulses, this premature atrial stimulus may reach the junction when it is still *refractory*. In such cases the PAC may not be conducted to the ventricles and no QRS complex will

Fig. 12-1. Premature atrial contractions. **A,** Note the PAC after the fourth sinus beat. **B,** Blocking of the PAC occurs after the fourth sinus beat. The premature P wave falls on the T wave of the preceding beat and is not followed by a QRS complex.

Fig. 12-2. Atrial bigeminy. Every other beat is an atrial premature contraction.

appear. This situation will result in a *blocked PAC*. The ECG (Fig. 12-1, *B*) will show a premature P wave *not* followed by a QRS complex. Following the blocked P wave, there is a slight pause before the next normal beat resumes. The blocked PAC, therefore, produces a slight irregularity of the heartbeat. If you do not search carefully for these blocked PACs you will overlook them.

PACs may occur frequently (for example, five or more times/min) or sporadically. Two PACs occurring consecutively are referred to as "paired PACs." Sometimes , as shown in Fig. 12-2, each sinus beat is followed by a PAC. (This pattern is referred to as *atrial bigeminy*.)

Clinical Significance

PACs are very common. They may occur both in persons with normal hearts and in persons with organic heart disease. Finding PACs, therefore, does not imply that the person has cardiac disease. In normal subjects PACs may be seen with emotional stress, with excessive coffee drinking, or as a result of sympathomimetic drugs (epinephrine, isoproterenol, theophylline). PACs may produce palpitations—the patient may complain of feeling a skipped beat or an irregular pulse. PACs, as noted, may also be seen with any type of heart disease. Frequent PACs are sometimes the forerunner of atrial fibrillation or paroxysmal atrial tachycardia.

PAROXYSMAL ATRIAL TACHYCARDIA (PAT)

Paroxysmal atrial tachycardia (PAT)* is the second tachyarrhythmia we shall discuss. The first was sinus tachycardia (p. 166). *PAT is simply a run of three or more consecutive PACs.*

---

*As described later in this chapter (p. 182), most of the cases of so-called PAT are actually related to a *reentrant*-type mechanism involving the AV junction. Hence the terms "PAT" and "*AV junctional tachycardia*" are sometimes used synonymously.

In some cases, the run of PAT may be brief and self-limited. In other cases, it may be sustained for hours, days, or even weeks. Figs. 12-3 to 12-5 show several examples.

PAT has the following characteristics:
1. The heart rate with PAT is generally between 140 and 250 beats/min. Recall that with sinus tachycardia the heart rate in adults did not generally exceed 160 to 180 beats/min.
2. PAT is usually extremely regular. Each beat falls exactly on time, and the RR intervals between beats do not generally show any variability. This also contrasts with sinus tachycardia, in which there is generally some slight but discernible beat-to-beat variability.
3. P waves may or may not be visible. When seen, they are generally different from the P waves in a patient with normal sinus rhythm. The PR interval may be the same as, greater than, or less than the patient's usual PR interval.
4. The QRS complexes are usually of normal width, since intraventricular conduction is generally normal with PAT. (A wide QRS complex will be seen if the patient has an underlying bundle branch block or if the PAT induces a "rate-related" bundle branch block.)

Clinical Significance

PAT may be seen both in normal persons and in those with organic heart disease. It, therefore, does not necessarily imply that the patient has any significant heart disease. For example, healthy adults can have attacks of PAT that may break spontaneously or that occasionally require special treatment (as outlined below). PAT may also occur with heart disease of any type. One special condition associated with PAT is *ventricular preexcitation* seen in the Wolff-Parkinson-White or Lown-Ganong-Levine syndrome (Chapter 10).

Patients with PAT usually complain of light-headedness or palpitations. Occasionally

PAROXYSMAL ATRIAL TACHYCARDIA (PAT)

Fig. 12-3. This strip shows PAT (a run of more than three PACs). The rate is about 167 beats/min. Note the marked regularity of the rhythm. No P waves are visible.

PAROXYSMAL ATRIAL TACHYCARDIA

Fig. 12-4. PAT with a rate of about 200 beats/min.

Fig. 12-5. Paroxysmal atrial tachycardia treated with carotid sinus massage. The first 14 beats in this rhythm strip show PAT with a rate of about 150 beats/min. Carotid sinus massage resulted in abrupt termination of the tachycardia, with the appearance of normal sinus rhythm.

PAT produces syncope. A run of PAT in a patient with limited cardiac reserve may precipitate angina pectoris or congestive heart failure.

Treatment

Many times PAT will resolve spontaneously or after the patient is sedated. There are several methods of direct therapy. Most of these methods of treating PAT involve increasing the amount of vagal tone on the heart. Recall that the vagus nerve exerts a braking effect on the heart, slowing stimulus formation and conduction in the sinus node and the AV junction. Patients with PAT have an excessive number of stimuli traveling through the AV junction. Therefore, one approach to treating PAT is to increase vagal tone. There are several ways of doing this. The patient may try *Valsalva's maneuver* (straining and bearing down as if to have a bowel movement). *Carotid sinus massage* may also terminate an attack of PAT by increasing vagal tone (Fig. 12-5).

Numerous drugs can also be used to treat PAT. Verapamil, a calcium-blocking drug, is highly effective. Digitalis acts by increasing vagal tone at the AV junction. Edrophonium (Tensilon) also increases vagal tone. Propranolol (Inderal) blocks sympathetic stimuli. Phenylephrine (Neo-Synephrine), an intravenous vasoconstrictor, raises the blood pressure rapidly, causing a reflex increase in vagal tone similar to what occurs with carotid sinus massage. Quinidine or procainamide may also be useful.

It is essential to be familiar with the adverse effects and contraindications of any drug prior to its use. The clinical pharmacology of antiarrhythmic agents is discussed in many texts (see Bibliography). In general, most patients will respond to one of the above drugs. Often, therapy is effective within minutes. Occasionally, PAT requires more immediate therapy. Younger patients and those without significant underlying cardiovascular disease may tolerate heart rates up to 250 beats/min with complaints only of palpitations or light-headedness. However, in patients with limited cardiac reserve, heart rates above 160 beats/min (or even less) may have disastrous consequences. These patients may develop anginal pain. They may also have congestive heart failure or hypotension. In such emergency circumstances, when PAT is associated with angina, congestive heart failure, or hypotension and when initial therapy with vagal maneuvers and drugs fails, electrical cardioversion may be required.

Electrical cardioversion is the use of a direct current (DC) electric shock to treat certain tachyarrhythmias. The DC shock is administered with special paddles placed on the chest wall. In treating some arrhythmias, such as ventricular flutter or ventricular fibrillation, an *unsynchronized* DC shock is given. In treating PAT and other supraventricular arrhythmias, such as atrial fibrillation and atrial flutter, it is essential to give a synchronized DC shock. The shock is synchronized so it does not occur during the *vulnerable period* of ventricular repolarization (simultaneous with the apex of the T wave). It has been noted that DC shocks given to the heart during the vulnerable period may produce ventricular fibrillation. Therefore, in treating PAT, *synchronized* DC shock must be given. The details of electrical cardioversion lie outside the scope of this book. (See DeSilva et al., 1980.)

AV JUNCTIONAL RHYTHMS

With PACs and PAT the ectopic pacemaker is located somewhere in the atria outside the sinus node. Under certain circumstances, the AV junction may also function as an ectopic pacemaker, producing an AV junctional rhythm. In older textbooks, the term "AV nodal" or "nodal" rhythm is used to refer to AV junctional rhythm. The terms *"AV junctional," "junctional," "AV nodal,"* and *"nodal"* are all synonymous.

In Chapter 4 we described the basic mechanism of AV junctional rhythms and the pattern seen with AV junctional escape beats. When the AV junction is the cardiac pacemaker, the atria are stimulated in a *retrograde* fashion from bottom to top. An arrow representing the spread of atrial depolarization with junctional rhythm points upward, just the opposite of the direction of atrial depolarization when normal sinus rhythm is present. This retrograde stimulation of the atria will produce an upright (positive) P wave in lead aV_R and a downward (negative) P wave in lead II (Fig. 4-5), just the opposite of the pattern seen with normal sinus rhythm (Fig. 4-3). The ventricles will be normally depolarized (unless a bundle branch block is present) with AV junctional rhythm, resulting in a narrow QRS complex.

In some cases of AV junctional rhythm the atria will be stimulated before the ventricles. In other cases the stimulus may reach the ventricles first. Finally, in still other cases the atria and the ventricles will be stimulated simultaneously. If the atria are stimulated first, the P wave will precede the QRS complex. (A retrograde P wave preceding the QRS may also occur with some ectopic atrial beats. However, the distinction between ectopic atrial and AV junctional beats is usually not of clinical importance.) If the ventricles are first to be stimulated, the QRS complex will precede the P wave. If atrial and ventricular depolarization are simultaneous, the P wave will be "buried" in the QRS complex and no apparent P wave will be seen.

To summarize, AV junctional beats can be recognized on the ECG by one of the following three patterns (Fig. 12-6):

1. Retrograde P waves (positive in lead aV_R, negative in lead II) preceding the QRS complex
2. Retrograde P waves following the QRS complex
3. Absent P waves (buried in the QRS), so the baseline between QRS complexes is flat

AV junctional rhythms can be considered in two general classes—slow escape rhythms and tachycardias—depending on the rate. The *slow* junctional escape rhythms are less than 60 beats/min. The junctional *tachycardias* have rates between 100 and 250 beats/min.

AV JUNCTIONAL BEATS

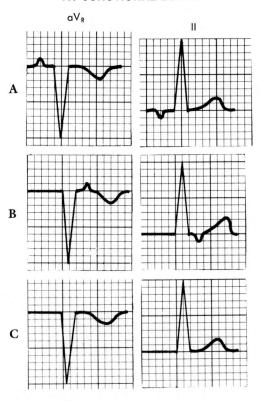

Fig. 12-6. AV junctional beats produce P waves that point upward in lead aV_R and downward in lead II—just the opposite of what is seen in sinus rhythm. The P wave may precede the QRS complex, **A,** follow it, **B,** or occur simultaneously with it, **C.** In the last instance no P wave will be visible.

AV Junctional Escape Rhythms

AV junctional escape beats were mentioned previously in the section on sinus arrest (p. 168). An AV junctional escape beat (Fig. 11-7) is simply a beat that comes after a pause because the normal sinus pacemaker fails to function. The AV junctional escape beat, therefore, is a "safety beat." Following this escape beat, the normal sinus pacemaker may resume function. However, if this does not occur, a slow AV junctional escape rhythm may continue. An AV junctional escape rhythm is simply a consecutive run of AV junctional beats. The heart rate is usually slow, between 30 and 60 beats/min.

Fig. 12-7 shows an example of an AV junctional escape rhythm. It is not surprising that the basic rate of the AV junction is slower than that of the sinus node. If the AV junction had a faster inherent rate, it would compete with the sinus node for control of the heartbeat.

AV junctional escape rhythms can be seen in a number of clinical settings—digitalis toxicity (Chapter 16), toxic reactions to beta-blockers or calcium-channel blockers (diltiazem, verapamil), acute myocardial infarction, hypoxemia, hyperkalemia. Treatment depends on the cause (for example, stopping the digitalis, oxygenating the patient, and so on). If the heart rate becomes excessively slow with an AV junctional rhythm, then drugs such as atropine (a vagal blocker) or isoproterenol (a sympathomimetic stimulator) may be used acutely to increase the heart rate.

AV Junctional Tachycardias

As mentioned, the AV junction can also be the site of ectopic stimuli producing premature AV junctional contractions (PJCs) and junctional tachycardia.

PJCs are simply premature beats formed in the AV junction. They resemble premature atrial contractions (PACs), except that the P waves, when seen, will be retrograde with a PJC (Figs. 12-8 and 12-9). If no P wave is seen before the premature beat, then there is no way of telling if it is a PAC (with P wave lost in the preceding T wave) or a PJC (with the P wave buried in the QRS complex). The distinction is purely academic. PACs and PJCs have the same clinical significance, and treatment is the same.

An AV junctional tachycardia, analogous to PAT, is simply a run of three or more consecutive PJCs (Figs. 12-10 and 12-11). AV junctional tachycardia and PAT can be considered clinically as a single entity. They have the same clinical significance and treatment.

JUNCTIONAL ESCAPE RHYTHM

Fig. 12-7. This strip shows a slow junctional escape rhythm at 43 beats/min with no visible P waves.

Fig. 12-8. Note the retrograde P waves (positive in lead aV_R, negative in lead II) on the ECG of a patient with junctional premature beats. The P wave polarity is the reverse of what is seen with normal sinus rhythm.

Fig. 12-9. The junctional escape beat *(JE)* comes after a pause and is followed by a junctional premature contraction *(JPC)*. Note the retrograde (inverted) P wave preceding the JPC in lead II.

JUNCTIONAL TACHYCARDIA

Carotid sinus massage

Fig. 12-10. Note the retrograde (inverted) P waves preceding the QRS complexes in this lead II strip from a patient with junctional tachycardia.

JUNCTIONAL TACHYCARDIA

Fig. 12-11. The heart rate is about 150 beats/min. This lead II strip shows retrograde (inverted) P waves *(arrow)* that are barely visible and are buried in the ST-T complexes.

Current evidence indicates that most cases of PAT are actually due to reentry (p. 175, footnote) involving the AV junction. (The terms "*AV junctional*" and "*AV nodal*" are sometimes used synonymously in connection with reentrant tachycardias.) A minority of cases of atrial tachycardia are due to an "automatic" atrial focus, firing at a rapid rate. For a detailed discussion of the diagnosis and therapy of reentrant versus automatic supraventricular tachycardias, see Josephson and Kastor (1977).

Not uncommonly you will see a tracing like the one in Fig. 12-3, showing a regular tachycardia with a rate of about 200 beats/min. No P waves are seen, and it is impossible to tell whether the rhythm is PAT or an AV junctional tachycardia. The treatment in this case is the treatment outlined previously for PAT.

The differential diagnosis of PAT and AV junctional tachycardia from other tachyarrhythmias is described in detail in Chapter 18.

REVIEW OF CHAPTER 12

Stimuli that pace the heart can arise not only in the sinus node but in other cardiac tissues—the atria, the AV junction, or the ventricles.

The terms *"ectopy," "ectopic pacemaker,"* and *"ectopic contraction* or *beat"* are used to describe these stimuli that arise in areas of the heart outside the sinus node. There are two major categories of ectopic beats:

1. *Premature ectopic beats* are extra beats that come before the next normal beat is expected. Examples are PACs, PJCs, and PVCs.
2. *Escape beats* are usually AV junctional or ventricular beats that are *not* premature but come after a pause in the normal rhythm.

PACs show the following:

1. The PAC usually has a slightly different-shaped P wave and/or slightly longer or shorter PR interval than the preceding P waves and PR intervals. Sometimes the P wave of the PAC is hidden in the T wave of the preceding beat.
2. The QRS complex of the PAC is usually identical or similar to the QRS complex of the preceding normal beat.
3. Occasionally a PAC is *blocked,* that is, it cannot penetrate the AV junction. In such cases, you will see a premature P wave that is *not* followed by a QRS complex.

PAT is a run of three or more consecutive PACs. It shows the following features:

1. The heart rate is generally between 140 and 250 beats/min.
2. The rhythm is usually extremely regular.
3. P waves may or may not be visible, and the shape of the P wave and the length of the PR interval may differ from the patient's usual pattern.

AV junctional rhythm shows the following features:

1. The P wave, when seen, is negative (downward) in lead II and positive (upward) in lead aV_R, just the reverse of the pattern seen with normal sinus rhythm. These are called *retrograde* P waves.
2. These retrograde P waves may precede or follow the QRS complex.
3. In some cases, retrograde P waves may be buried within the QRS complex. If this occurs, then the baseline between the QRS complexes remains completely flat.

AV junctional rhythms may be categorized as junctional escape rhythms and junctional tachycardias. AV junctional escape rhythm is a run of AV junctional beats with a slow rate, generally between 40 and 60 beats/min. AV junctional tachycardia, in contrast, is a run of three or more consecutive PJCs. AV junctional tachycardia has the same clinical significance as PAT.

Review Questions—Chapter 12

True or false (1 to 4):
1. PAT is sinus rhythm with a rate of 140 to 250 beats/min.
2. PAT is invariably a sign of serious organic heart disease.
3. PAT is usually extremely regular.
4. PAT is defined as a run of three or more consecutive PACs.
5. Why might the patient whose rhythm strip is shown below complain of occasional palpitations?

6. What is the beat marked **X**?

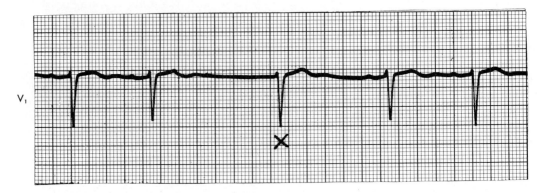

7. a. What is the approximate heart rate?
    b. What arrhythmia is present?

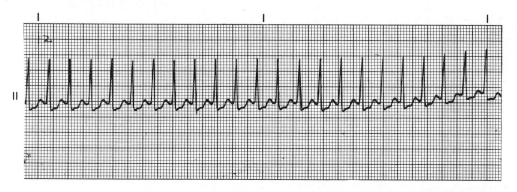

Answers

1. False. PAT is an ectopic rhythm with the pacemaker outside the sinus node.
2. False. PAT frequently occurs in normal hearts.
3. True.
4. True.
5. Palpitations might have been caused by occasional PACs. Note that the fifth beat here is a PAC (or possibly a PJC, since the P wave of the premature beat is not seen).

6. Junctional escape beat. Note that the beat comes after a pause in normal rhythm and is not preceded by a P wave.
7. a. Approximately 210 beats/min. (Count the number of QRS cycles in 6 sec and multiply by 10.)
    b. PAT; the arrhythmia here was treated with carotid sinus massage.

13 Supraventricular Arrhythmias—II

Atrial Flutter and Atrial Fibrillation

Atrial flutter and atrial fibrillation (Fig. 13-1) are two distinct but related arrhythmias. Like PAT, atrial flutter and atrial fibrillation are *ectopic* atrial rhythms. With all three arrhythmias, the atria are *not* stimulated from the sinus node but from an ectopic site. In PAT the atria are stimulated at a rate generally between 140 and 250 beats/min. In atrial flutter, the atrial rate is even faster, generally between 250 and 350 beats/min. Finally, with atrial fibrillation, the atrial depolarization rate is between 400 and 600 beats/min. You can consider these three ectopic atrial tachyarrhythmias on a continuum from PAT to atrial flutter to atrial fibrillation, with the *atrial* rate becoming progressively more rapid in each case.

ATRIAL FLUTTER

With both atrial flutter and atrial fibrillation there are no true P waves on the ECG. Instead, with atrial flutter we see characteristic flutter waves (F waves) (Fig. 13-2) while in atrial fibrillation we see fibrillatory waves (f waves). As shown in Fig. 13-1, flutter waves have a characteristic *sawtooth* shape.

As mentioned, the atria in atrial flutter are being stimulated about 300 times/min. What

Fig. 13-1. Atrial flutter and fibrillation. Notice the sawtooth waves with atrial flutter *(F)* and the irregular fibrillatory waves with atrial fibrillation *(f)*.

happens to the ventricles? With atrial flutter (and atrial fibrillation) the ventricular (QRS) rate will vary depending on the ability of the AV junction to conduct stimuli from the atria to the ventricles. If the ventricles respond to each flutter wave, then the ventricular rate will be around 300 beats/min. Most commonly the ventricular rate in atrial flutter is about 150 beats/min, 100 beats/min, or 75 beats/min. Atrial flutter with a ventricular response of 150 beats/min is called 2:1 flutter because of the ratio of the atrial rate (300 beats/min) to the ventricular rate (150 beats/min). Atrial flutter with a ventricular rate of 100 beats/min is 3:1 flutter and with a rate of 75 beats/min is usually 4:1 flutter. As

ATRIAL FLUTTER

Fig. 13-2. A, Note the variable appearance of flutter waves in different leads. In lead I the waves are barely apparent while in leads II and III the classic "sawtooth" waves appear. The ventricular rate is about 160 beats/min, and the flutter rate is about 320 beats/min; thus 2 : 1 conduction is present. **B,** Carotid sinus massage produces marked slowing of the ventricular rate by increasing vagal tone.

mentioned, atrial flutter with a ventricular rate equal to the atrial rate, 300 beats/min, or 1:1 flutter is very rare. Characteristically patients with atrial flutter will increase or decrease their ventricular rate by stepwise fractions of the atrial rate (Fig. 13-3). Thus a patient may change abruptly from atrial flutter with a ventricular response of 75 to 100 beats/min, to 150 beats/min, or even to 300 beats/min. In some patients the ventricular response with atrial flutter will be more variable.

Clinical Significance

Atrial flutter is rarely seen in people with normal hearts. This is in contrast to atrial fibrillation (described later), which may occur transiently in normal individuals. Atrial flutter is not specific for any particular type of heart disease but occurs, for example, in patients with valvular heart disease, acute myocardial infarction or chronic ischemic heart disease, cardiomyopathy, hypertensive heart disease, lung disease, and pulmonary emboli as well as after cardiac surgery.

Treatment

Treatment of atrial flutter depends on the clinical condition. In some patients atrial flutter will revert spontaneously to normal sinus rhythm. In other patients who are hypoxic, treatment with oxygen may help restore normal sinus rhythm.

Patients in atrial flutter are frequently treated with digitalis. Digitalis has two major effects on atrial flutter. It slows conduction through the AV junction, thereby slowing and stabilizing the ventricular rate, and it tends to increase the rate of atrial depolarization. Increasing the atrial rate may convert atrial flutter to atrial fibrillation. Thus digoxin administered to a patient in atrial flutter may convert the patient to atrial fibrillation with a slower and more stable ventricular rate. Rarely patients may convert to normal sinus rhythm from atrial flutter following digitalization. In other cases, a second drug (such as quinidine) is added to help convert atrial flutter to normal sinus rhythm. Quinidine is an antiarrhythmic drug that is useful in treating both atrial flutter and atrial fibrillation. In selected cases either verapamil, a calcium channel–blocking drug, or a beta-blocking drug such as propranolol (Inderal) may be used orally or intravenously to slow the ventricular response during atrial flutter.

In many patients atrial flutter will persist despite pharmacologic therapy with digitalis and quinidine. Fortunately, atrial flutter is one of the arrhythmias most easily treated with electrical cardioversion. As described previously with PAT, a synchronized DC shock is given with the patient properly anesthetized. Of all the atrial arrhythmias, atrial flutter is probably the easiest to cardiovert electrically. Therefore, some cardiologists rec-

ATRIAL FLUTTER

Fig. 13-3. Note the variable ventricular rate in this patient with atrial flutter.

ommend synchronized DC shock as the treatment of choice in the patient with atrial flutter.

Another way of treating atrial flutter is with very rapid pacing of the atria by means of a temporary pacing wire (*overdrive* pacing, p. 269). The details of this therapy, however, lie outside the scope of this book.

To summarize, atrial flutter is an atrial tachyarrhythmia in which the atria are stimulated (depolarized) at a rate of 250 to 350 beats/min, with a ventricular response that is often some fraction of the atrial rate (½, ¼, and so on). Atrial flutter may be treated with special drugs (digitalis, quinidine), synchronized DC shock, or rapid atrial pacing.

ATRIAL FIBRILLATION

Atrial fibrillation is one of the most commonly seen arrhythmias. In atrial fibrillation the atria are stimulated (depolarized) at a very rapid rate, up to 600 times/min. This fibrillatory activity produces a characteristic irregular, wavy pattern in place of the normal P waves. These irregular waves, seen in Fig. 13-4, are called *fibrillatory* or *f waves*. In some cases, the f waves are relatively coarse (Fig. 13-5). In other cases, fine fibrillation is seen

ATRIAL FIBRILLATION

Fig. 13-4. Irregular undulation of the baseline because of fibrillatory (f) waves. There are no true P waves, and the ventricular (QRS) rate is irregular.

RAPID ATRIAL FIBRILLATION

Fig. 13-5. Coarse fibrillatory waves with a rapid ventricular response. This patient had hyperthyroidism. (The commonly used term "rapid atrial fibrillation" is actually a misnomer since "rapid" refers to the ventricular rate rather than the atrial rate. The same is true for "slow atrial fibrillation.")

(Fig. 13-6). Atrial fibrillation, therefore, is characterized by rapid oscillatory depolarization of the atria, producing irregular undulations of the ECG baseline without true P waves.

Because of the rapid atrial depolarization rate, the AV junction in patients with atrial fibrillation is being bombarded by innumerable stimuli from the atria. If every stimulus (each f wave) penetrated the AV junction, the ventricles would beat at a rate of 600 times/min, with obvious consequences to the patient. Fortunately, the AV junction is refractory to most of these impulses and allows only a fraction of these atrial stimuli to reach the ventricles. In patients with a normal AV junction who suddenly develop atrial fibrillation, the ventricular rate is generally 110 to 180 beats/min. Fig. 13-6 shows an example of atrial fibrillation with a ventricular rate of about 140 beats/min. Characteristically, the ventricular rate with atrial fibrillation is haphazardly irregular. This irregular ventricular rate results from the AV junction being stimulated in an apparently random fashion by the rapidly fibrillating atria.

To summarize, there are two ECG characteristics of atrial fibrillation. First, you will see the irregular, wavy baseline produced by the rapid f waves. Second, the ventricular

ATRIAL FIBRILLATION

Fig. 13-6. Fibrillatory waves may be hard to find. In this tachyarrhythmia no P waves are evident. The ventricular rate is about 140 beats/min and irregular. Although no clear fibrillatory waves are visible here, the rhythm is nevertheless atrial fibrillation.

ATRIAL FIBRILLATION

Fig. 13-7. A very irregular ventricular rate is present here. Although no clear P waves can be seen, this rhythm (like the one in Fig. 13-6) is nevertheless atrial fibrillation with a rapid ventricular response.

(QRS) rate is usually quite irregular. When the ventricular rate is very fast (Fig. 13-7), it may be difficult to distinguish the f waves. However, in such cases the diagnosis of atrial fibrillation can be made by finding a very irregular ventricular rate in the absence of definite P waves.

Clinical Aspects

In some patients, atrial fibrillation occurs *paroxysmally* and may last for only minutes, hours, or days. In others the atrial fibrillation is *chronic* and may persist for months or years.

Atrial fibrillation may occur both in normal persons and in patients with a variety of cardiac diseases. Paroxysmal atrial fibrillation is occasionally precipitated by emotional stress, excessive alcohol consumption, or vomiting spells in otherwise healthy people. In such cases the paroxysmal atrial fibrillation often spontaneously reverts to normal sinus rhythm or is converted easily with digitalis alone.

Atrial fibrillation is also one of the most common arrhythmias seen in patients with organic heart disease. Common pathologic causes include coronary artery disease, hypertensive heart disease, and valvular heart disease. Patients with coronary artery disease may develop paroxysmal atrial fibrillation in the course of an acute myocardial infarction. However, in most cases the atrial fibrillation develops as a consequence of *chronic* ischemic myocardial disease, presumably resulting in fibrosis and dilation of the atria. Patients with hypertensive heart disease typically develop left ventricular and left atrial enlargement as a result of years of sustained high blood pressure. Dilation of the atria predisposes this group of patients to atrial fibrillation. Atrial fibrillation is also commonly caused by valvular heart disease, particularly where there is mitral valve involvement. For example, severe mitral stenosis or mitral regurgitation will produce marked atrial enlargement, predisposing to atrial arrhythmias.

Atrial fibrillation may also occur in other conditions. For example, patients with thyrotoxicosis (hyperthyroidism) may develop atrial fibrillation, often with an extremely rapid ventricular rate (Fig. 13-5). Atrial fibrillation (or flutter) is not uncommon following cardiac surgery. Atrial fibrillation may also occur with chronic pericarditis, pulmonary emboli, cardiomyopathies, and other forms of heart disease.

Clinical Consequences

What happens physiologically when a patient develops atrial fibrillation? Normally after the P wave the atria contract, pumping blood into the ventricles. With atrial fibrillation, normal atrial depolarization is lost and the atria fibrillate (quaver) instead of contracting synchronously. In these circumstances the normal atrial "kick" is lost, and the result is decreased cardiac output since ventricular filling is decreased.

Hemodynamically, therefore, the most significant effect of atrial fibrillation is decreased cardiac output. This decreased cardiac output will be most marked in patients with underlying cardiac impairment. The degree of decreased output will also depend on the ventricular rate in atrial fibrillation. The faster the ventricular rate is in atrial fibrillation, the more decreased the cardiac output will be. Thus the patient in atrial fibrillation at a rate of 180 beats/min is more likely to be hypotensive or in congestive heart failure than would be the case with a rate of 100 beats/min.

To summarize, decreased cardiac output in atrial fibrillation reflects two major factors: (1) the loss of normal atrial contractility (atrial kick) and (2) the rapid ventricular rate. The drop in cardiac output with atrial fibrillation (as with any tachyarrhythmia) can produce one (or more) of the following three clinical problems: (1) congestive heart failure, (2) hypotension and even shock, and (3) myocardial ischemia. Initial clinical assessment of the patient in atrial fibrillation must focus on these three areas. Is the patient showing signs of congestive failure (difficulty breathing, rales in the chest, edema of the feet)? Is the patient's blood pressure low? Is there evidence of myocardial ischemia with symptoms of anginal chest pain and/or ECG signs of acute ischemia or actual infarction (ST segment depressions or elevations, new Q waves, and so on)? Patients in atrial fibrillation associated with pulmonary edema, hypotension, or acute myocardial ischemia require emergency therapy.

Atrial Thrombi and Embolization

Up to this point we have stressed the decreased cardiac output seen with atrial fibrillation. A second problem caused by atrial fibrillation is the tendency of some patients with chronic atrial fibrillation to develop atrial clots (thrombi) that may dislodge into the arterial circulation, causing peripheral emboli. Such arterial emboli can cause cerebrovascular accident, occlusion of the blood supply to the legs, and other complications. Not all patients with chronic atrial fibrillation develop atrial thrombi. This problem is most common in patients with rheumatic mitral valve disease. Atrial thrombi in these patients are probably formed as a consequence of the combined effects of the stagnation of blood in the fibrillating atria and the underlying rheumatic inflammation of the atria, which serves as a site for thrombus formation.

The risk that an atrial thrombus will break off and embolize is also increased when a patient in atrial fibrillation is converted to normal sinus rhythm. The sudden resumption of normal atrial contraction may cause dislodgment of part of the atrial clot. For this reason patients in chronic atrial fibrillation, particularly with underlying rheumatic valvular disease, are generally anticoagulated for at least 10 to 14 days prior to and following cardioversion.

To summarize, the major clinical effects of atrial fibrillation are the result of decreased cardiac output and the increased potential for atrial thrombus formation and peripheral embolization.

Treatment

We will not discuss the details of treating atrial fibrillation but instead will focus more broadly on the general clinical approach to patients with this arrhythmia. There are two ways of treating atrial fibrillation. The first is pharmacologically, with drugs like digitalis and quinidine. The second is with electrical cardioversion, the same as that described for PAT and atrial flutter. Treatment with drugs generally takes hours or days to convert atrial fibrillation to sinus rhythm. Treatment with electrical cardioversion, if successful, is immediately effective. However, patients in chronic atrial fibrillation (present for months or years) may not convert to normal sinus rhythm with any therapy. This is particularly true in cases of chronic rheumatic heart disease with extremely dilated atria that are not capable of normal depolarization.

There are two major clinical questions to ask in approaching patients with atrial fibrillation. First, is the arrhythmia causing a significant decrease in cardiac output, as indicated by myocardial ischemia, hypotension, or congestive heart failure? Second, is the atrial fibrillation paroxysmal or chronic? As a general rule, patients in paroxysmal atrial fibrillation that is producing myocardial ischemia, shock, or pulmonary edema should be considered candidates for electrical cardioversion if they do not respond promptly to drug therapy. In these cases the longer the rapid heart rate persists the greater will be the chance of irreversible myocardial damage.

In most cases atrial fibrillation does not require immediate cardioversion. Drug therapy alone can be used initially to control the arrhythmia. The mainstay of treating rapid atrial fibrillation is digitalis. Digitalis acts by slowing conduction of stimuli through the AV junction. In atrial fibrillation, as noted, the junction is being bombarded by innumerable stimuli from the atria, which are fibrillating 400 to 600 times/min. The prime clinical concern in patients with rapid atrial fibrillation is to slow the ventricular rate. In patients with atrial fibrillation and a rapid ventricular rate, digitalis given intravenously (or even orally) can generally slow the ventricular rate below 100 beats/min in a matter of hours. Some patients with paroxysmal atrial fibrillation may actually convert to normal sinus rhythm after being given just digitalis. In other cases it is necessary to add a second drug, such as quinidine, to try to restore normal atrial depolarization.

The usual sequence in treating rapid atrial fibrillation pharmacologically is to slow the ventricular response with digitalis, which blocks the AV junction. If sinus rhythm is not restored after the patient has been digitalized, then quinidine can be started. Quinidine alone may sometimes increase conduc-

tion through the AV junction (because of the drug's vagolytic effect). Therefore, quinidine should never be given to a patient in atrial fibrillation unless the ventricular rate has first been slowed (usually to less than 100 beats/min) with digitalis.

As in the case of atrial flutter, either verapamil or a beta-blocking drug can be used in selected cases to help control the ventricular response of atrial fibrillation. Furthermore, patients with large left atria (for example, greater than 5.0 cm on the echocardiogram) often revert to atrial fibrillation even if electrical cardioversion is initially successful.

General Approach to the Patient

At the same time that you are starting to treat any patient with atrial fibrillation, you should be thinking of the cause of this arrhythmia. Search for evidence of coronary artery disease, hypertensive heart disease, cardiomyop-

Fig. 13-8. Atrial fibrillation with PVCs.

Fig. 13-9. Atrial fibrillation with complete heart block. The ventricular rate is very slow and regular because of the complete AV block.

athy, valvular disease, or pericardial disease. A thyroid blood level should be obtained in patients with unexplained atrial fibrillation, since hyperthyroidism is a treatable cause of this arrhythmia. Remember that some patients, particularly young adults, may go into paroxysmal atrial fibrillation without underlying heart disease.

Atrial Fibrillation and Other Arrhythmias

Atrial fibrillation may occur with other arrhythmias, just as you can have sinus rhythm with PVCs, PACs, and so on. Fig. 13-8 shows an example of atrial fibrillation with PVCs. Atrial fibrillation can also occur in the presence of complete heart block (Fig. 13-9). In such cases, the atrial fibrillation occurs with a very slow and regular ventricular response. In any patient with atrial fibrillation and a very slow ventricular rate, always think of possible digitalis toxicity (Chapter 16).

Occasionally, it may be difficult to decide whether atrial fibrillation or atrial flutter is present. The coarse atrial fibrillatory waves may resemble flutter waves. In such cases the arrhythmia is often referred to as flutter-fibrillation and has the same clinical significance and treatment as atrial fibrillation.

REVIEW OF CHAPTER 13

PAT, atrial flutter, and *atrial fibrillation* are three supraventricular tachycardias that can be considered on a continuum.

The atrial rate of *PAT* is generally 140 to 250 beats/min while that of atrial flutter is 250 to 350 beats/min and that of atrial fibrillation, 400 to 600 beats/min.

Atrial flutter shows the following:

1. Characteristic sawtooth flutter waves occur instead of P waves.
2. The ventricular rate may vary. For example, QRS complexes may occur with every fourth flutter wave. This is called 4:1 flutter. With 2:1 flutter, there is one QRS complex for every two flutter waves, and the ventricular rate is half the atrial rate. A 1:1 atrial flutter with a ventricular rate about 300 beats/min is rare.

Atrial flutter rarely, if ever, occurs in normal hearts and is most often seen in patients with valvular heart disease, ischemic heart disease, lung disease, cardiomyopathy, pulmonary emboli, and after cardiac surgery.

Atrial flutter may be treated with synchronized DC shock (cardioversion), with drug therapy, or with rapid atrial pacing.

Atrial fibrillation shows the following:

1. Rapid irregular undulations of the baseline (fibrillatory waves) occur instead of P waves.
2. A ventricular rate that is usually grossly irregular is seen. When the patient is given digitalis, the ventricular rate will slow.

In some cases, atrial fibrillation occurs chronically. In other cases, it is paroxysmal. Atrial fibrillation occasionally occurs in normal people. Common causes of atrial fibrillation are coronary artery disease, hypertensive heart disease, and rheumatic valvular heart disease. Atrial fibrillation may also occur with hyperthyroidism, cardiomyopathy, cardiac surgery, pulmonary emboli, chronic pericarditis, and other conditions.

Paroxysmal atrial fibrillation may often be converted to normal sinus rhythm with DC cardioversion or with drug therapy (digitalis, quinidine).

Atrial fibrillation may occur with other arrhythmias, such as PVCs, complete heart block, and so on. Atrial fibrillation with a very slow ventricular rate (50 beats/min or less) may indicate digitalis toxicity.

Review Questions—Chapter 13

1. Answer the following questions about the rhythm strips shown below:
   a. What is the atrial rate?
   b. What is the ventricular rate?
   c. What is this arrhythmia?

2. Answer the following questions about the rhythm strips shown below:
   a. What is the *average* heart rate?
   b. What is the rhythm?

3. The atrial rate with atrial flutter is *(faster, slower)* than the atrial rate with atrial fibrillation.
4. The atrial rate with atrial flutter is *(faster, slower)* than the atrial rate with PAT.
5. The ventricular rate with atrial fibrillation is always greater than 100 beats/min (true or false).

Answers

1. a. About 300 beats/min.
   b. About 75 beats/min.
   c. Atrial flutter with 4:1 AV conduction.
2. a. About 70 beats/min. (Count the number of RR cycles in 6 sec and multiply by 10.)
   b. Atrial fibrillation.
3. Slower.
4. Faster.
5. False.

14 Ventricular Arrhythmias

The three preceding chapters have focused on *supra*ventricular arrhythmias—rhythm disturbances arising in the sinus node, the atria, or the AV junction, with normal ventricular depolarization. Now we will discuss another major ECG topic, the ventricular arrhythmias. Ectopic (non-sinus) beats frequently arise in the ventricles themselves, producing premature ventricular contractions, ventricular tachycardia, and sometimes ventricular fibrillation.

PREMATURE VENTRICULAR CONTRACTIONS (PVCs)

Premature ventricular contractions (PVCs)* are premature beats arising in the ventricles, analogous to premature atrial contractions (PACs) and premature junctional contractions (PJCs), which are *supra*ventricular premature beats. Recall that with PACs and PJCs the QRS complex was usually of normal width because the stimulus spreads normally through the bundle branches into the ventricles. With PVCs, on the other hand, the premature beat arises in either the right or the left ventricle. Therefore, the ventricles will not be stimulated simultaneously, and the stimulus will spread through the ventricles in an aberrant direction. Thus the QRS complex will be wide with PVCs just as it is with a bundle branch block pattern. Figs. 14-1 to 14-3 show examples.

PVCs have two major characteristics:
1. They are premature and occur before the next normal beat is expected.
2. They are aberrant in appearance. The QRS complex is abnormally wide (usually 0.12 sec or more). The T wave and the QRS complex usually point in opposite directions.

Features

There are several features of PVCs that are of clinical importance.

Frequency. The frequency of PVCs refers to how many PVCs are seen per minute or per other unit of time. The frequency may range from one isolated PVC to many. As we will discuss, the difference between an occasional PVC and multiple PVCs may be the difference between no treatment and emergency therapy.

PVCs may occur in various combinations. For example, two PVCs occurring consecutively (Fig. 14-4) are referred to as a *pair,* or *couplet.* Three PVCs in a row are, by definition, *ventricular tachycardia,* discussed later in this chapter (Fig. 14-5). Sometimes, as shown in Fig. 14-6, *A,* PVCs occur so frequently that each normal beat is followed by a PVC. This produces a distinctive repetitive grouping of one normal beat–one PVC, with the sequence repeated several times. Such a pattern is called *ventricular bigeminy. Ventricular trigeminy* (Fig. 14-6) refers to the sequence of two normal beats with a PVC.

Coupling interval. The term "coupling interval" is frequently used and refers to the interval between the PVC and the preceding normal beat. In many cases, where there are multiple

---

*In the ECG literature the terms "ventricular premature beat," "ventricular premature depolarization," and "ventricular extrasystole" are also used.

Fig. 14-1. A premature ventricular contraction is recognized because it comes before the next normal beat is expected and has a wide aberrant shape. (Also note the long PR interval in the normal sinus beats, indicating first-degree AV block.)

Fig. 14-2. Note the wide aberrant shapes of premature ventricular contractions compared to the more narrow ones of PACs.

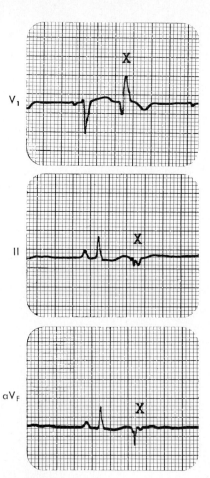

Fig. 14-3. Note that the same premature ventricular contraction (**X**) recorded simultaneously in three different leads shows different shapes. Compare this with Fig. 14-9, illustrating multiform PVCs that show different shapes in the same lead.

Monitor lead

Fig. 14-4. Two premature ventricular contractions (**V**) are termed "paired PVCs." These also show the R on T phenomenon. (See text and Fig. 14-10.)

VENTRICULAR TACHYCARDIA

Fig. 14-5. Note the two short bursts of ventricular tachycardia, defined as three or more consecutive PVCs.

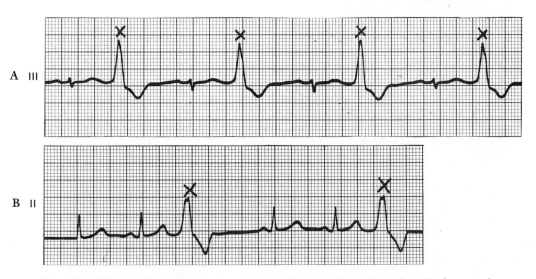

Fig. 14-6. Ventricular premature contractions. **A,** Ventricular bigeminy. Each normal sinus beat is followed by a PVC (marked with an **X**). **B,** Ventricular trigeminy. After every two sinus beats a PVC occurs.

PVCs, there is *fixed coupling,* the coupling interval being approximately the same for each PVC (Fig. 14-6). At other times PVCs may show a *variable coupling interval.* Clinically, fixed and variably coupled PVCs are generally treated in the same fashion.

Compensatory pause. As you may have noticed, PACs, and PVCs are usually followed by a pause before the next normal beat. The pause following a PVC is usually longer than the pause following a PAC, but there are exceptions. A fully compensatory pause (Fig. 14-7)

indicates that the interval between the normal QRS complexes immediately before and immediately after the PVC is exactly twice the basic RR interval. A fully compensatory pause is more characteristic of PVCs than of PACs. Sometimes a PVC will fall almost exactly between two normal beats, and in such cases the PVC is said to be *interpolated* (Fig. 14-8).

Uniform and multiform PVCs. PVCs are premature beats arising from an ectopic focus in the ventricles. The terms *uniform* and *multiform* are used to describe the appearance of

FULLY COMPENSATORY PAUSE

Fig. 14-7. Some PVCs cause a fully compensatory pause—the interval between the two sinus beats that surround the PVC (R_3 and R_4 in this case) being exactly two times the normal interval between sinus beats (R_1 and R_2). Notice that the P waves come on time, except that the third P wave is interrupted by the PVC and therefore does not conduct normally through the AV junction. The next (fourth) P wave also comes on time. The fact that the sinus node continues to pace despite the PVC results in the fully compensatory pause.

INTERPOLATED PVC

Fig. 14-8. Sometimes a PVC (marked X here) will fall between two normal beats, in which case it is *interpolated.*

PVCs in a lead. Uniform PVCs, as the name implies, have the same appearance in any lead and arise from the same focus (Fig. 14-6). (They will, of course, have different shapes in different leads, just as any normal beat can.) In contrast, multiform PVCs have different morphologies in the same lead (Fig. 14-9). Multiform PVCs often, but not always, arise from different foci. Uniform PVCs are uni*focal* whereas multi*form* PVCs are not necessarily multi*focal*. Uniform PVCs may occur in healthy people or in those with underlying organic

heart disease. Multiform PVCs usually indicate organic heart disease.

R on T phenomenon. The "R on T," or "PVC on T," phenomenon refers to PVCs that are timed so they fall near the peak* of the T wave of the preceding normal beat (Fig. 14-10). PVCs falling on the T wave in this way are significant because they may precipitate ventricular tachycardia or ventricular fibrillation, par-

---

*Or at the nadir of a negative T wave.

MULTIFOCAL PVCs

Fig. 14-9. Multiform PVCs here have different shapes in the same lead. (Compare with Fig. 14-3.)

R ON T PHENOMENON

Monitor lead

Fig. 14-10. A PVC (marked X) falling near the peak of the T wave of the preceding beat may predispose to ventricular tachycardia or ventricular fibrillation. PVCs exhibiting this R on T (PVC on T) timing should be treated, particularly when they occur in the setting of acute MI.

ticularly in the course of acute myocardial infarction. Recall from our discussion of synchronized DC cardioversion (p. 177) that the peak of the T wave is a time during which an external stimulus is especially likely to produce ventricular tachycardia or fibrillation. However, ventricular tachycardia and ventricular fibrillation commonly occur without a preceding "R on T" beat, and not every "R on T" beat will precipitate a ventricular tachyarrhythmia.

Clinical Significance

PVCs are among the most commonly seen arrhythmias. They may occur both in normal people and also in those with serious organic heart disease. They may be a stable and benign finding, or they may be the precursors of cardiac arrest and sudden death from ventricular fibrillation. Clearly, the physician needs certain ground rules to help decide which PVCs require treatment and which do not. A few general principles will be discussed here.

As mentioned, PVCs are not uncommon in normal people in all age groups. Young adults, for example, may have PVCs caused by anxiety or excessive caffeine. Certain drugs, such as epinephrine, isoproterenol (Isuprel), and aminophylline (all used in asthmatics), may provoke PVCs in normal hearts. Nevertheless, finding frequent PVCs should always prompt a careful search for underlying cardiac disease (heart murmurs, abnormal chest x-ray findings, and so on) and a careful drug history. Occasional unifocal PVCs in an otherwise healthy person are not usually a source of concern. PVCs are common in subjects with mitral valve prolapse (click-murmur syndrome). Finding that the PVCs disappear or decrease in frequency when the patient exercises is always reassuring, although this may also occur with PVCs caused by organic heart disease. On the other hand, PVCs that increase in frequency during exercise are often serious and generally re-

quire further evaluation, particularly if ventricular tachycardia occurs with exertion.

PVCs can also be seen with virtually any type of heart disease. For example, they may be seen in patients with valvular heart disease, hypertensive heart disease, or ischemic heart disease with or without myocardial infarction. PVCs are the most common arrhythmia seen with acute myocardial infarction and may be the forerunners of ventricular tachycardia and ventricular fibrillation.

PVCs, as noted, can be caused by the toxic effects on the heart of numerous drugs (such as epinephrine, isoproterenol, and aminophylline, which are cardiac stimulants). Ventricular ectopy is also an important sign of digitalis toxicity (discussed in Chapter 16). Any patient who develops PVCs while taking digitalis should be suspected of having digitalis toxicity. PVCs may be seen with electrolyte disturbances, such as hypokalemia, and in patients with lung disease or hypoxemia from any cause.

Treatment

Treatment of PVCs depends on several considerations. In every case, a search should be made for possibly reversible causes of the PVCs. Elimination of caffeine, certain drugs, anxiety, and so on may be effective therapy in patients with occasional PVCs. Judicious administration of oxygen to hypoxemic patients or treatment of anemia, hypokalemia, or hypomagnesemia may be sufficient in appropriate cases. Withholding digitalis and checking the serum digoxin level are mandatory in any patient who develops PVCs while taking digitalis.

PVCs occurring during acute myocardial infarction are of particular concern because of the increased risk of ventricular tachycardia and ventricular fibrillation in this setting. As a general rule, patients with frequent PVCs (greater than five/min), paired PVCs (two in a row), multifocal PVCs, or PVCs showing an R on T phenomenon should be treated immediately with an intravenous drug such as lidocaine (Xylocaine) or procainamide (Pronestyl). Some cardiologists believe that even a single PVC occurring in a patient with an acute myocardial infarction should be similarly treated. In addition, some cardiologists recommend prophylactic administration of lidocaine to certain patients with acute myocardial infarction because ventricular fibrillation may occur without any "warning" arrhythmia.

Drug Therapy

The use of antiarrhythmic drugs in patients with frequent PVCs who do not have acute myocardial infarction or ischemia is controversial and a matter of current debate and research. As noted above, frequent PVCs may be seen in otherwise healthy people. Even in patients with underlying heart disease, there is no evidence that suppression of isolated PVCs with drugs improves survival. Perhaps most important is the fact that all the drugs (such as quinidine, procainamide, and disopyramide) used to treat PVCs all have important and sometimes life-threatening side effects. Furthermore, not only do these drugs fail to suppress the ventricular ectopy, they sometimes also actually make the situation worse by paradoxically increasing the number of PVCs. In some patients treatment with "antiarrhythmic" drugs can provoke a possibly fatal arrhythmia such as *torsades de pointes* (p. 209).

For more complete discussion of these complex therapeutic issues the reader is referred to the Bibliography. It should be emphasized again that whenever you are confronted by a patient with frequent PVCs it is always important to search for potentially reversible causes (in particular, hypoxemia, hypokalemia, hypomagnesemia, and certain drugs). Correcting metabolic problems or drug effects may obviate the need to treat the patient with additional, potentially toxic, medications.

VENTRICULAR TACHYCARDIA

PVCs are important primarily because they may be the precursors of sustained ventricular tachycardia and ventricular fibrillation, which are life-threatening arrhythmias. *Ventricular tachycardia is, by definition, simply a run of three or more consecutive PVCs.* This is exactly analogous to atrial tachycardia, which is a run of three or more consecutive PACs. Examples of ventricular tachycardia are shown in Figs. 14-5 and 14-11 to 14-13. Ventricular tachycardia may occur as a single isolated burst, may recur paroxysmally, or may persist for a long run. The heart rate is generally between 100 and 200 beats/min. Very rapid ventricular tachycardia with a sine-wave appearance is sometimes referred to as *ventricular flutter* and usually leads to ventricular fibrillation.

Sustained ventricular tachycardia is a life-threatening arrhythmia for two major reasons. First, most patients are not able to maintain an adequate blood pressure with this rapid a heart rate and quickly become hypotensive. Second, sustained ventricular tachycardia may degenerate into ventricular fibrillation (Fig. 14-14), producing cardiac arrest.

Treatment

There are two aspects to the treatment of ventricular tachyarrhythmias. The first is preventive. Treatment of malignant PVCs in patients with recent MI may be prophylactic against future bouts of ventricular tachycardia or particularly ventricular fibrillation. The second is suppressive. Patients with acute MI who are having frequent PVCs or intermittent runs of ventricular tachycardia generally require emergency administration of an intravenous antiarrhythmic drug, such as lidocaine, to attempt to suppress the ventricular ectopy.

Occasionally you will be required to treat a patient having a long run of ventricular tachycardia who is becoming hypotensive. In such cases you can try giving the patient a sharp punch to the midsternum with your clenched fist. This treatment, termed *thump version* (Fig. 14-13) (p. 236, footnote), may restore a normal heart rhythm by itself in a case of ventricular tachycardia. While thump version is being tried, the electrical cardioverter should be charged up; if the thump does not restore normal rhythm, the patient should be given an immediate DC shock. Immediately preceding or following electrical cardioversion the patient should be started on intravenous medication to suppress further ectopy and the cause of the ventricular tachycardia should be carefully sought.

Causes

The etiologic factors of ventricular tachycardia are the same as those discussed earlier with PVCs. The same list of reversible causes of PVCs also applies in evaluating patients with ventricular tachycardia.

Differential Diagnosis

Ventricular tachycardia is one of the major tachyarrhythmias. In preceding chapters we also mentioned several other important tachycardias, including sinus tachycardia, paroxysmal atrial tachycardia, atrial fibrillation, and atrial flutter. These are all examples of *supra*ventricular tachycardias. The differentia-

PAROXYSMAL VENTRICULAR TACHYCARDIA

monitor- continuous strip

Fig. 14-11. The monitor lead shows bursts of VT.

VENTRICULAR TACHYCARDIA TERMINATED BY DC SHOCK

Fig. 14-12. **A,** Long run of VT. **B,** Normal sinus rhythm restored after direct current cardioversion.

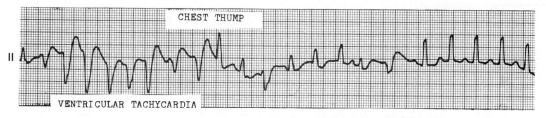

Fig. 14-13. VT terminated by a thump on the chest ("thump version").

VENTRICULAR FIBRILLATION

Fig. 14-14. VF may produce both coarse and fine waves. Immediate defibrillation should be performed.

tion of ventricular tachycardia from these supraventricular tachyarrhythmias is described in Chapter 18.

VENTRICULAR FIBRILLATION

In ventricular fibrillation (Figs. 14-14 and 14-15) the ventricles do not beat in any coordinated fashion but instead fibrillate or twitch asynchronously and ineffectively. There is no cardiac output, and the patient becomes unconscious immediately. Ventricular fibrillation is one of the three major ECG patterns seen with cardiac arrest. The other two are *asystole* and *electromechanical dissociation* (Chapter 17).

The ECG in ventricular fibrillation shows characteristic fibrillatory waves with an irregular pattern that may be either coarse or fine (Fig. 14-14).

Ventricular fibrillation requires immediate defibrillation with an unsynchronized DC shock. Patients who have had runs of ventricular tachycardia or ventricular fibrillation should also be given an immediate dose of an intravenous drug such as lidocaine to suppress further ventricular ectopy. Another antiarrhythmic agent, bretylium tosylate (Bretylol), has also been effective in treating and preventing ventricular fibrillation.

Ventricular fibrillation may occur in patients with heart disease of any type. It may be preceded by warning arrhythmias, such as PVCs or ventricular tachycardia, or it may occur spontaneously. Ventricular fibrillation may also occur in normal hearts, owing to the toxic effects of drugs such as epinephrine, during anesthesia, with lightning stroke, and so on.

ACCELERATED IDIOVENTRICULAR RHYTHM

Figs. 14-16 and 14-17 show examples of a distinctive arrhythmia that has been called "accelerated idioventricular rhythm" (AIVR) or "slow ventricular tachycardia." With typical ventricular tachycardia, the heart rate is generally faster than 100 to 110 beats/min. With AIVR, the ventricular rate is usually between 50 and 100 to 110 beats/min. The ECG with AIVR shows wide QRS complexes without P waves. (The cutoff between AIVR and ventricular tachycardia based on heart rate is arbitrary, and different authors use slightly different rate criteria.)

AIVR is particularly common with acute myocardial infarction. The arrhythmia is generally short and self-limited, lasting for minutes or less and generally requiring no specific therapy. Treatment (for example, with lidocaine) is indicated if AIVR is associated with actual ventricular tachycardia (Fig. 14-17).

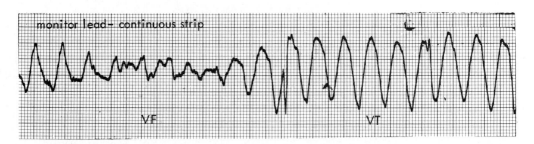

Fig. 14-15. Ventricular fibrillation *(VF)* and ventricular tachycardia *(VT)* occurring together.

In some cases (Fig. 14-16) AIVR occurs as a benign escape rhythm that competes with the underlying sinus mechanism. When the sinus rate slows, AIVR appears, and when the sinus rate speeds up, the arrhythmia disappears. In contrast, other cases of AIVR are initiated by very premature beats (Fig.14-17) rather than by escape beats. This latter type of AIVR is more likely to be associated with actual ventricular tachycardia.

"TORSADES DE POINTES": A SPECIAL FORM OF VENTRICULAR TACHYCARDIA

In recent years, a special type of ventricular tachycardia has been recognized called "torsades de pointes," a French term meaning "twisting of the points." Fig. 14-18 shows an example of this distinctive form of ventricular tachycardia. Note how the vector of the QRS complexes appears to rotate cyclically, point-

ACCELERATED IDIOVENTRICULAR RHYTHM

Fig. 14-16. AIVR in a case of inferior wall myocardial infarction. The first four beats show the typical pattern, followed by a return of sinus rhythm, then the reappearance of AIVR.

Fig. 14-17. Accelerated idioventricular rhythm *(AIVR)* and ventricular tachycardia *(VT)* occurring together. Note the similarity between them, but the rate in AIVR is slower.

"Torsades de pointes"
ventricular tachycardia

Fig. 14-18. Note the shifting polarity and amplitude of the QRS complexes during a bout of ventricular tachycardia. This is the hallmark of torsades de pointes. There is also QT prolongation (0.52 sec) in the normal sinus beats.

ing downward for several beats and then twisting and pointing upward in the same lead.

Torsades de pointes is important because of its diagnostic and therapeutic implications. As shown in Fig. 14-18, torsades de pointes classically occurs in the setting of delayed ventricular repolarization, evidenced by prolongation of the QT interval or the presence of prominent U waves. Reported causes include

1. Drug toxicity, particularly that due to quinidine (quinidine syncope, p. 142) and related antiarrhythmic agents (disopyramide [Norpace] and procainamide [Pronestyl, Procan SR]) as well psychotropic drugs (phenothiazines and tricyclic antidepressants)
2. Electrolyte imbalance, including hypokalemia, hypomagnesemia, and hypocalcemia, which prolong repolarization

3. Miscellaneous factors such as complete heart block, hereditary QT prolongation syndrome, liquid protein diets, and myocardial ischemia

Recognition of torsades is critical because the use of drugs conventionally recommended in treating ventricular tachycardia (such as quinidine or procainamide) may worsen the arrhythmia by delaying ventricular repolarization. Therapy therefore should include removing or correcting causative factors (drug toxicity, electrolyte imbalance). In emergency settings, a temporary pacemaker may be inserted to accomplish "overdrive" suppression of the arrhythmia by increasing the underlying heart rate and thereby decreasing ventricular repolarization time. Drug therapy with bretylium or isoproterenol may be useful in selected cases. For further discussion of this important new topic, readers are referred to the Bibliography.

REVIEW OF CHAPTER 14

PVCs have the following characteristics:

1. They are premature and occur before the next normal beat is expected.
2. They have an aberrant shape. The QRS complex is abnormally wide, usually 0.12 second (three small time boxes) or more in duration, and the T wave and QRS complex usually point in opposite directions.

There are several other features of PVCs that are important.

PVCs may occur with varying *frequency*. Two in a row are called a *couplet*. Three in a row are *ventricular tachycardia*. When a PVC occurs regularly after each normal beat, this is called *ventricular bigeminy*. When the rhythm is two normal beats followed by a PVC, this is *ventricular trigeminy*.

A PVC is often followed by a compensatory pause before the next beat.

Uniform PVCs have the same shape in a single lead. *Multiform* PVCs have different shapes in the same lead.

When a PVC occurs simultaneously with the apex of the T wave of the preceding beat, this is called an *R on T phenomenon*. It may be the forerunner of ventricular tachycardia or ventricular fibrillation.

PVCs may occur both normally and in patients with organic heart disease.

Treatment of PVCs depends on several considerations. Look for reversible causes (hypoxemia, congestive heart failure, digitalis toxicity or toxicity due to other drugs, hypokalemia, hypomagnesemia, and so on). Frequent PVCs in the presence of acute MI should be promptly suppressed.

Ventricular tachycardia is a run of three or more PVCs.

Ventricular fibrillation occurs when the ventricles stop beating and, instead, fibrillate or twitch in an ineffective fashion. It is one of the three major ECG patterns seen with cardiac arrest; the other two are *asystole* and *electromechanical dissociation* (Chapter 17).

Accelerated idioventricular rhythm (AIVR) is a ventricular arrhythmia that resembles a slow ventricular tachycardia with a rate between 50 and 100 to 110 beats/min. It is commonly seen with myocardial infarction and is usually self-limited.

Torsades de pointes is the name of a recently described form of ventricular tachycardia in which the QRS complexes in the same lead appear to twist periodically and turn in the opposite direction. This arrhythmia is generally seen in the setting of delayed ventricular repolarization (increased QT interval or prominent U waves) due to drugs such as quinidine or a variety of other factors.

Review Questions—Chapter 14

1. What is the arrhythmia shown below?

2. Which two arrhythmias does the rhythm strip below show?

3. Name three potentially treatable causes of PVCs.

True or false (4 to 7):

4. The QRS complex of a PVC is always wide.
5. PVCs falling on the T wave of the preceding beat are usually serious.
6. Ventricular tachycardia is a run of three or more consecutive PVCs.
7. Ventricular fibrillation produces cardiac arrest.
8. Define "ventricular bigeminy."

Answers

1. Ventricular tachycardia.
2. Atrial fibrillation with PVCs.
3. Hypoxemia, digitalis toxicity, anemia, and so on (see p. 204).
4. True.
5. True. "R on T" phenomenon may precipitate ventricular fibrillation or ventricular tachycardia.
6. True.
7. True. Asystole and electromechanical dissociation are the two other major ECG patterns that may occur with cardiac arrest (Chapter 17).
8. Ventricular bigeminy is characterized by a PVC following each normal beat (Fig. 14-6, *A*).

15 AV Heart Block

Heart block is the general term for atrioventricular (AV) conduction disturbances. Normally, the AV junction acts like an apparent bridge between the atria and the ventricles. The PR interval, as mentioned earlier, is primarily a measure of the lag in AV conduction between the initial stimulation of the atria and the initial stimulation of the ventricles. The normal PR interval is between 0.12 and 0.2 second. Heart block occurs when there is impaired conduction through the AV junction, either transiently or permanently. The mildest form of heart block is called *first-degree heart block*. Here the PR interval is simply prolonged above 0.2 second. *Second-degree heart block* is an intermediate grade of AV conduction disturbance. The most extreme form of heart block is called *third-degree* or *complete heart block*. Here the AV junction does not conduct any stimuli between the atria and ventricles. These three degrees of heart block are described in this chapter, along with the related topic *AV dissociation*.

FIRST-DEGREE HEART BLOCK

In first-degree heart block the PR interval is prolonged above 0.2 second and is constant from beat to beat (Fig. 15-1).

First-degree heart block does not produce any symptoms or any significant change in cardiac function. There are numerous causes, and most factors that produce first-degree AV block can also produce second- and third-degree block. For example, digitalis, which has a vagal effect on the AV junction, can produce any degree of heart block. Other drugs such as quinidine, any of the numerous beta-blocking agents, and the calcium-channel blockers (verapamil and diltiazem) can also cause severe depression of AV conduction.

Patients with ischemic heart disease may develop heart block of any degree. This may occur with chronic myocardial ischemia over a long time or with an acute myocardial infarction. Varying degrees of heart block are particularly common with inferior wall infarction because the right coronary artery, which generally supplies the inferior wall, also usually supplies the AV junction. In addition, acute inferior MI is often associated with increased vagal tone. Heart block during inferior wall infarction tends to be transient.

Hyperkalemia may cause first-degree heart block. Other signs of hyperkalemia (as mentioned in Chapter 10) include peaking of the T waves and widening of the QRS complexes. First-degree AV block may occur with acute rheumatic fever. Occasionally first-degree AV block may be seen in normal persons.

SECOND-DEGREE AV BLOCK

Second-degree AV block is somewhat more complicated because there are two types—Mobitz type I (also called Wenckebach block) and Mobitz type II. Despite this imposing nomenclature, the two types of second-degree block are actually not too difficult to understand.

FIRST DEGREE AV BLOCK

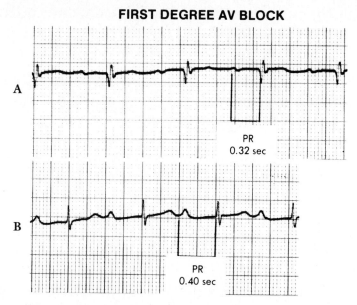

Fig. 15-1. With first-degree AV block the PR interval is uniformly prolonged above 0.2 second with each beat. **A** and **B** are from different patients.

Mobitz Type I (Wenckebach) AV Block

With the Wenckebach pattern, each stimulus from the atria to the ventricles has a more difficult time passing through the AV junction. Finally, a point is reached where the stimulus is not conducted at all. This blocked beat is followed by relative recovery of the AV junction, and the whole cycle starts again.

The characteristic ECG picture of Wenckebach block, therefore, is a progressive lengthening of the PR interval from beat to beat until finally a beat is dropped. The dropped beat is a P wave that is not followed by a QRS complex, indicating failure of the AV junction to conduct the stimulus from the atria to the ventricles. Fig. 15-2 diagrammatically depicts the Wenckebach phenomenon, and Fig. 15-3 shows an actual example of this pattern. The number of P waves oc-

curring before a beat is dropped is variable. In some cases it is two or three or more. What characterizes the Wenckebach pattern is the general sequence of progressive lengthening of the PR interval followed by a dropped beat.

As you can see from the examples, the Wenckebach cycle also produces a distinct clustering of QRS complexes separated by a pause that results from the dropped beat. Any time you see an ECG with this type of *group beating*, suspect a Wenckebach block and look for the diagnostic pattern of lengthening PR intervals.

Clinically patients with the Wenckebach type of AV block are usually without symptoms unless the ventricular rate is very slow. The pulse rate is irregular.

Common causes of Wenckebach block include digitalis toxicity and ischemic heart dis-

WENCKEBACH (MOBITZ TYPE I) SECOND-DEGREE AV BLOCK

Fig. 15-2. The PR interval lengthens progressively with successive beats until one P wave is not conducted at all. Then the cycle repeats itself.

WENCKEBACH (MOBITZ TYPE I) SECOND-DEGREE AV BLOCK

Fig. 15-3. Notice the progressive increase in PR intervals, with the third P wave in each sequence not followed by a QRS complex. Wenckebach block produces a characteristically irregular rhythm with grouping of the QRS complexes.

MOBITZ TYPE II SECOND-DEGREE AV BLOCK

Fig. 15-4. With Mobitz type II block there is a series of nonconducted P waves followed by a P wave that is conducted. In this diagrammatic example 3:1 AV block is present, with three P waves for each QRS complex. The QRS is wide (0.12 sec). (See also Fig. 20-7.)

ease. Digitalis should therefore be withheld in any patient who develops Wenckebach block. Wenckebach block is also not uncommon with acute inferior wall infarction. In such cases the heart block is usually transient and generally does not require any specific treatment except for observation, since these patients may progress into complete heart block. Of note, Wenckebach AV block has also been described in athletes at rest, due to a physiologic increase in vagal tone.

Mobitz Type II AV Block

Mobitz type II AV block is a rarer and more severe form of second-degree AV block. In most cases of Mobitz type II AV block, the QRS complexes of the conducted beats are wide (≥ 0.12 sec). The characteristic features of Mobitz type II AV block are shown in Fig. 15-4. As you can see, in Mobitz type II AV block there is a series of nonconducted P waves, followed by a P wave that is conducted. For example, with 3:1 block every third P wave is conducted to the ventricles. With 4:1 block every fourth P wave is followed by a QRS complex. Fig. 20-8 shows 2:1 block involving the His-Purkinje system rather than just the AV node.*

Mobitz type II AV block is generally a sign of severe conduction system disease. Since patients with this form of block often progress into complete heart block, cardiologists generally consider this an indication for a pacemaker. Unlike Wenckebach (Mobitz type I) AV block, Mobitz type II AV block is not usually seen with digitalis excess or with inferior wall infarction. However, Mobitz type II AV block is occasionally seen with anterior wall myocardial infarction, and these patients often progress into complete heart block. Therefore, cardiologists generally treat a patient with an anterior wall myocardial infarction who develops Mobitz type II AV block by inserting a pacemaker.

THIRD-DEGREE (COMPLETE) HEART BLOCK

First- and second-degree heart blocks are examples of *incomplete* block because the AV junction does conduct stimuli, albeit intermittently, to the ventricles. With complete heart block, there is no transmission of stimuli from the atria to the ventricles. Instead, the atria and the ventricles are paced independently. With complete heart block, atrial and ventricular depolarization are completely independent. The atria generally continue to be paced by the sinus node. The ventricles, however, are paced by an escape pacemaker located somewhere below the point of block in the AV junction. The ventricular rate with complete heart block may be lower than 30 beats/min or as high as 60 beats/min. The atrial rate is generally faster than the ventricular rate.

Examples of complete heart block are shown in Figs. 15-5 and 15-6. The ECG with complete heart block has the following characteristics:

1. P waves are present, with a regular atrial rate that is faster than the ventricular rate.
2. QRS complexes are present, with a slow (usually fixed) ventricular rate.
3. The P waves bear no relation to the QRS complexes, and the PR intervals

---

*A point of common confusion: It should be noted that 2:1 AV block per se does not always indicate a Mobitz type II block. Not uncommonly 2:1 AV block is due to a Wenckebach (Mobitz I) mechanism in which the block simply occurs after every other P wave. In such cases careful search of a long rhythm strip will often reveal 3:2, 4:3, etc. types of Wenckebach in addition to the 2:1 periods. Furthermore, in most (but not all) cases of AV Wenckebach the QRS complex is of normal duration. In contrast, when 2:1 block is due to a Mobitz II mechanism the His-Purkinje system is involved and the QRS duration is usually prolonged. Thus, when you see 2:1 block with a narrow QRS, it most likely represents AV Wenckebach. On the other hand, 2:1 block with a wide QRS and without other evidence of Wenckebach periodicity is likely Mobitz II block which carries a more serious prognosis for progression to complete heart block.

are completely variable since the atria and ventricles are electrically disconnected.

4. Complete heart block occasionally occurs in a patient whose basic atrial rhythm is atrial fibrillation or atrial flutter. In these patients the ventricular rate is slow and almost completely regular (Fig. 13-9).

With complete heart block the QRS complexes may be either of normal width (Fig. 15-5) or abnormally wide (Fig. 15-6) with the appearance of a bundle branch block pattern. The width of the QRS complexes depends in part on the location of the blockage in the AV junction. If the block is in the first part of the junction (AV node), the ventricles will be stimulated normally by a junctional pacemaker and the QRS complexes will be narrow (Fig. 15-5) unless the patient has an underlying bundle branch block. However, if the block is lower in the AV junction (bundle of His), the ventricles will be paced by an *idioventricular pacemaker* producing wide QRS complexes resembling a bundle branch block pattern (Fig. 15-6). As a general clinical rule, complete heart block with wide QRS complexes tends to be less stable than complete heart block with narrow QRS complexes since the ventricular rate is usually slower.

THIRD-DEGREE (COMPLETE) AV BLOCK

Fig. 15-5. Complete heart block is characterized by independent atrial *(P)* and ventricular (QRS) activity. The atrial rate is always faster than the ventricular rate. The PR intervals are completely variable. Some P waves fall on the T wave, distorting the shape of the T wave. Other P waves may fall in the QRS complex and be "lost." Note that the QRS complexes are of normal width, indicating that the ventricles are being paced from the AV junction. Compare this with Fig. 15-6, an example of complete heart block with wide QRS complexes because the ventricles are being paced from below the AV junction (idioventricular pacemaker).

THIRD-DEGREE (COMPLETE) AV BLOCK

Fig. 15-6. Another example of complete heart block, showing a slow idioventricular rhythm and a faster independent atrial (sinus) rhythm.

Complete heart block can occur for a number of reasons. It is most commonly seen in older patients who have chronic degenerative changes in their conduction systems *not* related to an acute myocardial infarction. Such chronic degenerative conduction disease is the most common cause of complete heart block. Digitalis intoxication, which can cause first- and second-degree heart block, can also lead to complete heart block (Chapter 16). Complete heart block may sometimes be seen acutely as a complication of myocardial infarction. The course and therapy of complete heart block with myocardial infarction depend to a large extent on whether the infarct is anterior or inferior. As mentioned before, transient AV conduction disturbances are commonly seen with acute inferior wall infarctions because of the common blood supply to the AV junction and inferior wall (via the right coronary artery) in most cases. Occlusion of the right coronary artery with inferior infarction also often leads to temporary ischemia of the AV junction, sometimes resulting in complete heart block. (In addition, acute inferior infarction often causes an increase in vagal tone.) Complete heart block occurring with inferior wall myocardial infarction is often a transient and reversible complication that may respond to atropine and does not require a temporary pacemaker.

With acute anterior myocardial infarction and complete heart block, the situation is more serious. Patients with anterior wall infarction who develop complete heart block generally have extensive myocardial damage. The idioventricular escape rhythm that develops is usually slow and unstable. Therefore, if complete heart block occurs with an acute anterior MI, the cardiologist will generally insert a temporary pacemaker (and subsequently a permanent one).

Regardless of its cause, complete heart block is a serious and potentially life-threatening arrhythmia. If the ventricular rate becomes too slow, the cardiac output will drop and the patient may faint. Fainting spells associated with complete heart block are referred to as *Stokes-Adams attacks*. In some patients, complete heart block is a chronic and persistent finding. In others the heart block may occur transiently and be recognized only with continuous ambulatory ECG monitoring (using a Holter apparatus) for a period of 24 hours or longer.

Complete heart block resulting from digitalis toxicity or acute inferior myocardial infarction is often transient and can be treated medically without the insertion of a pacemaker. However, patients with chronic complete heart block, particularly those with angina, congestive heart failure, or Stokes-Adams attacks, require an implanted (permanent) pacemaker (Chapter 20).

BIFASCICULAR BLOCKS AND COMPLETE HEART BLOCK

Cardiologists have been interested in developing criteria to predict which patients with acute myocardial infarction (particularly anterior wall infarcts) will go on to develop complete heart block. If high-risk patients can be identified, they can be treated with prophylactic pacemakers. Current information suggests that certain high-risk patients can be identified. Specifically, it has been found that patients with an acute anterior wall myocardial infarction who develop complete heart block often develop other conduction disturbances before the onset of the complete heart block. These warning signals include (1) new left bundle branch block, (2) new right bundle branch block with left axis deviation, or (3) new right bundle branch block with right axis deviation. These are all examples of *bifascicular blocks*.

Recall from Chapter 7 that the ventricular conduction system is trifascicular, consisting of the right bundle branch and the left bundle branch, which further divides into left anterior and left posterior fascicles. Blockage of just the left anterior fascicle produces left an-

BIFASCICULAR BLOCK (RIGHT BUNDLE BRANCH BLOCK WITH LEFT ANTERIOR HEMIBLOCK)

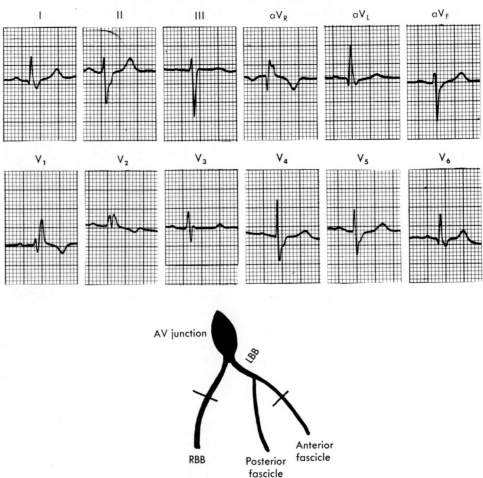

Fig. 15-7. Note that the chest leads show the typical RBBB pattern (rSR' in lead V_1 and qRS in V_6). The extremity leads show marked left axis deviation (mean QRS axis about −60°), consistent with left anterior hemiblock. Thus a bifascicular block, involving the right bundle and the anterior fascicle of the left bundle, is present (as shown in the diagram).

terior hemiblock with left axis deviation. Blockage of just the left posterior fascicle produces left posterior hemiblock with right axis deviation. Bifascicular block indicates blockage of any two of the three fascicles. For example, right bundle branch block with left anterior hemiblock produces an ECG pattern showing a right bundle branch block with marked left axis deviation (Figs. 8-20 and 15-7). Right bundle branch block with left posterior hemiblock is recognized by a right bundle branch block pattern with right axis deviation (provided other causes of right axis deviation are excluded). Similarly, a complete left bundle branch block may indicate blockage of both the anterior and the posterior fascicles.

Bifascicular blocks are significant because they make ventricular conduction dependent on the single remaining fascicle. Additional damage to this third remaining fascicle may completely block AV conduction, producing complete heart block (trifascicular block). Therefore, the acute development of bifascicular block during an acute anterior wall infarction is a warning signal of possible impending complete heart block. If bifascicular block occurs in the setting of acute anterior infarction (Fig. 8-20), cardiologists generally insert a temporary pacemaker as a prophylactic measure.

An important distinction must be made between *acute* bifascicular blocks occurring with anterior wall infarctions (Fig. 8-20) and *chronic* bifascicular blocks (Fig. 15-7). Many people without any symptoms at all may have ECGs resembling Fig. 15-7. Patients with chronic bifascicular block do not generally require a pacemaker, unless they develop high-degree AV block. The risk of complete heart block in patients with chronic bifascicular block seems to be quite low. In contrast, patients with acute anterior infarction who develop bifascicular block have a poor prognosis and a strong likelihood of developing complete heart block.

AV DISSOCIATION

AV dissociation is a distinct arrhythmia, mentioned here because it is often confused with complete heart block.

With AV dissociation the sinus node and AV junction get "out of synch"; thus the sinus node loses its normal control of the ventricular rate. As a result the atria and ventricles are paced independently—the atria from the sinus node, the ventricles from the AV junction. This is similar to what occurs with complete heart block. *However, with AV dissociation the ventricular rate is slightly faster than the atrial rate.* Occasionally, the atrial and ventricular rates are almost the same (*isorhythmic* AV dissociation).

AV dissociation usually occurs when the

AV DISSOCIATION (AVD)

Fig. 15-8. AV dissociation is characterized by independent atrial and ventricular rhythms, with the ventricular rate usually the same as (or slightly faster than) the atrial rate. Note that the first and fifth P waves are hidden in the T waves and that the fourth and eighth P waves are lost in the QRS complex. (See Question 141, p. 321.)

sinus node has been depressed by increased vagal tone, for example, with acute myocardial infarction, by certain drugs (such as digitalis), or in other pathologic states. Occasionally AV dissociation occurs in normal people.

An example of AV dissociation is shown in Fig. 15-8. The ECG shows P waves with a variable PR interval because the ventricular (QRS) rate is slightly faster than the atrial rate. At times the P waves may merge with the QRS complex and become imperceptible for several beats. If the sinus rate speeds up sufficiently (or the AV junctional rate slows), the stimulus may be able to penetrate the AV junction, reestablishing sinus rhythm.

There are two major differences between AV dissociation and complete heart block:

1. The atrial (P wave) rate with AV dissociation is nearly the same as or somewhat slower than the ventricular (QRS) rate. With complete heart block, the ventricular rate is usually much slower than the atrial rate.
2. With AV dissociation, although the atria and ventricles beat independently, a stimulus from the atria can penetrate the AV junction if it comes at the right time. With complete heart block, however, the atria and ventricles beat independently because there is a block somewhere in the AV junction, and stimuli *cannot* pass from the atria to the ventricles. Thus, with AV dissociation the sinus node and AV junction are only desynchronized while with complete heart block they are electrically disconnected.

In contrast to complete heart block* therefore, AV dissociation is a minor, usually transient, arrhythmia. Generally no special treatment is required. If it is caused by a drug, the drug may be stopped.

---

*There is understandable confusion among students and clinicians regarding the term *AV dissociation*. This confusion arises because the term is actually used in two related, though not identical, ways in the ECG literature. As used in this chapter, the term AV dissociation refers to a distinct arrhythmia which is different from complete heart block. Some authors use the term AV dissociation in a more general sense to refer to any arrhythmia in which the atria and ventricles are paced from separate sites. This second definition will obviously also include complete heart block as well as some cases of ventricular tachycardia where the atria remain in sinus rhythm (pp. 252 and 261).

REVIEW OF CHAPTER 15

There are three types of AV heart block:

1. *First-degree AV block*—the PR interval is uniformly prolonged beyond 0.2 second.
2. *Second-degree AV block*—there are two subtypes:
   a. *Wenckebach (Mobitz type I) AV block*—increasing prolongation of the PR interval occurs until a P wave is blocked and not followed by a QRS complex. This produces a distinctive clustering of QRS complexes separated by a pause resulting from the dropped beat. The QRS clustering is known as *group beating*.
   b. *Mobitz type II AV block*—a series of P waves occurs without QRS complexes, followed by a P wave and a QRS complex; for example, with 3:1 block, every third P wave is conducted and followed by a QRS complex. The conducted P waves have the same PR interval.
3. *Third-degree (complete) AV block*—this shows the following:
   a. The atria and ventricles beat independently because stimuli cannot pass through the AV junction.
   b. The atrial rate is faster than the ventricular rate.
   c. The PR interval constantly changes.

Complete heart block with acute anterior wall infarction is sometimes preceded by the sudden appearance of *bifascicular block* (right bundle branch block with left anterior or posterior hemiblock or complete left bundle branch block). However, asymptomatic patients with chronic bifascicular block usually do not require any special therapy.

The significance of complete heart block with acute myocardial infarcts depends on the location of the infarct. Complete heart block occurring with acute inferior wall infarction is not uncommon, is usually transient, and can often be managed without a pacemaker. In contrast, complete heart block with acute anterior wall infarcts is usually associated with a poor prognosis and generally requires a pacemaker.

Complete heart block must be distinguished from *AV dissociation*. With AV dissociation, the atria and ventricles beat independently; however, the ventricular rate is about the same as or faster than the atrial rate. AV dissociation is a minor, usually transient, arrhythmia.

Review Questions—Chapter 15

True or false (1 to 5):
1. With first-degree AV block, the heart rate will be very slow.
2. Bifascicular block always leads to complete heart block.
3. The PR interval is constant in complete heart block.
4. Digitalis toxicity may cause complete heart block.
5. Complete heart block may occur with atrial fibrillation.
6. The rhythm strip below shows which of the following?
   a. Wenckebach type second-degree AV block.
   b. Complete heart block.
   c. 3:1 AV block.
   d. AV dissociation.
   e. Blocked premature atrial contraction.

7. In the rhythm strip below
   a. What is the approximate atrial (P wave) rate?
   b. What is the approximate ventricular (QRS) rate?
   c. Is the PR interval constant?
   d. What is the ECG abnormality shown?

Answers

1. False. The heart rate may be slow, fast, or normal.
2. False.
3. False.
4. True. Digitalis toxicity may cause any degree of AV block.
5. True. See Fig. 13-9.

6. a. Wenckebach block. Note the succession of P waves, with increasing PR intervals, followed by a dropped (nonconducted) P wave in the fifth beat.
7. a. 100 beats/min.
   b. 42 beats/min.
   c. No.
   d. Complete heart block.

16 Digitalis Toxicity

This chapter focuses on the arrhythmias and conduction disturbances caused by digitalis intoxication. There are several reasons for discussing this topic in an introductory textbook. The most important reason is that digitalis is a frequently prescribed drug and digitalis toxicity is a common clinical problem. Furthermore, digitalis toxicity can cause fatal arrhythmias. Early recognition of digitalis toxicity, therefore, should be a preoccupation of everyone in clinical medicine. Finally, because digitalis toxicity can produce virtually any arrhythmia and all degrees of heart block, this topic provides a convenient review of material presented in previous chapters.

CLINICAL BACKGROUND

Digitalis refers to a class of cardiac drugs with specific effects on the mechanical and electrical function of the heart. The two most commonly used digitalis preparations are digoxin and digitoxin.

Digitalis is used in clinical practice for two major reasons. First, it is used in patients with congestive heart failure to increase the strength of myocardial contraction. This is its *mechanical* action. Second, digitalis also affects the *electrical* function of the heart, making it a useful drug in treating certain arrhythmias. The antiarrhythmic action of digitalis results primarily because it slows conduction through the AV junction. Consequently, digitalis is extremely useful in treating such supraventricular arrhythmias as paroxysmal atrial tachycardia (PAT), atrial fibrillation, and atrial flutter, where there is excessive transmission of stimuli from the atria to the ventricles through the AV junction.

Unfortunately, although digitalis has wide use in the treatment of heart failure and certain arrhythmias, it also has a relatively low margin of safety. The difference between therapeutic and toxic concentrations of digitalis is very narrow. This is the reason for the high prevalence of digitalis toxicity.

SIGNS OF DIGITALIS TOXICITY

Digitalis toxicity can produce general systemic symptoms as well as specific cardiac arrhythmias and conduction disturbances. The most common extracardiac symptoms of digitalis intoxication include anorexia (loss of appetite), nausea, and vomiting. Visual effects (changes in color perception) and mental changes have also been reported. In this section, we will concentrate on the arrhythmias and conduction disturbances produced by digitalis excess.

As a general clinical rule, *virtually any arrhythmia and all degrees of heart block can be produced by digitalis intoxication*. Of all the arrhythmias we have discussed, atrial fibrillation and atrial flutter with a rapid ventricular response are *least* likely to be caused by digitalis toxicity. However, there remain a number of arrhythmias that are commonly seen with digitalis toxicity.

Ventricular Arrhythmias

Premature ventricular contractions (PVCs) are often the first sign of digitalis toxicity.

Isolated PVCs may occur at first. Ventricular bigeminy (Fig. 16-1), with each normal beat followed by a PVC, is common. Ventricular tachycardia and fatal ventricular fibrillation may occur if the ventricular ectopy is not recognized and treated (see p. 208).

Bidirectional Ventricular Tachycardia

Bidirectional ventricular tachycardia (Fig. 16-2) resembles ventricular tachycardia, except that each successive beat in any lead alternates in direction. This distinct tachyarrhythmia should always raise the question of digitalis intoxication.

AV Junctional (Nodal) Rhythms

AV junctional rhythms are frequently a sign of digitalis toxicity. Most AV junctional rhythms resulting from excessive digitalis have a rate of less than 120 beats/min.

Fig. 16-1. Ventricular bigeminy caused by digitalis toxicity. Ventricular ectopy is one of the most common signs of digitalis toxicity. The underlying rhythm in **A** is atrial fibrillation. In **B** each normal QRS complex is followed by a PVC.

BIDIRECTIONAL TACHYCARDIA

Fig. 16-2. This digitalis-toxic arrhythmia is a special type of ventricular tachycardia with QRS complexes that alternate in direction from beat to beat. No P waves are present.

PAROXYSMAL ATRIAL TACHYCARDIA WITH BLOCK

Fig. 16-3. This rhythm strip shows PAT (atrial rate about 200 beats/min) with 2:1 block, producing a ventricular rate of about 100 beats/min.

Sinus Bradycardia and Sinoatrial (SA) Block

Sinus bradycardia may be one of the earliest signs of digitalis excess. SA block with sinus arrest may also occur.

Paroxysmal Atrial Tachycardia With AV Block (PAT With Block)

PAT with block is another tachyarrhythmia that has not been discussed in earlier chapters. (An example appears in Fig. 16-3.) PAT with block shows the following: an atrial tachycardia with P waves occurring at a rate usually between 150 and 250 beats/min and, because of the AV block, a slower ventricular rate. Most commonly 2:1 AV block is present, so the ventricular rate will be half the atrial rate. Digitalis toxicity is the most common, but not the only, cause of this arrhythmia. Superficially PAT with block may resemble atrial flutter; however, in PAT with block the baseline between P waves is isoelectric. Furthermore, when atrial flutter is present the atrial rate is faster (usually 250 to 350 beats/min).

AV Heart Block and AV Dissociation

Because digitalis slows conduction through the AV junction, it is not surprising that toxic doses of digitalis can result in any degree of AV heart block.

First-degree AV block. In first-degree AV block there is uniform prolongation of the PR interval greater than 0.2 second. Some degree of PR lengthening may be expected with digitalis therapy. More marked widening of the PR interval suggests early digitalis toxicity.

Second-degree AV block. With higher doses of digitalis, first-degree AV block may progress to second-degree AV block of the Mobitz type I (Wenckebach) variety.

Complete heart block. Third-degree, or complete, heart block may also occur with digitalis toxicity.

In addition digitalis toxicity may cause AV dissociation (see p. 221).

Atrial Fibrillation With Slow Ventricular Rate

As mentioned, atrial fibrillation and atrial flutter with a rapid ventricular response are the two arrhythmias least likely to be caused by digitalis toxicity. However, digitalis toxicity can occur in patients with atrial fibrillation or flutter. In such cases the toxicity is often shown by marked slowing of the ventricular rate (less than 50 beats/min) (Fig. 16-4) and/or the appearance of PVCs. (In some cases the earliest sign of digitalis toxicity in a patient with atrial fibrillation may be a subtle *regularization* of the ventricular rate.)

Fig. 16-4. Atrial fibrillation with an excessively slow ventricular rate because of digitalis toxicity. Atrial fibrillation with a rapid ventricular rate is rarely caused by digitalis toxicity. However, in patients with underlying atrial fibrillation, digitalis toxicity is often manifested by excessive slowing or regularization of the ventricular (QRS) rate.

• • •

The spectrum of digitalis toxicity arrhythmias and conduction disturbances is obviously broad. It is simpler to list the patterns *not* caused by digitalis toxicity. Although digitalis may be responsible for any degree of AV heart block, it does not produce intraventricular conduction disturbances (bundle branch block patterns).

As a general rule digitalis toxicity should be suspected in any patient with a bradyarrhythmia (sinus bradycardia, SA block, second- or third-degree heart block, atrial fibrillation with a slow ventricular rate, slow AV junctional rhythms). Also look for digitalis toxicity in any patient with ventricular ectopy (PVCs, ventricular bigeminy, ventricular tachycardia, ventricular fibrillation). Bidirectional ventricular tachycardia and PAT with block are two special arrhythmias often associated with digitalis toxicity. Of all the arrhythmias mentioned above, ventricular ectopy and AV junctional rhythms are probably the most common ECG signs of digitalis toxicity.

Because of its frequency and potential lethality, digitalis toxicity should be suspected in any patient taking digitalis who has an unexplained arrhythmia until you can prove

otherwise. The list below summarizes the most common arrhythmias and conduction disturbances seen with digitalis toxicity.

1. Ventricular ectopy: isolated PVCs, ventricular bigeminy, ventricular tachycardia, ventricular fibrillation
2. Bidirectional ventricular tachycardia
3. AV junctional (nodal) rhythms
4. Sinus bradycardia and SA block
5. AV heart block (first, second, third degree) and AV dissociation
6. Atrial fibrillation with a slow ventricular response
7. PAT with block

FACTORS PREDISPOSING TO DIGITALIS TOXICITY

There are a number of factors that significantly increase the hazard of digitalis intoxication.

Hypokalemia. A low serum potassium concentration makes certain digitalis-induced arrhythmias (particularly ventricular ectopy and PAT with block) more likely. Hypokalemia is not uncommon in digitalized patients because these patients frequently receive diuretics for treatment of heart failure and edema. Diuretics, such as furosemide (Lasix) and bumetanide (Bumex), the thiazides (Diuril, Hydrodiuril), and ethacrynic acid (Edecrin), result in urinary potassium loss. Therefore, most patients on digitalis and a potassium-wasting diuretic will require potassium supplementation. Serum potassium concentration must be checked periodically in all patients on digitalis and in every patient suspected of having digitalis toxicity.

Hypomagnesemia and hypercalcemia. Hypomagnesemia is seen in a variety of settings—including alcoholism, intestinal malabsorption, and diuretic therapy. Hypercalcemia is seen with hyperparathyroidism, certain tumors, and some other conditions.

Hypoxemia and chronic lung disease. Hypoxemia and chronic lung disease also increase the risk of digitalis toxicity.

Myocardial infarction. Patients with acute myocardial infarction appear to be more sensitive to digitalis, and lower doses are recommended in the first few days for these patients.

Old age. Elderly patients are, in general, more sensitive to digitalis.

Renal insufficiency. Digoxin, the most widely used preparation of digitalis, is excreted primarily in the urine. Therefore any degree of renal insufficiency, as measured by increased blood urea nitrogen (BUN) and creatinine concentration, requires a lower maintenance dose of digoxin.

TREATMENT OF DIGITALIS TOXICITY

The first step in treatment is prevention. Before starting any patient on digitalis, you should have a baseline ECG, serum electrolytes, and BUN and creatinine measurements. (Serum magnesium blood levels are usually not required unless clinically indicated.) In addition, take into consideration the patient's age, pulmonary status, and whether the patient is having an acute myocardial infarction. Early signs of digitalis toxicity, such as PVCs, sinus bradycardia, or increasing AV block, should be carefully checked. Furthermore,

concomitant quinidine administration increases the digoxin level in patients taking both drugs. A similar effect occurs with verapamil.

Definitive treatment of digitalis toxicity depends on the particular arrhythmia seen. In cases of minor arrhythmias, such as occasional PVCs, sinus bradycardia, first-degree or Wenckebach AV block, or AV junctional rhythms, stopping the digitalis and observing the patient are usually adequate. More serious arrhythmias, such as ventricular tachycardia, may require suppression with an intravenous drug (for example, lidocaine or procainamide). Potassium chloride should be given to raise the serum potassium level well within normal limits (unless complete heart block is present). Patients with complete heart block from digitalis toxicity may require a temporary pacemaker to tide them over while the effect of the digitalis dissipates, particularly if they have symptoms of syncope, hypotension, or congestive heart failure. In other cases, complete heart block can be managed conservatively while the digitalis wears off. PAT with block can often be treated with potassium chloride. Another drug that may be useful in treating certain digitalis toxic arrhythmias (ventricular ectopy, PAT with block) is phenytoin (Dilantin), a drug better known for its use in treating seizure disorders. The doses and methods of administering these drugs are described in some of the references listed in the Bibliography.

Finally, it is important to mention that electrical cardioversion of arrhythmias in patients who are digitalis toxic is extremely hazardous and may precipitate fatal ventricular tachycardia and fibrillation. Therefore, you should avoid trying to electrically cardiovert patients who have PAT with block, atrial fibrillation, atrial flutter, and so on and who are suspected of having digitalis toxicity as well.

SERUM DIGOXIN LEVELS

The concentration of digoxin (or digitoxin) in the serum can be measured by means of radioimmunoassay. For digoxin, the most widely used digitalis preparation, therapeutic concentrations range between 0.5 and 2 ng/ml in most laboratories. Concentrations exceeding 2 ng/ml are associated with a high incidence of digitalis toxicity. In ordering a test of digoxin levels in a patient, it is important to recognize that therapeutic levels do not rule out the possibility of digitalis toxicity. Some patients, as mentioned, are more sensitive to digitalis. In other patients factors such as hypokalemia may produce digitalis toxicity despite a "therapeutic" serum level. Conversely, still other patients, particularly those in atrial fibrillation with a rapid ventricular response, will require higher levels of digitalis to control their ventricular rate. A high digitalis level, therefore, does not necessarily indicate digitalis toxicity. However, patients with high digitalis levels should be examined for evidence of digitalis excess, including extracardiac symptoms (for example, gastrointestinal symptoms) and all the cardiac effects that have been discussed.

DIGITALIS TOXICITY AND DIGITALIS EFFECT

Do not confuse digitalis toxicity (which refers to the arrhythmias and conduction disturbances produced by this drug) with digitalis effect. *Digitalis effect* (p. 140) refers to the distinct scooping of the ST-T complex seen in some patients taking digitalis. The presence of digitalis effect does not imply digitalis toxicity.

REVIEW OF CHAPTER 16

Digitalis toxicity can produce almost any arrhythmia and all degrees of AV heart block. The following arrhythmias commonly occur with digitalis toxicity:
1. Ventricular ectopy (PVCs)—isolated PVCs may occur at first, often followed by ventricular bigeminy (each normal beat followed by a PVC). Finally, fatal ventricular tachycardia and ventricular fibrillation may occur if the digitalis toxicity is not recognized and treated.
2. Bidirectional ventricular tachycardia—this arrhythmia resembles conventional ventricular tachycardia, except that each successive beat in any lead points in the opposite direction.
3. AV junctional (nodal) rhythms.
4. Sinus bradycardia and SA block—actual sinus arrest may also occur.
5. PAT with block (paroxysmal atrial tachycardia with AV block).
6. AV heart block—first-degree AV block occurs initially and may be followed by second-degree Wenckebach-type AV block. Complete heart block or AV dissociation may also occur.
7. Atrial fibrillation or flutter with a slow ventricular response—when patients with atrial fibrillation or flutter are given excess digitalis, the ventricular rate may slow to 50 beats/min or less and often becomes very regular.

Atrial fibrillation or atrial flutter with a rapid ventricular response rarely occur as a result of digitalis toxicity. In addition, digitalis toxicity does not produce bundle branch blocks.

Factors such as renal failure, hypokalemia, hypercalcemia, hypomagnesemia, hypoxemia, old age, and acute myocardial infarction may predispose to digitalis toxicity. Concomitant administration of quinidine or verapamil will also increase serum digoxin levels.

Digitalis toxicity should not be confused with digitalis effect. *Digitalis effect* refers to the shortening of the QT interval and scooping of the ST-T complex produced by *therapeutic* doses of digitalis.

Review Questions—Chapter 16

1. Name three factors that may potentiate digitalis toxicity.

True or false (2 to 5):

2. PVCs are a common manifestation of digitalis toxicity.
3. Atrial fibrillation with a rapid ventricular response is a common manifestation of digitalis toxicity.
4. Left bundle branch block may be caused by digitalis toxicity.
5. Complete heart block may be caused by digitalis toxicity.
6. The rhythm strip shown below is from a patient with digitalis toxicity. Identify the arrhythmia.

Answers

1. Hypokalemia, hypoxemia, acute myocardial infarction, renal failure. See p. 230 for other answers.
2. True.
3. False.
4. False.
5. True.
6. Atrial fibrillation with an excessively slow ventricular rate (possibly resulting from complete heart block).

17 Cardiac Arrest

In the preceding chapters the major disorders of heart rhythm (arrhythmias) and atrioventricular conduction (heart block) have been systematically discussed. In this chapter, instead of presenting entirely new ECG patterns, we will review some of the topics mentioned earlier, placing them in a special clinical perspective. The subject of this chapter is the recognition of life-threatening arrhythmias causing cardiac arrest. *Cardiac arrest occurs when the heart stops contracting effectively and ceases to pump blood.*

CLINICAL ASPECTS

The patient in cardiac arrest loses consciousness within seconds and may even have a convulsion as a result of inadequate blood flow to the brain. Irreversible brain damage will usually occur within 4 minutes and often sooner. Furthermore, shortly after the heart stops pumping, spontaneous breathing will also cease, so in those cases where the patient is found without a palpable pulse or respiration, the term *"cardiopulmonary arrest"* is used. In other cases, when respirations stop first (primary respiratory arrest), cardiac activity will stop very shortly thereafter.

The diagnosis of cardiac arrest should be made clinically even before the patient is connected to an electrocardiograph. Cardiac arrest should be recognized immediately in any unconscious person who does not have palpable pulses. The patient, therefore, is quickly examined by trying to feel for pulses in the carotid arteries in the neck. In addition, the patient with cardiac arrest will become cyanotic (bluish gray) from lack of oxygenated blood (hypoxemia). No heart tones will be audible with a stethoscope on the chest, and the blood pressure will, of course, be unobtainable. The arms and legs become cool, and if the brain becomes severely hypoxic, the pupils will become fixed and dilated. Seizure activity may occur. *The absence of pulses in an unconscious person, however, is the major diagnostic sign of cardiac arrest.*

Once cardiac arrest is recognized, treatment must be immediately started. The basic method of *cardiopulmonary resuscitation* (CPR) has been described by the National Academy of Sciences. In capsule form, the initial treatment of any cardiac arrest consists of the following four steps:

A—Establish an *A*irway.

B—*B*reathe for the patient, either by the mouth-to-mouth method or by manually compressing a rubber Ambu (automatic manual breathing unit) bag, forcing air into the patient's nose or mouth.

C—Maintain *C*irculation by external cardiac compression (rhythmic compression of the lower sternum with the heels of the palms).

D—Begin *D*efinitive treatment with whatever intravenous or intracardiac drugs are needed, with electrical defibrillation, with a temporary pacemaker when indicated, and so on.

While the above steps are being done by two or more rescuers, another rescuer can raise the patient's lower extremities to a vertical position and keep them elevated for 15

234

seconds. This brings blood back to the circulation. The details of CPR, including drug dosages, technique of intracardiac injections, use of defibrillators, and so on, lie outside the scope of this book but are fully discussed in the references in the Bibliography. In this chapter, we will concentrate primarily on the particular ECG patterns seen during a cardiac arrest and on the clinical implications of these patterns. It is important to reemphasize that initial treatment of the patient with ventilation and external cardiac compression should *never* be delayed and must be started before the patient is connected to the electrocardiograph.

THE THREE BASIC ECG PATTERNS IN CARDIAC ARREST

There are only three basic ECG patterns seen with cardiac arrest, and they have been mentioned in earlier chapters. Cardiac arrest may be associated with ventricular fibrillation (or related arrhythmias such as ventricular tachycardia or torsades de pointes [Chapter 14]),

ventricular standstill (asystole), or electromechanical dissociation. We will review each of these patterns again briefly, stressing the clinical implications of each pattern in cardiac arrest (Figs. 17-1 to 17-7).

Ventricular Fibrillation

In ventricular fibrillation (VF) the ventricles do not contract but instead twitch or fibrillate in a completely ineffective way. There is no cardiac output, and the patient loses consciousness within seconds. The characteristic ECG pattern, with its unmistakable oscillatory waves, is illustrated in Fig. 17-1.

Of the three basic ECG patterns in cardiac arrest, VF is the most common one seen initially. It may appear spontaneously. However, as noted in Chapter 14, VF is often preceded by other ventricular arrhythmias, such as premature ventricular contractions and ventricular tachycardia. Fig. 17-2 shows ventricular tachycardia degenerating into VF during a cardiac arrest.

Treatment of VF was mentioned earlier.

Fig. 17-1. Ventricular fibrillation causing cardiac arrest.

VT   VF

Fig. 17-2. Ventricular tachycardia *(VT)* and ventricular fibrillation *(VF)* recorded during cardiac arrest.

The patient should be immediately defibrillated using a DC *defibrillator (cardioverter)* to administer a DC shock to the heart by means of paddles placed on the chest wall (p. 177). Fig. 17-7, *D,* shows an example of a successful defibrillation.

The drug bretylium tosylate (Bretylol) may also be helpful in treating or preventing VF. Drugs such as lidocaine or procainamide (Pronestyl) are not effective in directly treating VF but may be used prophylactically to prevent further episodes once normal sinus rhythm is restored.

Success in defibrillating any patient depends on a number of factors. Perhaps the most important is haste. The less delay in defibrillation, the greater will be the chance of success.

*In fact, if a defibrillator is immediately available, a defibrillatory shock should be given to any patient in cardiac arrest, even before connection is made to the electrocardiograph.** The reason for this priority is that the most common cause of cardiac arrest is VF, as mentioned before. (Even if the patient has ventricular standstill, the second most likely arrhythmia in cardiac arrest, DC shock will not be harmful.) Success in treating VF also depends on

keeping the patient well oxygenated by artificial ventilation and by periodically administering sodium bicarbonate intravenously to counteract the acidosis that develops during the arrest. In some cases, epinephrine given intravenously, via endotracheal tube, or by direct intracardiac injection may make it easier to defibrillate a patient. Sometimes it may take repeated shocks before the patient is successfully defibrillated. In other cases, all attempts will fail. Finally, it is important to stress that external cardiac compression must be continued between attempts at defibrillation.

Ventricular Standstill (Asystole)

Ventricular standstill and escape rhythms were described in Chapter 11. The normal pacemaker of the heart is the sinus node, located in the right atrium. Failure of the sinus node to function (sinus arrest) will lead to ventricular standstill (asystole) if no other subsidiary pacemaker (for example, in the atria, AV junction, or ventricles) takes over. In such cases the ECG will record a *straight-line pattern,* as seen in Fig. 17-3, indicating asystole.*

Treatment of ventricular standstill also re-

---

*At this point it should be mentioned that sometimes a strong thump on the sternum with your fist ("thump version") may itself restore normal rhythm, particularly if the patient is having runs of ventricular tachycardia. Therefore, if the patient's ECG monitor shows ventricular tachycardia a single chest thump can be administered. Fig. 14-13 illustrates successful "thump version."

*Whenever you see a straight-line pattern, always check to see that all the electrodes are connected to the patient. They often become disconnected during a cardiac arrest, leading to the mistaken diagnosis of asystole.

Fig. 17-3. Complete ventricular standstill (asystole) producing a straight-line pattern during cardiac arrest.

quires continued external cardiac compression. Sometimes spontaneous cardiac electrical activity will resume. Drugs such as epinephrine and calcium injected intravenously or directly through the chest wall into a cardiac chamber (intracardiac stick) may help stimulate cardiac activity. Finally, if all else fails, patients with ventricular standstill will require a *temporary pacemaker,* inserted as an emergency at the bedside. As described in Chapter 20, a temporary pacemaker is simply a special catheter wire electrode usually inserted through a vein *(transvenous* pacemaker) into the right ventricle and connected to a battery outside the body. In a dire emergency, the pacemaker wire is sometimes inserted directly into the heart through the chest wall *(transthoracic* temporary pacemaker). In recent years a new type of temporary pacemaker has become available that does not require intravenous insertion. This *external* pacemaker utilizes special electrodes, which can be pasted on the chest wall.

Temporary pacemakers are different from permanent pacemakers (Chapter 20), in which the pacemaker battery is inserted surgically under the skin of the chest wall. As mentioned above, electrical defibrillation of

patients with a straight-line pattern on the ECG will not do any harm. However, it will also not be of help in treating ventricular standstill.

Not uncommonly in ventricular standstill, you will also see *occasional* QRS complexes appearing at infrequent intervals against the background of the basic straight-line rhythm. These are *escape beats* (Chapter 11) and represent the attempt of intrinsic cardiac pacemakers to restart the heart's beat. Examples of escape rhythms with underlying ventricular standstill are shown in Fig. 17-4. In some cases the escape beats are narrow (Fig. 17-4, *A*), indicating their origin from either the atria or the AV junction. In other cases, they come from a lower focus in the ventricles, producing a slow *idioventricular* rhythm with wide QRS complexes (Fig. 17-4, *B*). In cases where a slow escape rhythm appears during a cardiac arrest, drugs such as atropine (a vagal blocker) and isoproterenol or epinephrine (sympathetic stimulators) may be given intravenously to speed up the heart rate.

These escape beats should not be confused with *artifacts* produced by cardiac compression. Artifacts are large wide deflections that occur with each cardiac compression (Fig.

Fig. 17-4. Escape rhythms with underlying ventricular standstill: **A,** junctional escape rhythm with narrow QRS complexes; **B,** idioventricular escape rhythm with wide QRS complexes. Treatment should include the use of intravenous atropine and, if needed, isoproterenol in an attempt to speed up these bradycardias, which cannot support the circulation.

Fig. 17-5. External cardiac compression artifacts. External cardiac compression during a resuscitation produces artifactual ECG complexes (marked *C*), which may be mistaken for actual QRS complexes: **A,** ventricular standstill with external cardiac compression; **B,** straight-line pattern interrupted by external cardiac compression artifacts and two escape beats *(QRS)*; **C,** ventricular fibrillation with cardiac compression.

17-5). Their size varies with the strength of the compression, and their direction varies with the lead in which they appear (negative in leads I, II, III, and aV_F and positive in leads aV_R and aV_L). They should not be mistaken for spontaneous electrical activity of the heart.

Electromechanical Dissociation

The large majority of patients with cardiac arrest will have an ECG showing either ventricular fibrillation or ventricular standstill (sometimes with escape beats). Occasionally, however, the ECG of a patient in cardiac arrest will continue to show identifiable QRS complexes. The actual heart rhythm in such cases may be a sinus rhythm, AV junctional (nodal) rhythm, or heart block. However, despite the presence of regularly recurring QRS complexes and even P waves on the ECG, the patient is unconscious and does not have a palpable pulse or blood pressure. In other words, the patient has cardiac electrical activity but no mechanical heart contractions to effectively pump blood. The term *"electromechanical dissociation"* (EMD) is used in such cases.

EMD can arise in a number of settings.

When assessing a patient with EMD, it is essential to consider the potentially *reversible* causes first. One of the most important of these is pericardial effusion (in which the pericardial sac fills up with an excessive amount of blood or other fluid). This serves to mechanically "choke off" the heart, preventing it from adequately filling and emptying. The term *"pericardial tamponade"* ("tamp" meaning "to plug up") is used to describe situations where pericardial effusion produces decreased cardiac output and ultimately cardiac arrest. Pericardial tamponade can be treated by removal of some of the fluid from the pericardial sac with a special needle inserted through the chest wall (pericardiocentesis). Because the disease process is primarily extracardiac (involving the pericar-

Fig. 17-6. Sinus rhythm with electromechanical dissociation (EMD). Although the ECG showed sinus rhythm, the patient had no pulse or blood pressure. In this case the EMD was a result of depression of myocardial function after a cardiac arrest. (Pericardial tamponade may also cause EMD.)

dium), the ECG generally shows relatively normal electrical activity, despite the impaired mechanical function of the heart. (While on the subject of pericardial effusion, recall from Chapter 10 the major ECG pattern seen with pericardial effusion: low voltage complexes.) Tension pneumothorax and massive pulmonary embolism are two other causes of EMD, both also potentially reversible.

Probably the most common setting in which EMD occurs is where the myocardium has sustained severe generalized injury that *may not be reversible* (for example, myocardial infarction). In such cases, even though the heart's conduction system may be intact enough to generate a relatively normal rhythm, there is not enough functional ventricular muscle to respond to this electrical signal with an adequate contraction. Sometimes the myocardial depression will be temporary and reversible and the patient may respond to intracardiac injections of calcium (the ion essential for cardiac contraction), to the administration of intravenous fluids (to expand the circulatory volume), or to an infusion of inotropic agents (dopamine, dobutamine, or epinephrine). If the heart rate is relatively slow, then drugs like atropine and isoproterenol (Isuprel) are given to increase heart rate and cardiac output. During this time, of course, it is necessary to continue external cardiac compression since the heart's

own intrinsic rhythm is not producing any cardiac output because of the EMD.

Fig. 17-6 shows an example of EMD in which the ECG shows sinus rhythm, yet no pulse or blood pressure was present secondary to severe depression of myocardial contractility.

• • •

The three basic ECG patterns seen with cardiac arrest—ventricular fibrillation, ventricular standstill, and electromechanical dissociation—have all been described separately. However, during the course of resuscitating any patient, it is not unusual to see two or even all three of these ECG patterns at different times during the arrest. For example, consider the following hypothetical, but typical, example of a patient who is found in the hospital bed, unconscious and without palpable pulse or spontaneous respiration. CPR is immediately begun by the hospital staff. In addition, for the reasons described previously (p 236), the patient is given an electrical shock from the defibrillator even before being connected to an electrocardiograph. The first ECG pattern seen, in this case, is a straight line, indicating complete asystole. Following external cardiac compression, artificial ventilation, intravenous injections of epinephrine, calcium, and bicarbonate, ventricular fibrillation is seen on the ECG. The patient is immediately defibrillated again. This is followed

ECG shows ventricular standstill (asystole)

External cardiac compression started
Intracardiac calcium and epinephrine given
Intravenous bicarbonate given

ECG now shows ventricular fibrillation (VF)

400 ws of direct current (DC)
shock given by electrical defibrillator

ECG now shows sinus rhythm with VPCs

Intravenous lidocaine given here to
suppress ventricular premature contractions
(V) and to prevent further episodes of
ventricular fibrillation

A   asystole

B   external cardiac compression   R

C   ventricular fibrillation

D   ventricular fibrillation   D.C. 400 w s

E   R   R   R   R

F   V

G   V   V

Fig. 17-7. ECG history of cardiac arrest and successful resuscitation. The left panel shows the ECG sequence during an actual cardiac arrest. The right panel shows sequential therapy appropriate for the different ECG patterns. Initially, **A** and **B**, there is ventricular standstill (asystole) with a straight-line pattern, treated by external cardiac compression. This is followed, **C** and **D**, by ventricular fibrillation. Sinus rhythm, **E** to **G**, appears after defibrillation with 400 watt-seconds of direct current electric shock. *C* is an external cardiac compression artifact; *R* is an R wave from the spontaneous QRS complex; *V* is a ventricular premature contraction.

by the appearance of normal sinus rhythm. Intravenous lidocaine is given to prevent ventricular tachyarrhythmia. However, despite the normal rhythm, no pulse can be felt, indicating electromechanical dissociation. Intravenous calcium is therefore given (along with a careful intravenous fluid challenge and dopamine), and the pulse becomes palpable. In this case electromechanical dissociation probably represented a reversible depression in myocardial function and circulation following the cardiac arrest. Had the electromechanical dissociation persisted despite adequate heart rate and administration of calcium and fluids, the next step might have been an attempted pericardiocentesis in the hope of finding a treatable cause of the EMD (namely, pericardial tamponade).

Fig. 17-7 shows an actual example of the ECG history of a cardiac arrest.

CLINICAL CAUSES OF CARDIAC ARREST

Cardiac arrest resulting from any of the three mechanisms—ventricular fibrillation (and related arrhythmias), ventricular standstill, or electromechanical dissociation—may occur in numerous settings. Cardiac arrest can result from any type of organic heart disease. For example, a patient with an acute MI may have a cardiac arrest for several reasons: Myocardial ischemia and increased ventricular irritability may precipitate ventricular fibrillation. Damage to the conduction system may result in ventricular standstill. Finally, electromechanical dissociation may occur with extensive myocardial injury. Occasionally, actual rupture of the ventricular wall will occur, leading to fatal pericardial tamponade. Lightning or electric shock may produce cardiac arrest in normal hearts. Cardiac arrest may also occur during surgical procedures. Drugs such as epinephrine may produce ventricular fibrillation. Quinidine and related drugs can lead to torsades de pointes (described in Chapter 14). Excessive digitalis can also lead to fatal ventricular arrhythmias. Recognition of arrhythmias caused by digitalis intoxication was discussed in the preceding chapter. Marked elevation of the serum potassium concentration (Chapter 10) will ultimately lead to cardiac arrest with ventricular standstill. A very low serum potassium concentration may lead to a fatal ventricular arrhythmia, particularly in a patient taking digitalis. Hypokalemia (as well as hypomagnesemia and hypocalcemia) can also lead to torsades de pointes. Obviously, this is only a partial list of the possible clinical settings of cardiac arrest.

Following successful resuscitation of the patient in cardiac arrest, an intensive search for the clinical cause must be started. A 12-lead ECG, along with serum cardiac enzymes, will help diagnose MI. Complete blood count and serum electrolytes should be checked, as well as an arterial blood gas sample. A portable chest x-ray unit can be brought to bedside. In addition, a pertinent medical history should be obtained from every available source, with particular attention to drug usage (digitalis, quinidine, and so on) and previous cardiac problems.

REVIEW OF CHAPTER 17

Cardiac arrest occurs when the heart stops pumping blood. The diagnosis should be made clinically even before the patient is connected to an electrocardiograph. The major clinical sign of cardiac arrest is absence of pulses in an unconscious patient.

Cardiac arrest may be associated with one or more of the three following rhythms:

1. *Ventricular fibrillation*—The ECG may also show runs of typical ventricular tachycardia or torsades de pointes (p. 209).
2. *Ventricular standstill (asystole)*—The ECG shows a straight-line pattern. Occasional junctional or ventricular escape beats may interrupt the basic straight-line pattern.
3. *Electromechanical dissociation* (EMD)—This is characterized by regularly recurring QRS complexes, sometimes even P waves, that are not associated with a palpable pulse or blood pressure. It is usually caused by diffuse myocardial injury. However, other causes include pericardial tamponade, tension pneumothorax, and massive pulmonary embolism.

During the course of resuscitating any patient, you may see any or all of the above patterns.

In addition, the ECG in cardiac arrest will show distinctive *artifacts* caused by external cardiac compression. These cardiac compression artifacts are wide complexes that should not be mistaken for the intrinsic electrical activity of the heart.

The treatment of cardiac arrest is described in the text.

Review Questions—Chapter 17

1. Would a pacemaker be of any value in treating a patient with cardiac arrest and EMD?
2. The rhythm strip below was obtained from a patient during the course of a cardiac arrest.
   a. What is the basic rhythm?
   b. What are the complexes marked X caused by?

Answers

1. No. By definition, patients with EMD have relatively normal electrical activity. The problem is that this electrical activity is not associated with adequate mechanical (pumping) action, usually because of diffuse myocardial injury, pericardial tamponade, or severe intravascular volume losses. A pacemaker would not be of help in this situation because the patient already has adequate electrical stimulation.
2. a. Idioventricular escape rhythm.
   b. External cardiac compression artifacts.

18 Bradycardias and Tachycardias
Review and Differential Diagnosis

The preceding chapters have described the major arrhythmias and AV conduction disturbances. There are several ways of classifying these abnormalities. In this section we will simply divide them into two groups, bradycardias and tachycardias, and discuss the differential diagnosis of each group.

BRADYCARDIAS (BRADYARRHYTHMIAS)

We have mentioned several arrhythmias and conduction disturbances associated with a slow heart rate. The term *"bradycardia"* or *"bradyarrhythmia"* is used here to refer to arrhythmias and conduction abnormalities producing a heart rate of less than 60 beats/min. Fortunately, the differential diagnosis of a patient with a slow pulse is relatively simple since there are only a handful of possible causes. Specifically, we can cite five general types of bradyarrhythmias:

1. Sinus bradycardia, including SA block
2. AV junctional (nodal) escape rhythm
3. AV heart block (second or third degree) or AV dissociation
4. Atrial fibrillation (or flutter) with slow ventricular response
5. Idioventricular escape rhythm

Sinus bradycardia. Sinus bradycardia (Fig. 18-1) is sinus rhythm with a rate less than 60 beats/min. Each QRS is preceded by a P wave, and the P wave is negative in lead aV_R and positive lead II, indicating that the sinus node is

the pacemaker. Some patients may have a sinus bradycardia as slow as 40 beats/min or less.

Sinus bradycardia may be related to a decreased firing rate of the sinus node or to actual SA block. The most extreme example is sinus node arrest (Chapter 11).

AV junctional escape rhythm. With a slow junctional escape rhythm (Fig. 18-2) either the P waves are *retrograde* (inverted in lead II, upright in lead aV_R) or else no P waves are apparent if the atria and ventricles are stimulated simultaneously.

AV heart block (second or third degree) or AV dissociation (Fig. 18-3). A slow ventricular rate of 60 beats/min or less (even as low as 20 beats/min) is the rule with complete heart block, owing to the slow intrinsic rate of the junctional or idioventricular pacemaker. Patients with second-degree AV block (either Wenckebach or Mobitz type II) usually also have a bradycardia because of the dropped beats (Figs. 15-3 and 15-4). AV dissociation, which is often confused with complete heart block (pp. 222 and 261), is usually also associated with a heart rate of less than 60 beats/min.

Atrial fibrillation or flutter with a slow ventricular rate (Fig. 18-4). Paroxysmal atrial fibrillation is generally associated with a rapid ventricular rate. The ventricular rate may become excessively slow (less than 50 to 60 beats/min) if too much digitalis has been administered (Chapter 16) or if the patient has underlying disease of the AV junction. In such cases

SINUS BRADYCARDIA

Fig. 18-1. Sinus bradycardia with a slight sinus arrhythmia.

AV JUNCTIONAL RHYTHM

Fig. 18-2. The heart rate is about 43 beats/min. The baseline between complexes is perfectly flat (no P waves evident).

COMPLETE HEART BLOCK

Fig. 18-3. The atrial (P wave) rate is about 80 beats/min. The ventricular (QRS) rate is about 43 beats/min. The atria and ventricles are beating independently, so the PR intervals are variable. The QRS complex is wide because the ventricles are paced by an idioventricular pacemaker.

ATRIAL FIBRILLATION WITH A SLOW VENTRICULAR RATE

Fig. 18-4. Regularization and excessive slowing of the ventricular rate with atrial fibrillation are sometimes a sign of digitalis toxicity.

the ECG shows the characteristic atrial fibrillatory waves with a slow ventricular (QRS) rate. The f waves may be very fine and easily overlooked.

Idioventricular escape rhythm. In some cases, where the SA nodal and AV junctional escape pacemakers fail to function, a very slow pacemaker in the ventricular conduction (His-Purkinje) system may take over. This rhythm is referred to as an idioventricular escape rhythm. The rate is usually very slow (<45 beats/min) and the QRS complexes are wide without any preceding P wave (see Fig. 17-4, *B*).

Clinical Significance

With the exception of sinus bradycardia, which may be a normal variant, the other bradycardias are all abnormal.* The possible causes of AV junctional rhythms, heart block, and atrial fibrillation were all described in earlier chapters. *It is worth reemphasizing that in any patient with a bradycardia the possibility of digitalis intoxication must always be considered.* Sinus bradycardia, AV junctional rhythm, second- and third-degree AV block, and atrial fibrillation or flutter with an excessively slow ventricular response are all common signs of digitalis toxicity.

Patients with any of the bradycardias listed may have no symptoms or may complain of light-headedness or fainting resulting from decreased cardiac output. Treatment depends on the particular arrhythmia and the clinical setting.

To summarize, most patients with an ECG heart rate of less than 60 beats/min will have one of the five following arrhythmias: sinus bradycardia (including SA block), AV junctional rhythm, AV heart block (or AV dissociation), atrial fibrillation or flutter with a very slow ventricular rate, idioventricular escape rhythm.*

TACHYCARDIAS (TACHYARRHYTHMIAS)

At the opposite end of the spectrum are those patients with rapid heart rates. The term *"tachycardia"* or *"tachyarrhythmia"* refers to rhythm disturbances producing a heart rate faster than 100 beats/min. The differential diagnosis of tachycardias is somewhat more complicated than the straightforward list of bradycardias. Still, the possible list of tachyarrhythmias is not long, and the correct diagnosis can generally be deduced in a rational fashion.

---

*Occasionally normal subjects (in particular, athletes with increased vagal tone at rest) may show junctional rhythms or even AV Wenckebach.

*Bradycardia can also be due to a wandering atrial pacemaker (Fig. 18-14).

ATRIAL FIBRILLATION WITH A RAPID VENTRICULAR RATE

Fig. 18-5. The ventricular rate is about 130 beats/min (13 QRS cycles/6 sec). Note the characteristic haphazardly irregular rhythm.

In approaching tachyarrhythmias we must first make a basic distinction between *supraventricular tachycardia* (SVT) and *ventricular tachycardia* (VT). These terms have already been defined (Chapters 11, 12, and 14). There are five major SVTs: sinus tachycardia, paroxysmal atrial tachycardia (PAT) (including AV junctional tachycardia), atrial fibrillation, atrial flutter, and multifocal atrial tachycardia. In each of these tachyarrhythmias the pacemaker is located in either the atria or the AV junction, above the ventricles (hence *supra*ventricular). This is in contrast to VT, where the stimulus starts in the ventricles themselves. VT (as defined in Chapter 14) is simply a run of three or more consecutive premature ventricular contractions (Fig. 14-5). With VT the QRS complexes are always wide because the ventricles are not being stimulated simultaneously. The rate of VT is usually between 100 and 200 beats/min. With SVT, the ventricles are stimulated normally (simultaneously), so the QRS complex will be narrow (unless a bundle branch block is also present).

The first step in analyzing a tachyarrhythmia is to look at the width of the QRS complex. If the QRS complex is narrow (0.1 sec or less), then you are dealing with SVT and not VT. If the QRS complex is wide, then consider the rhythm to be VT unless it can be proved otherwise.

Differential Diagnosis of SVTs

Let us begin with the differential diagnosis of SVTs. The heart rate is greater than 100 beats/min, and the QRS complexes are narrow. The four most common supraventricular arrhythmias have already been mentioned. They are (1) sinus tachycardia, (2) PAT (including AV junctional tachycardia), (3) atrial fibrillation, and (4) atrial flutter. A fifth possibility, discussed below, is *multifocal atrial tachycardia*.

The characteristics of these four arrhythmias have already been described in previous chapters. *Sinus tachycardia* in adults generally produces a heart rate between 100 and 180 beats/min. Finding an SVT with a rate of 180 beats/min or more means that you are almost certainly dealing with one of the other three arrhythmias listed. *PAT* (or AV junctional tachycardia) and *atrial fibrillation* can be distinguished on the basis of regularity. PAT is usually an almost perfectly regular tachycardia with a ventricular rate between 140 and 250 beats/min. Of all the arrhythmias, PAT is the most regular. Atrial fibrillation, on the other hand, is distinguished by its irregularity. Remember that with rapid atrial fibrillation (Fig. 18-5) the fibrillatory waves may not be clearly visible but the diagnosis of atrial fibrillation can be made in almost every case by noting the absence of P waves and the haphazardly irregular QRS

Fig. 18-6. This strip shows atrial flutter with 2:1 conduction.

Fig. 18-7. Four look-alike supraventricular tachyarrhythmias: **A,** sinus tachycardia; **B,** atrial fibrillation; **C,** paroxysmal atrial (junctional) tachycardia (PAT); **D,** atrial flutter with 2:1 block. When the ventricular rate is about 150 beats/min, these four arrhythmias may be difficult if not impossible to tell apart. In this example of sinus tachycardia the P waves can barely be seen. Note the irregularity of the atrial fibrillation. In PAT the rate is very regular without evident P waves. In atrial flutter the F waves cannot be seen clearly.

complexes. *Atrial flutter* (Fig. 18-6) is characterized by sawtooth flutter waves between QRS complexes. However, when atrial flutter is present with 2:1 block (when the atrial rate is 300 beats/min and the ventricular response is 150 beats/min), the flutter waves are often hidden. Atrial flutter at 150 beats/min, therefore, can be confused with sinus tachycardia, PAT, or atrial fibrillation (Fig. 18-7). Atrial fibrillation can be excluded because atrial flutter with 2:1 conduction is generally very regular.

Nevertheless, the differential diagnosis of sinus tachycardia, PAT with a ventricular rate of 150 beats/min, atrial fibrillation, and atrial flutter can be a problem (Fig. 18-7). Recall that at a rate of 150 beats/min the P waves with sinus tachycardia and PAT may be hidden. One way of separating these possibilities is to use carotid sinus massage (CSM).* Pressure on the carotid sinus produces a reflex increase in vagal tone. The effects of CSM on sinus tachycardia, PAT, and atrial flutter are described next.

Sinus tachycardia. Sinus tachycardia generally slows slightly with CSM. However, there is

---

*However, carotid sinus massage is not without risks, particularly in elderly patients. For details regarding this maneuver, readers are referred to the Bibliography.

no abrupt change in heart rate. Slowing of sinus tachycardia may make the P waves more evident. Sinus tachycardia generally begins and ends gradually, not abruptly.

PAT. PAT and AV junctional tachycardia usually have an *all or none* response to CSM. In successful cases, PAT will break suddenly and sinus rhythm will resume following CSM (Fig. 12-5). In other cases, CSM has no effect, and the tachycardia continues at the same rate.

Atrial flutter. CSM will often increase the degree of block in atrial flutter, converting flutter with a 2:1 response to 3:1 or 4:1 flutter with a ventricular rate of 100 or 75 beats/min. Slowing of the ventricular rate will unmask the characteristic flutter waves (Fig. 13-2).

• • •

The final SVT, which we have not yet discussed, is *multifocal atrial tachycardia* (MAT). An example of MAT is shown in Fig. 18-8. This tachyarrhythmia is characterized by multiple ectopic foci stimulating the atria. To diagnose MAT, it is necessary to find three or more P waves with different shapes. The PR intervals often will vary. This arrhythmia is most commonly seen in patients with chronic lung disease. Because the ventricular rate is irregular and rapid, MAT is most likely to be mistaken for atrial fibrillation.

MULTIFOCAL ATRIAL TACHYCARDIA

Fig. 18-8. The P waves show variable shapes or variable PR intervals, or both.

Differential Diagnosis of VT

Tachycardias are divided into SVTs and VT. This section describes the differential diagnosis of VT. A tachycardia with widened QRS complexes indicates two possible diagnoses. The first and more important is VT, a life-threatening arrhythmia. As noted, VT is a consecutive run of three or more PVCs at a rate generally between 100 and 200 beats/min. It is usually very regular. The second possible cause of a tachycardia with widened QRS complexes is so-called "SVT with aberration." The term *"aberration"* simply means that some abnormality in ventricular activation is present and causing widened QRS complexes.

Differential Diagnosis of SVT with Aberrancy from VT

There are only two major mechanisms for aberrancy with an SVT: (1) a bundle branch block pattern and (2) the Wolff-Parkinson-White (WPW) preexcitation syndrome.

SVT with bundle branch block. If a patient develops any of the five major SVTs listed above in association with a bundle branch block, the ECG will show a wide-complex tachycardia that may be mistaken for VT. For example, a patient with sinus tachycardia, atrial fibrillation, atrial flutter, PAT, or MAT who also has a right or left bundle branch block will show a wide-complex tachycardia.

Fig. 18-9, *A,* gives an example of atrial fibrillation with a rapid ventricular response occurring with LBBB. Fig. 18-9, *B,* gives an example of actual VT. There is an obvious resemblance, making it difficult to tell these patterns apart. The major distinguishing feature is the irregularity of the atrial fibrillation as opposed to the regularity of the VT. However, in some cases VT may be irregular.

It is also important to recognize that in some cases of SVT with aberration the bundle branch block is seen only during the episodes of tachycardia. Such rate-related bundle branch blocks are said to be "tachycardia dependent."

Fig. 18-9. Supraventricular tachycardia with bundle branch block compared to ventricular tachycardia. **A,** Atrial fibrillation with LBBB pattern. **B,** Ventricular tachycardia. It may be difficult and sometimes impossible to tell from the ECG if a patient has actual ventricular tachycardia or a supraventricular tachycardia with bundle branch block.

Fig. 18-10. A, Atrial fibrillation with the Wolff-Parkinson-White (WPW) syndrome may lead to a wide-complex tachycardia with very rapid rate. Note that some of the RR intervals are less than 0.20 second. Irregularity is due to the underlying atrial fibrillation. **B,** After converison to sinus rhythm the classic WPW triad is visible: relatively short PR interval, wide QRS, and delta wave (*arrow* in V₃).

SVT with WPW syndrome. The second mechanism responsible for a wide-complex tachycardia is SVT with the WPW syndrome (described in Chapter 10). As noted, patients with WPW preexcitation have an accessory pathway (bundle of Kent) connecting either atrium with either ventricle, thus bypassing the AV junction. Such patients are especially prone to developing PAT with a narrow (normal) QRS complex, for the reason described on p. 155. On occasion, however, particularly if atrial fibrillation (or atrial flutter) develops, a wide-complex tachycardia may result from conduction down the bypass tract at very high rates. This kind of wide-complex tachycardia will also, obviously, mimic VT. An example of WPW with atrial fibrillation is shown in Fig. 18-10.

The possible diagnosis of WPW with atrial fibrillation should be strongly suspected if you encounter a wide-complex tachycardia that is irregular and has a very high rate (very short RR intervals). In particular, RR intervals of 0.20 second or less are rarely seen with conventional atrial fibrillation and are also rare with ventricular tachycardia. They relate to the ability of the bypass tract (in contrast to the AV junction) to conduct impulses in extremely rapid succession (Fig. 18-10, *A*).

The recognition of WPW with atrial fibrillation is of considerable clinical importance because digitalis may, paradoxically, enhance conduction down the bypass tract. As a result the ventricular response may increase, leading to possible myocardial ischemia and in some cases to ventricular fibrillation. A similar effect has been reported with verapamil.

• • •

There are two important clues that may be helpful in differentiating SVT with aberration from VT. The first is the *presence of AV dissociation* and the second is the *shape of the QRS in lead V_1*.

Recall from Chapter 15 that in AV dissociation, the atria and ventricles are paced from separate sites, with a faster ventricular rate. Some, but not all, patients with VT also show AV dissociation; in other words, the ventricles are paced from an ectopic site at a rapid rate while the atria continue to be paced independently by the sinus node. In such cases you may be able to see P waves occurring at a slower rate than the rapid wide QRS complexes, as shown in Fig. 18-11. Some of the P waves may be "buried" in the QRS complexes and be difficult to discern. Unfortunately, not all cases of VT show AV dissociation. Therefore, the absence of AV dissociation does not exclude VT. However, the presence of AV dissociation in a patient with wide complexes at a rapid rate is diagnostic of VT. Furthermore, in some cases of VT with AV dissociation, the sinus node may transiently "capture" the ventricles, producing a beat with normal QRS duration ("cap-

Fig. 18-11. Ventricular tachycardia with AV dissociation. Note the independent atrial rate (75/min) and ventricular rate (140/min). (From Goldberger, E.: Treatment of cardiac emergencies, ed. 4, St. Louis, 1985, The C.V. Mosby Co.)

ture beat") or a "fusion beat," in which case the sinus beat and ventricular beat coincide to produce a hybrid complex. Fig. 18-12 illustrates capture and fusion beats in a case of VT.

The second important clue in the differential diagnosis of SVT from VT with aberration is the shape of the QRS complex in lead V_1 (Wellens et al., 1978). It has been noted that if V_1 shows an RS ($\wedge_\Gamma$) or R wave ($\wedge$) then VT is likely to be present. An RSR′ ($\neg\sqrt{}$) with R′ > R is suggestive but not diagnostic of SVT while an RSR′ ($\wedge\wedge$) with R > R′ suggests VT.

There are, however, cases where it may be impossible to distinguish between VT and SVT with aberration. In such cases clinical judgment must be used. For example, if the patient is hypotensive, then the tachycardia should be treated as VT (Table 2).

Clinical Significance

As mentioned earlier, the first question to ask in looking at any tachyarrhythmia is whether the rhythm is VT or not. If VT is present, then emergency treatment is required as described in Chapter 14.

With SVT the therapy depends on the clinical setting. In the case of sinus tachycardia (Chapter 11) treatment is directed at the underlying cause (for example, fever, sepsis,

Table 2. Differential Diagnosis of Tachycardias*

Narrow QRS Complexes	Wide QRS Complexes

A. Supraventricular tachycardia
   1. Sinus tachycardia
   2. Paroxysmal atrial tachycardia or AV junctional tachycardia
   3. Atrial fibrillation
   4. Atrial flutter
   5. Multifocal atrial tachycardia
	A. Ventricular tachycardia
	B. Supraventricular tachycardia with aberration
	   1. Bundle branch block
	   2. Wolff-Parkinson-White syndrome

*Ventricular rate greater than 100 beats/min

Fig. 18-12. Ventricular tachycardia with AV dissociation producing fusion *(F)* and capture *(C)* beats. Leads I and II were recorded simultaneously. (Courtesy Dr. Robert Engler.)

congestive heart failure, hyperthyroidism, and so on.) Similarly treatment of MAT should be directed at the underlying problem (usually chronic pulmonary disease). Electrical cardioversion should not be used in MAT, since it is not likely to be helpful and may induce serious ventricular arrhythmias. The calcium channel–blocking drug verapamil can be used to slow the ventricular response in MAT.

In treating the other three major SVTs (PAT, rapid atrial fibrillation, and atrial flutter), a decision must first be made whether initially to treat with electrical cardioversion or with drug therapy. There are no absolute rules for making such decisions. In assessing any patient with an SVT, you should ask the following three key questions relating to the effects of the tachycardia on the heart and circulation:

1. Is the patient's blood pressure abnormally low?
2. Is the patient having anginal chest pain?
3. Is the patient in severe congestive heart failure?

Patients in shock or with angina, pulmonary edema associated with rapid atrial fibrillation, atrial flutter, or PAT require emergency therapy. If they do not respond promptly to initial drug administration, then electrical cardioversion should be considered.

Another major question to ask about any patient having a tachyarrhythmia (or any arrhythmia for that matter) is whether the pa-

Fig. 18-13. Brady-tachy (sick sinus) syndrome. This rhythm strip shows supraventricular tachycardia (probably atrial flutter) followed by a sinus pause, an AV junctional escape beat (*J*), and then sinus rhythm.

Fig. 18-14. Wandering atrial pacemaker. Note the variability in P wave configuration caused by the shifting of pacemaker site. (From Phibbs, B.: The cardiac arrhythmias, ed. 3, St. Louis, 1978, The C.V. Mosby Co.)

tient is taking digitalis. Some arrhythmias, such as PAT with block, may be digitalis toxic rhythm disturbances for which electrical cardioversion is contraindicated (Chapter 16). Finally, in the case of atrial fibrillation you should check to see whether the arrhythmia is chronic or acute, remembering that although chronic atrial fibrillation can sometimes be converted to normal sinus rhythm the rhythm generally reverts to atrial fibrillation.

SICK SINUS SYNDROME AND THE BRADY-TACHY SYNDROME

We continue this discussion of arrhythmias with mention of an interesting group of patients who have bradyarrhythmias and sometimes alternating attacks of brady- and tachyarrhythmias.

The term *"sick sinus syndrome"* has been coined to describe patients who develop sinus node dysfunction that causes marked sinus bradycardia, sinus arrest, or junctional escape rhythms, which may lead to symptoms of light-headedness and even syncope.

In some patients with the sick sinus syndrome, these bradycardic episodes alternate with periods of tachycardia (for example, PAT, atrial fibrillation, or even VT). Sometimes the bradycardia will occur immediately after spontaneous termination of the tachycardia. The term *"brady-tachy syndrome"* has been used to describe this subset of patients with sick sinus syndrome who have tachyarrhythmias as well as bradyarrhythmias (Fig. 18-13).

Diagnosis of the sick sinus syndrome and, in particular, the brady-tachy variant often requires monitoring the patient's heartbeat over several hours or even days. A single ECG strip may be normal or may reveal only the bradycardic or tachycardic episode. Only long-term monitoring may reveal both sides of these patients' problem: the bradyarrhythmias and tachyarrhythmias. The use of continuous ECG (Holter) monitoring in evaluating elderly patients with light-headedness and syncope has shown a surprisingly high frequency of sick sinus syndrome. Treatment generally requires a permanent pacemaker to prevent sinus arrest and drugs, such as digitalis, quinidine, verapamil, or a beta-blocker, to control the tachycardias after the pacemaker has been inserted.

WANDERING ATRIAL PACEMAKER

We conclude this chapter by mentioning one relatively rare arrhythmia, wandering atrial pacemaker. Wandering pacemaker, an arrhythmia not mentioned up to this point, is somewhat difficult to classify. As shown in Fig. 18-14, it is characterized by multiple P waves of varying configuration with a relatively normal or somewhat slow heart rate. This pattern reflects shifting of the pacemaker between the sinus node, other atrial sites, and sometimes the AV junction. Wandering atrial pacemaker may be seen in a variety of settings. Occasionally it develops in normal subjects, and it may be seen with digitalis excess as well as with a variety of different types of organic heart disease.

Wandering atrial pacemaker is distinct from MAT (p. 249), another arrhythmia with multiple different P waves. In wandering atrial pacemaker, the rate is normal or slow. In MAT, it is rapid.

REVIEW OF CHAPTER 18

Arrhythmias can be grouped into *bradycardias* (with a heart rate *slower* than 60 beats/min) and *tachycardias* (with a heart rate *faster* than 100 beats/min).

Bradycardias include five major arrhythmias: (1) sinus bradycardia, (2) AV junctional (nodal) rhythm, (3) second- or third-degree heart block or AV dissociation, (4) atrial fibrillation (or flutter) with a slow ventricular rate, and (5) idioventricular escape rhythm. Digitalis toxicity may be responsible for any of these arrhythmias.

Tachycardias can be subdivided into (1) those with a *narrow* QRS complex and (2) those with a *wide* QRS complex.

The narrow–QRS complex tachycardias are always *supraventricular* tachycardias (SVT). The five most common SVTs are (1) sinus tachycardia, (2) paroxysmal atrial tachycardia (or AV junctional tachycardia), (3) rapid atrial fibrillation, (4) atrial flutter, and (5) multifocal atrial tachycardia (MAT). Carotid sinus massage is sometimes helpful in differentiating these arrhythmias at the bedside.

Tachycardias with a wide QRS complex may be either *ventricular* or any of the SVTs in association with a *bundle branch block* or *Wolff-Parkinson-White* pattern.

The term *sick sinus syndrome* describes patients with sinus node dysfunction who may develop marked sinus bradycardia, sometimes with sinus arrest or slow junctional rhythms, which may cause lightheadedness or syncope. Some patients with the sick sinus syndrome have periods of tachycardias alterating with the bradycardias *(brady-tachy syndrome)*.

Wandering atrial pacemaker is an arrhythmia characterized by multiple P waves of varying configuration, usually with a relatively normal or slow heart rate.

Review Questions—Chapter 18

1. Answer the following questions concerning the lead II rhythm strip below:
   a. Is the rhythm an SVT or a VT?
   b. Are there P waves present?
   c. What is this arrhythmia?

2. What is the most likely diagnosis for the arrhythmia shown below (monitor lead)?

3. A 40-year-old man complaining of occasional palpitations with a fast heartbeat is found to have runs of SVT with a rate of 200 beats/min on his Holter monitor tracing. The rhythm is very regular. What is the most likely diagnosis?

Answers

1. a. SVT because of narrow QRS complexes.
   b. No. Baseline shows irregular, fibrillatory pattern.
   c. Atrial fibrillation.

2. VT.

3. PAT. The rate is too fast for sinus tachycardia and too regular for atrial fibrillation.

19 Limitations and Uses of the ECG

Throughout this book, we have stressed the clinical uses of the ECG. The purpose of this review chapter is threefold: to underscore some important limitations of the ECG, to reemphasize its utility, and to review some common pitfalls in its interpretation.

Like most clinical tests, the ECG yields both *false-positive* and *false-negative* results. A false-positive result is an apparently abnormal ECG in a normal subject. For example, prominent precordial voltage may occur in the absence of LVH (p. 81). Furthermore, Q waves may occur as a normal variant and therefore do not always indicate heart disease (p. 113). False-negative results, on the other hand, occur when the ECG fails to show evidence of some cardiac abnormality. For example, some patients with acute MI may not show diagnostic ST-T changes, or patients with chronic coronary artery disease may not show ST depressions during stress testing.

The diagnostic accuracy of any test is determined by the percentages of these false-positive and false-negative results. The *sensitivity* of a test is a measure of the percentage of patients with a particular abnormality that can be identified by an abnormal test result. For example, a test with 100% sensitivity will not have any false-negative results. The more false-negative results, the less sensitive is the test. The *specificity* of a test is a measure of the percentage of false-positive results. The more false-positive test results, the less specific is the test. As noted above, both the sensitivity and the specificity of the ECG in diagnosing a variety of conditions, including myocardial

infarction, are limited. It is of great importance for those in clinical practice to be aware of these diagnostic limitations.

Following is a list of a number of important problems that *cannot* be excluded simply because the ECG is normal or shows only nondiagnostic abnormalities:

1. Prior MI
2. Acute MI*
3. Severe coronary artery disease†
4. Significant LVH
5. Significant RVH
6. Intermittent arrhythmias (such as ventricular tachycardia, complete heart block)
7. Acute pulmonary embolism
8. Pericarditis

Despite these important limitations, the ECG is an extremely useful test that often helps in the diagnosis of specific cardiac conditions and sometimes can aid in the evaluation and management of general medical problems (such as electrolyte disorders). The following list indicates some of the particular areas in which the ECG may be helpful:

1. Significant hyperkalemia, a life-threatening electrolyte abnormality, virtually always produces ECG changes, beginning with T wave peaking, loss of P waves, QRS widening, and finally asystole (p. 142).

---

*The pattern of acute MI may also be masked in patients with LBBB, Wolff-Parkinson-White preexcitation, or electronic pacemakers.

†A normal exercise tolerance test also does not exclude severe coronary artery disease.

259

2. LVH is seen in most patients with severe aortic stenosis.

3. Most patients with an atrial septal defect show an RBBB pattern.

4. Persistent ST elevations several weeks after an MI should suggest a ventricular aneurysm.

5. Low QRS voltage in a patient with elevated central venous pressure (distended neck veins) suggests possible pericardial tamponade.

6. Elevated central venous pressure in a patient with ECG evidence of acute inferior wall infarction suggests associated right ventricular infarction (Chapter 8).

7. Frequent PVCs and nonspecific ST-T changes, particularly in a younger patient, should prompt a search for mitral valve prolapse (click-murmur syndrome).

8. Unexplained atrial fibrillation should prompt a search of occult mitral valve disease or hyperthyroidism.

9. A new RBBB pattern, particularly in association with sinus tachycardia, should suggest the possibility of pulmonary embolism.

10. Most patients with acute MI show diagnostic ECG changes (new Q waves, ST elevations, hyperacute T waves, ST depressions, or T wave inversions). However, in the weeks and months following acute MI these changes may become less apparent and, in some cases, disappear.

11. The combination of left atrial enlargement and right ventricular hypertrophy on the ECG should suggest the possibility of mitral stenosis.

12. The combination of low voltage and sinus bradycardia should suggest possible hypothyroidism.

13. The combination of low voltage and poor precordial R wave progression is commonly seen in chronic lung disease.

14. The triad of relatively low limb lead voltage, prominent precordial voltage, and poor R wave progression suggests an underlying cardiomyopathy (Chapter 10).

COMMON APPLICATIONS OF THE ECG

The ECG may also provide very important clues in the evaluation of certain major medical problems, such as syncope, coma, shock, and weakness.

Syncope

Syncope (fainting) can result from primary cardiac factors as well as from a variety of noncardiac causes. The noncardiac causes include vasovagal syncope, orthostatic (postural) hypotension, brain dysfunction from vascular insufficiency or metabolic derangements (alcohol, hypoglycemia), and vagal hyperreactivity (carotid sinus syndrome). The cardiac causes can be divided into mechanical obstructions (aortic stenosis, primary pulmonary hypertension, atrial myxoma) and electrical problems (brady- or tachyarrhythmias).

Patients with syncope resulting from aortic stenosis generally show LVH on their resting ECG. Primary pulmonary hypertension is most common in young adult women. The ECG generally shows RVH. The presence of frequent PVCs may be a clue to intermittent ventricular tachycardia. Complete heart block in a patient with syncope constitutes the Stokes-Adams syndrome (p. 219). In some cases, serious arrhythmias may be recorded only on longer rhythm strips or when 24-hour Holter monitoring is performed. Syncope in a patient with ECG evidence of bifascicular block (such as RBBB with left anterior hemiblock) should prompt a search for intermittent second- or third-degree heart block. Syncope in patients taking quinidine may be caused by drug toxicity. These patients often have QT prolongation or prominent U waves and thus are prone to torsades de pointes (quinidine syncope, p. 210), which may occur despite the fact that the serum quinidine level is in the "therapeutic" or even "sub-therapeutic" range.

Coma

An ECG should be obtained on all comatose patients. If coma is from MI with subsequent cardiac arrest, diagnostic ECG changes related to the infarct are usually seen. Subarachnoid hemorrhage may cause very deep T wave inversions (Fig. 9-10), simulating the changes of MI. Patients with coma associated with hypercalcemia will often show a short QT interval. Myxedema coma generally presents with ECG evidence of sinus bradycardia and low voltage. Widening of the QRS in a comatose patient should raise the possibility of drug overdose (phenothiazine or tricyclic antidepressant) or of hyperkalemia.

Shock

An ECG should always be obtained promptly on any patient with hypotension because MI is a major cause of shock (cardiogenic shock). In other cases, hypotension may be caused by a brady- or tachyarrhythmia. Finally, some patients with shock from noncardiac causes (for example, hypovolemia) may develop myocardial ischemia and sometimes infarction as a consequence of their initial problem.

Weakness

An ECG should be obtained on all patients with unexplained weakness. Elderly patients, in particular, may have relatively "silent" MIs with minimal or atypical symptoms, such as the onset of fatigue or general weakness. A prolonged QT interval may be an important clue to unsuspected hypocalcemia, an important metabolic cause of weakness. Hypokalemia may cause weakness along with characteristic ECG changes, including ST depression, T wave flattening, and prominent U waves. In other cases weakness may result from a brady- or tachyarrhythmia.

COMMON PITFALLS IN ECG INTERPRETATION

You can minimize errors in interpreting ECGs by taking care to analyze *all* the points listed on p. 276 in Chapter 21. Many mistakes result from the failure to be systematic. Other mistakes result from confusing ECG patterns that are "look-alikes."

Following are some of the most common pitfalls (caveats) in ECG interpretation:

1. *Failure to look for standardization mark.* Many an ECG is mistakenly thought to show "high" or "low" voltage when, in fact, the voltage is normal but the standardization marker is set at $2\times$ or $\frac{1}{2}\times$.

2. *Atrial flutter with 2:1 block (conduction).* This is one of the most commonly missed diagnoses. The rhythm is often misdiagnosed as either sinus tachycardia (mistaking part of a flutter wave for a P wave) or paroxysmal atrial tachycardia (PAT). When you see a narrow-complex tachycardia with a ventricular rate of about 150/min, you should strongly suspect atrial flutter.

3. *Wolff-Parkinson-White (WPW) pattern.* WPW is frequently mistaken for bundle branch block, hypertrophy, or infarction because the preexcitation results in a wide QRS and may also cause increased QRS voltage, T wave inversions, and pseudoinfarction Q waves.

4. *AV dissociation vs complete heart block.* In AV dissociation the atria and ventricles become "desynchronized," with the QRS rate the same as or slightly faster than the P wave rate (p. 222). In complete heart block the atria and ventricles also beat independently but the ventricular rate is much slower than the atrial (sinus) rate. AV dissociation is usually a minor arrhythmia, although it may reflect conduction disease or drug toxicity (for example, digitalis). Complete heart block is always a major arrhythmia and often requires pacemaker therapy.

5. *Normal variant vs pathologic Q waves.* Do not forget (p. 114) that Q waves may be a

normal variant as part of QS waves in leads aV_R, aV_L, aV_F, III, V_1, and occasionally V_2. Small q waves, as part of qR waves, may occur in leads I, II, III, aV_L, aV_F, and the left chest leads (V_4 to V_6). Such small "septal" q waves are less than 0.04 second in duration. On the other hand, small pathologic Q waves may be overlooked because they are not always very deep. In some cases it may not be possible to state definitively whether a Q wave is pathologic or not.

6. *AV Wenckebach.* In this commonly missed diagnosis an important clue is the appearance of "group beating" (p. 215). The QRS complexes become grouped in clusters due to the intermittent failure of conduction.

7. *Hidden ("buried") P waves.* These may lead to mistakes in the diagnosis of a number of arrhythmias, including blocked premature atrial contractions (PACs), PAT with block, and second- and third-degree (complete) AV block. It is important, therefore, to search in the ST segment and T wave for buried P waves.

8. *Multifocal atrial tachycardia (MAT) and atrial fibrillation.* These are often confused because the ventricular response in both is usually rapid and irregular. In MAT, look for multiple different P waves. In atrial fibrillation, be careful not to mistake the fibrillatory (f) waves for actual P waves.

9. *Left bundle branch block (LBBB).* This may be mistaken for infarction because it is associated with poor R wave progression and often ST segment elevation in the right chest leads.

10. *U waves.* These are sometimes overlooked. While small U waves are a physiologic finding, large U waves (which may be apparent in only the chest leads) are sometimes an important marker of hypokalemia or drug (for example, quinidine) toxicity. Large U waves may be associated with increased risk of *torsades de pointes,* a potentially lethal ventricular arrhythmia (p. 209).

11. *Severe hyperkalemia.* Severe hyperkalemia must always be considered immediately in any patient with an unexplained wide QRS, particularly if P waves are not apparent. Delay in making this diagnosis has proved fatal, because severe hyperkalemia may lead to asystole and cardiac arrest while the clinician is waiting for the report from the chemistry laboratory.

REVIEW OF CHAPTER 19

Like most clinical tests, the ECG yields both *false-positive* and *false-negative* diagnoses. For example, not all Q waves indicate MI and not all subjects with actual MI show diagnostic ECG changes. A normal or nondiagnostic ECG also does not exclude LVH, RVH, intermittent life-threatening brady- or tachyarrhythmias, pulmonary embolism, or pericarditis. Despite these limitations in sensitivity and specificity, the ECG does have major uses in a wide range of clinical situations. Besides its obvious utility in assisting cardiac diagnosis, the ECG may also help in evaluating some major medical problems (such as syncope, coma, weakness, and shock).

Review Questions—Chapter 19

1. Which arrhythmias can lead to syncope (fainting)?
   True or false   (2 and 3)
2. A normal exercise tolerance test excludes significant coronary disease.
3. The more false-positive results associated with a particular test, the less sensitive the test is.

Answers

1. Syncope can be caused by a variety of brady- or tachyarrhythmias (including excessive sinus bradycardia, AV junctional escape rhythm, second- or third-degree AV block, atrial fibrillation with an excessively slow ventricular response, ventricular tachycardia, paroxysmal atrial tachycardia, atrial fibrillation, or atrial flutter).

2. False.
3. False. The sensitivity of a test is a measure of how well the test can detect a given abnormality. False-positive results (abnormal results in normal subjects) will lower the specificity, not the sensitivity, of the test.

20 Pacemakers: An Introduction

The purpose of this chapter is to provide a brief overview of an important aspect of clinical electrocardiography, electronic cardiac pacemakers. Particular emphasis will be placed on different types of pacemakers, major indications for pacemaking, and recognition of pacemaker malfunction.

DEFINITIONS

Pacemakers are battery-powered devices designed to electrically stimulate the heart. Pacemakers are used primarily in cases where the patient's own heart rate is excessively slow (bradyarrhythmias, Chapter 18).

A pacemaker has two major components: a battery, which serves as the power source, and a wire electrode, which attaches to the heart chamber being stimulated (usually the right ventricle).

There are two basic types of pacemakers: *temporary* and *implanted (permanent) pacemakers.* In temporary pacemakers the pacing wire is connected to a battery outside the body. With long-term implanted pacemakers, the battery is inserted subcutaneously, usually under the chest wall. In both cases the pacemaker wire is usually threaded through a vein into the right ventricular cavity, so the pacemaker electrode can then stimulate the endocardium of the right ventricle (Fig. 20-1). Occasionally, *epicardial* pacemaker wires are used. In such cases the wire is sewn directly into the epicardium of the left or right ventricle, and the battery is implanted under the skin of the abdomen. In addition, atrial pacing can be performed under special circum-

stances. Finally, some of the more recent pacemakers are *dual chambered,* with electrodes in both the right atrium and the right ventricle.

PACEMAKER ECG PATTERNS

When a ventricular pacemaker fires, it produces a short vertical deflection (pacemaker spike) followed by a QRS complex (representing depolarization of the ventricle). Can you predict what the ECG will show with a functioning right ventricular pacemaker? The ECG should show an LBBB pattern (Fig. 7-8). Recall (p. 96) that the pacemaker is stimulating the right ventricle initially and therefore left ventricular depolarization will be delayed. Figs. 7-8 and 20-2 show examples of typical pacemaker tracings. The vertical line preceding each QRS complex is the pacemaker spike, followed by a wide QRS complex with an LBBB morphology (QS in V_1 and wide R wave in V_6). What pattern would you predict with an epicardial pacemaker stimulating the left ventricle? It would be that of an RBBB.

An atrial pacemaker will produce a spike followed by a P wave.

PACEMAKER BATTERIES

There are a variety of battery units that can be used to power implanted pacemakers. Early pacemaker batteries used mercury-zinc cells. However, because of their relatively short life span, these units have been supplanted by lithium batteries, which may last for 5 or more years. (Nuclear-powered pace-

Fig. 20-1. Implanted pacemaker generator (battery) with a wire electrode inserted through the left subclavian vein into the right ventricle.

Fig. 20-2. Pacemaker beats. The first QRS complex is from a normal sinus beat. It is followed by four pacemaker beats. Note the pacemaker spike *(S)* preceding each paced beat. Pacemaker beats are wide and resemble bundle branch block beats.

makers are also available for younger patients.) As the power cells of conventional pacemakers wear out, the pacemaker rate will usually start to slow.

VENTRICULAR PACING: FIXED RATE AND DEMAND PACEMAKERS

There are two modes of pacemaker function: (1) *fixed rate* and (2) *demand*. A fixed-rate pacemaker is one that fires at a specific preset rate, regardless of the patient's own heart rate. The earliest pacemakers were fixed-rate pacemakers. Currently, virtually all pacemakers are demand-type units. A demand pacemaker literally functions "on demand," that is, only when the patient's heart rate falls below a preset number. Therefore, a demand pacemaker has two distinct aspects: first, a *sensing* mechanism designed so the pacemaker will be inhibited when the heart rate is adequate; second, a *pacing* mechanism designed to trigger the pacemaker when no intrinsic QRS complexes occur within a predetermined time period. In contrast, fixed-rate pacemakers lack a sensing mechanism. Demand units can be temporarily converted to fixed-rate mode by placing a special magnet on the chest wall over the battery. The magnet test is routinely performed when the pacemaker rate is being checked. Some of the newer demand-type pacemakers are "programmable"; that is, the pacing rate can be adjusted once the pacemaker is implanted. Adjustment of rate is accomplished by placing a special magnet on the chest wall to activate a switch inside the pacemaker unit.

There are actually two types of demand ventricular pacemakers: QRS (R wave) inhibited and QRS (R wave) triggered. The function of both units is essentially the same—to pace the heart when the intrinsic rate falls below some preset value. However, the circuitry of QRS-inhibited and QRS-triggered pacemakers is different, resulting in different ECG patterns.

QRS-inhibited pacemakers emit pulses only when the spontaneous heart rate falls below the escape rate of the pacemaker (for example, 70/min) (Fig. 20-3). The QRS-inhibited pacemaker does not emit pulses when the patient's spontaneous heart rate is faster than the escape rate of the pacemaker. Each time the pacemaker senses a spontaneous QRS complex, formation of a pacemaker pulse will be inhibited. Therefore, a QRS-inhibited pacemaker will show pacemaker spikes only when the spontaneous heart rate is slower than the escape rate of the pacemaker. The spikes appear before each QRS complex.

The QRS-inhibited pacemaker also has a *refractory* period (for example, 0.4 sec), which begins whenever the pacemaker senses a QRS or emits a pulse. During the refractory period of the pacemaker, the pacemaker can neither stimulate the ventricle nor sense another R wave. However, if spontaneous ventricular beats or ventricular premature contractions occur during the refractory period, they will not be inhibited but will appear on the ECG. The refractory period is followed by an *alert* period, during which the pacemaker can sense an R wave. If no QRS is sensed by the end of the alert period, the pacemaker will emit another pulse. However, if a spontaneous QRS occurs, the pacemaker will be recycled into another refractory period and then into another alert period. The escape rate and the refractory period vary with different brands of QRS-inhibited pacemakers.

QRS-triggered pacemakers emit a pulse whenever the catheter tip senses a spontaneous QRS. The pulse is recorded on the ECG as a spike superimposed on the patient's own QRS (Fig. 20-4); hence, the term "QRS triggered." However, the pacemaker spike does not actually "capture the ventricles" because the heart is refractory to further depolarization immediately after the QRS complex. Therefore the QRS-triggered pacemaker is actually in a *standby* stage as long as adequate spontaneous ventricular activity is present. However, when the patient's

Fig. 20-3. QRS-inhibited pacing (lead II). In beats 1 and 2 the rhythm is regular sinus. In beat 3 the ventricular rate has slowed slightly so a pacemaker spike appears at approximately the same time as the regular stimulus spreads through the ventricles from the AV node. The result is a fusion beat. In beats 4 through 12 the pacemaker is functioning because the patient's spontaneous heart rate has slowed below the pacemaker escape rate (in this case, 70/min). Then the patient's spontaneous ventricular rate becomes more rapid, so beat 13 is a fusion beat and beat 14 again shows regular sinus rhythm. P waves merge into QRS complexes in beats 4 through 7 and then reemerge in beats 12 and 13. (From Goldberger, E.: Treatment of cardiac emergencies, ed. 4, St. Louis, 1985, The C.V. Mosby Co.)

Fig. 20-4. QRS-triggered pacing (lead II). In beats 1 through 4 the patient's spontaneous ventricular rate has slowed below the escape rate of the pacemaker, which has started to form stimuli at a regular rate of 70/min. In the meantime the patient's spontaneous heart rate is increasing (notice P waves emerging), so beats 5 through 8 are spontaneous regular sinus beats with pacemaker spikes occurring in the QRS complexes. Notice how the shapes of the QRS complexes and T waves of beats 5 through 8 are different from their shapes in beats 1 through 4. (From Goldberger, E.: Treatment of cardiac emergencies, ed. 4, St. Louis, 1985, The C.V. Mosby Co.)

heart rate slows below the escape rate of the pacemaker, the spikes will appear *before* each QRS, and the pacemaker will take over the function of pacing the heart. QRS-triggered pacemakers are a bit confusing at first examination because the pacemaker spikes that come with the patient's spontaneous beat tend to distort the QRS and ST-T complexes (Fig. 20-4). For this reason most of the pacemakers currently in use are QRS-inhibited rather than QRS-triggered devices.

DUAL-CHAMBER PACING

In recent years, there have been considerable advances in dual-chamber pacing, in which pacemaker wires are inserted into the right atrium as well as the right ventricle. In the most sophisticated models the circuitry permits sensing and pacing in both the atrium and the ventricle. Thus the atrial lead is able to sense the patient's intrinsic P waves and, when the atrial rate becomes too slow, to stimulate the right atrium. The circuitry is designed to allow for a physiologic delay between atrial stimulation and ventricular stimulation. This *AV delay* (interval between the atrial pacemaker spike and the ventricular pacemaker spike) is analogous to the PR interval seen in normal conduction.

With the type of dual-chamber pacemaker that allows for both atrial sensing and atrial pacing as well as ventricular sensing and pacing, a variety of ECG patterns may be seen depending on the patient's intrinsic electrical activity. A schematic of these pacemaker patterns is shown in Fig. 20-5.

Beats *1* to *5* show spontaneous atrial activity at a rate above the programmed atrial "escape" rate of the pacemaker. When these P waves are sensed by the atrial electrode, the atrial pacemaker will be inhibited. However, the spread of stimulus through the AV junction is slower than the programmed AV delay of the pacemaker; therefore, the ventricular pacemaker will produce a wide QRS complex preceded by a pacemaker spike *(V)*.

In beat 6 a spontaneous P wave is also present and conduction through the AV junction is delayed as in the five preceding beats; therefore, a ventricular pacemaker spike will occur, but in this beat the spontaneous QRS occurs at the same time as the

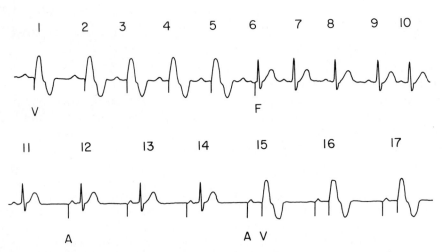

Fig. 20-5. Schematic of the different beats that may be seen with a properly functioning dual-chamber (DDD) pacemaker. (Adapted from Zipes, D.P.: In Current clinical applications of dual-chamber pacing. Proceedings of a symposium in Dallas, Tex., November 15, 1981, Minneapolis, 1982, Medtronic Inc.)

pacemaker spike, resulting in a so-called fusion beat *(F)*.

Beats *8* to *11* are normal beats, in which the atrial rate is above the escape rate of the atrial pacemaker and conduction through the AV junction is faster than the AV delay of the pacemaker; therefore, the pacemaker will be inhibited from discharging either atrial or ventricular stimuli.

In beats *12* to *14* the atrial rate has slowed; thus atrial pacemaker spikes *(A)* are now seen and the atrial electrode is pacing the atria. However, these paced P waves are conducted to the ventricles within the AV delay. Therefore, spontaneous QRS complexes occur.

In beats *15* to *17* the atrial rate has dropped below the programmed atrial pacemaker rate. In addition, the stimulus is delayed getting through the AV junction and this delay exceeds the programmed AV delay of the pacemaker. Therefore, paced stimuli are delivered to both the atrium and the ventricle. Note the pacemaker spikes preceding the P wave and the QRS complex in these last three beats of the series.

PROGRAMMABILITY

In the early days of cardiac pacing the pacemaker rate was not adjustable once the unit had been inserted. A major advance was the introduction of programmable pacemakers, in which the pacemaker rate could be externally changed. In newer pacemakers multiple other parameters in addition to the rate can be externally programmed—including the voltage of the pacemaker discharge, the sensitivity of the electrode to the intrinsic beats, the pacemaker refractory periods, and the duration of the pacemaker spike. For discussion of multiprogrammable pacemakers the reader is referred to the Bibliography.

INDICATIONS FOR CARDIAC PACING

There are a variety of indications for electronic pacemakers. As noted before, the major reason for implanting a pacemaker is the presence of a symptomatic bradyarrhythmia.

For example, permanent pacemakers are indicated in patients with syncope, light-headedness, weakness, or congestive failure caused by complete heart block, second-degree AV block, marked sinus bradycardia or sinus pauses (sick sinus syndrome), slow junctional rhythms, or atrial fibrillation or flutter with an excessively slow ventricular response.

Temporary pacemakers are often inserted during cardiac emergencies (such as MI), when an extremely slow heart rate occurs. For example, patients with acute *anterior* wall MI who develop complete heart block always require a temporary pacemaker (and a permanent pacemaker later on) because of the markedly slow heart rate that occurs. On the other hand, second-degree and even complete heart blocks are not uncommon with *inferior* wall MI because of excessive vagal tone or AV junctional ischemia. AV block with inferior infarction tends to be transient, and the heart rate is often adequate without an electronic pacemaker. However, other patients with inferior MI and second- or third-degree AV block, may require a temporary pacemaker if their heart rate becomes excessively slow, resulting in hypotension, angina, or congestive heart failure.

Temporary pacemakers are often employed after open heart surgery. Temporary pacemakers may also be required during cardiac arrest (p. 237), when the ECG shows asystole or a slow escape rhythm that does not respond to drug therapy. Occasionally temporary pacemakers are required in cases of digitalis toxicity, which may cause any of the major bradyarrhythmias.

As noted, temporary and permanent pacemakers are usually employed when the heart rate is too slow. Rarely, pacemakers are implanted to treat tachyarrhythmias (such as atrial or ventricular tachycardia). The use of pacing in the treatment of atrial flutter is mentioned on p. 189.

As described in Chapter 15, temporary pacemakers are often inserted prophylactically in patients with acute anterior wall MI who develop evidence of new bifascicular block (LBBB, RBBB with left anterior hemiblock, RBBB with left posterior hemiblock). Such patients have a high incidence of progressing to complete (trifascicular) heart block. On the other hand, as emphasized in Chapter 15, patients with *chronic* bifascicular block who are *without symptoms* do not require permanent pacemakers.

Dual-chamber pacing is helpful in maintaining physiologic timing between atrial systole (indicated by the P wave) and ventricular systole (indicated by the QRS). When ventricular pacing alone is used, such physiologic timing will be lost. In some patients, the loss of timed atrial contractions will cause a marked reduction in cardiac output. Dual-chamber pacing will produce a significant improvement in the cardiac performance of these patients. It may also be desirable in permitting a physiologic increase in ventricular rate during exercise in selected patients. For example, consider the patient with complete heart block and underlying sinus rhythm whose ventricular rate with a ventricular pacemaker is constant (say, 72/min) regardless of the atrial (P wave) rate. With a dual-chamber pacemaker the ventricular rate will be able to increase in tandem with the atrial rate during exercise, further increasing cardiac output.

Dual-chamber pacemakers, however, are not without their disadvantages. Atrial electrodes are more likely than ventricular electrodes to become dislodged. Furthermore, as noted below, dual-chamber pacemakers may induce tachycardias in some patients. In addition, dual-chamber pacemakers are considerably more expensive than simple ventricular pacemakers. Finally, atrial sensing or pacing is obviously of no use in the setting of atrial fibrillation or atrial flutter.

PACEMAKER MALFUNCTION

Pacemaker malfunctions occur when either the sensing or the pacing function is impaired.

For example, when the pacemaker battery runs down, the pacemaker rate generally slows and *failure to sense* may also occur. Failure to sense can be diagnosed by observing pacemaker spikes in spite of the patient's own adequate QRS rate (Fig. 20-6). The most common causes of failure to sense are dislodgment of the pacemaker wire or excessive fibrosis around the tip of the pacing wire.

Pacemaker malfunction can also result from *failure to pace*. Failure to pace is diagnosed either by observing pacemaker spikes without subsequent QRS complexes (failure to "capture") (Fig. 20-7) or by the complete absence of pacemaker spikes despite an excessively slow heart rate (Fig. 20-8). Failure to pace can also be caused by dislodgment of the pacemaker wire or by fibrosis around the tip of the pacing wire. In such cases, pacemaker spikes will occur without associated QRS complexes. In other cases (particularly with a broken electrode wire, a short-circuit in the pacing circuit, or electrical interference from the muscles of the chest wall), failure to pace will occur without any pacemaker spike.

Pacemaker malfunction in patients with temporary pacemakers should always prompt a search for loose connections between the battery and the pacing wire, a faulty battery, or a dislodged wire.

COMPLICATIONS OF PACEMAKER THERAPY

Pacemakers are not without potential harm. Therefore, careful thought should be given before inserting a temporary or, particularly, a permanent pacemaker. Infection may occur at the pacemaker site. The electrode may perforate the ventricular wall. The pacemaker itself may cause serious arrhythmias, particularly PVCs. Certain dual chamber pacemakers may initiate runs of supraventricular tachycardia ("endless loop" arrhythmias). Occasionally, the pacemaker will also pace the muscles of the chest wall or the diaphragm, resulting in patient discomfort.

Fig. 20-6. Pacemaker malfunction: failure to sense. Note that after the first two paced beats there is a series of sinus beats with first-degree AV block. Failure of the pacemaker unit to sense these intrinsic QRS complexes leads to inappropriate pacemaker spikes (*), which fall on T waves. Three of these spikes do not capture the ventricle because they occur during the refractory period of the cardiac cycle. (From Conover, M.H.: Understanding electrocardiography, ed. 4, St. Louis, 1984, The C.V. Mosby Co.)

Fig. 20-7. Pacemaker malfunction: failure to pace. Note that beats *1, 3,* and *4* show the pacemaker spikes *(s)* and normally paced QRS complexes and T waves. The remaining beats show only pacemaker spikes. *R* represents the patient's slow spontaneous QRS complexes. (From Goldberger, E.: Treatment of cardiac emergencies, ed. 4, St. Louis, 1985, The C.V. Mosby Co.)

Fig. 20-8. Pacemaker malfunction: failure to pace (no pacemaker artifact). The underlying rhythm is 2:1 AV block (Mobitz type II). Despite a slow heart rate, the pacemaker fails to function. (From Goldberger, E.: Treatment of cardiac emergencies, ed. 4, St. Louis, 1985, The C.V. Mosby Co.)

DIAGNOSIS OF MI WITH PACEMAKERS

The ECG diagnosis of MI may be difficult or impossible in patients with functioning pacemakers in which all beats are paced. In such cases (with a right ventricular electrode) the ECG will show an LBBB configuration. As described in Chapter 8, LBBB generally masks both the QRS and the ST-T changes of MI. Therefore, unless you see spontaneous QRS-T complexes, the dignosis of acute or prior MI may not be possible from the ECG alone.

Finally, it is important to recognize that pacemakers may also produce ECG changes simulating MI. Following periods of electronic pacemaking the ECG may show deep noninfarctional T waves in the patient's spontaneous beats. These *post-pacemaker T wave inversions* may be mistaken for primary ischemic ST-T changes.

APPENDIX: PACEMAKER CODE

A three-position pacemaker code is often used to describe what a particular pacemaker's functions and mode of response are. As shown below, the letter in the first position indicates the chamber(s) being paced—which may be the *atrium* (A), the *ventricle* (V), or *both* (D). The letter in the second position indicates the chamber(s) where sensing occurs—again the atrium (A), ventricle (V), or both (D). Finally, the letter in the third position refers to the mode of response of the pacemaker (p. 266). In the earlier, and in many current, pacemaker models the pacing mode was either *inhibited* (I) or *triggered* (T). The mode of response is labeled D *(double)* in the case of the newer, more advanced, *dual-chamber* pacemakers, which are engineered so the pacemaker responds to atrial electrical activity by delivering a ventricular spike (provided, or course, a spontaneous QRS has not already occurred). There is a fourth mode of response, designated R, which stands for *reverse*. A pacemaker in the reverse mode will pace during periods of tachycardia rather than bradycardia. Such pacemakers are used for their antiarrhythmic action (p. 269 and Bibliography).

The most widely used pacemakers today are VVI units; that is, they are single-chamber pacemakers that both pace (V) and sense (V) exclusively in the ventricle and are inhibited (I) by the patient's own QRS complexes.

The most versatile pacemakers are DDD units. These are dual-chamber pacemakers that can pace the atrium or ventricle (D) and sense in the atrium or ventricle (D). In addition, the mode of response is double (D): atrial pacing can be inhibited by the patient's P waves and a ventricular pacer spike may be triggered by the patient's P waves if a native QRS does not appear on time because of AV block.

The basic principles of a DDD (also called *universal* or *physiologic*) pacemaker have been explained. These pacemakers are dual chambered; that is, they have atrial and ventricular electrodes with sensing and pacing functions in both chambers. Furthermore, after an atrial beat is sensed, a ventricular spike will occur after a preset AV delay unless a spontaneous QRS occurs.

Other types of dual-chamber pacemakers (for example, DVI and VDD models) have also been developed. The specific uses and limitations of these dual chamber units are discussed in references in the Bibliography.

The three-letter pacemaker code has recently been expanded to five letters, reflecting the rapid advances in pacemaker electronics over the past few years. The fourth letter indicates the *programming* features of the pacemaker. The fifth letter indicates *special antiarrhythmic features* that are available in certain pacemakers. Further discussion of these technical areas lies outside the scope of this brief introduction.

Three-Position Pacemaker Code

Position	I	II	III
Category	Chamber(s) paced	Chamber(s) sensed	Mode of response(s)
Letters used	V–Ventricle	V–Ventricle	T–Triggered
	A–Atrium	A–Atrium	I–Inhibited
	D–Double*	D–Double	D–Double
			O–None
		O–None	R–Reverse

Double mode of response. This refers to dual-chamber pacemakers in which atrial pacing may be inhibited by the patient's own P waves and a ventricular spike may be triggered by the patient's P wave if AV block is present.

REVIEW OF CHAPTER 20

Pacemakers are battery-powered devices used to stimulate the heart electrically, particularly in cases where the patient's own heart rate is excessively slow. When the pacemaker wire is attached to the right ventricular endocardium, the ECG will show an LBBB pattern as a result of delayed left ventricular stimulation. Each QRS will be preceded by a pacemaker spike. Cardiac pacing can be done in a *fixed rate* or *demand* mode. Demand pacemakers are inhibited when the heart rate is faster than the escape rate of the pacemaker. There are two types of ventricular demand pacemakers: *QRS inhibited* and *QRS triggered*.

A temporary pacemaker is a unit with an external battery. Temporary pacing wires can be inserted during cardiac emergencies (for example, cardiac arrest caused by asystole or MI complicated by high-degree heart block or sinus arrest). An implanted permanent pacemaker, in which the battery is inserted subcutaneously, usually in the chest wall, is indicated for patients with symptomatic second- or third-degree AV block or other major bradyarrhythmias (such as sinus arrest or slow junctional escape rhythm) leading to inadequate cardiac output.

Dual-chamber (atrial and ventricular) pacemakers have been developed in recent years. These units may be helpful in maintaining physiologic timing between atrial and ventricular contractions, thus increasing cardiac output.

When the pacemaker battery starts to run down, the pacemaker rate will slow. Dislodgment of the pacemaker wire or excessive fibrosis around the tip of the wire can cause failure to sense or failure to pace. Pacing failure in permanent units can also be caused by electrode fracture, short-circuits, or electrical interference from skeletal muscles.

Pacemakers may obscure the ECG diagnosis of MI. Conversely, following electronic pacing of the ventricles, deep noninfarctional T wave inversions may appear in spontaneous QRS complexes *(post-pacemaker T wave pattern)*.

Review Questions—Chapter 20

1. The major indication for *permanent* pacemakers is
    a. History of multiple prior MIs.
    b. Symptomatic bradyarrhythmias.
    c. Digitalis toxicity.
    d. Ventricular bigeminy.
    e. Paroxysmal atrial tachycardia.
2. The following rhythm strip shows
    a. Failure to sense.
    b. Failure to pace.
    c. Normal pacemaker function with a PVC.
    d. Failure to sense and pace.

PVC

Answers

1. b.
2. b. This is an example of intermittent failure to pace, where the fourth pacemaker spike is not followed by a QRS. The two most common causes of failure to pace with a pacemaker spike that does not capture are dislodgment of the electrode wire and fibrosis around the pacing wire tip. Pacemaker failure may also occur in which no pacing spikes are seen (see p. 270).

21 How To Interpret an ECG

In Parts I and II we described the fundamentals of the normal ECG and the major abnormal patterns and arrhythmias. Part III is a collection of test questions to help you review these topics. We will conclude Part II with a brief summary of how to systematically approach any ECG.

ECG INTERPRETATION

Accurate interpretation of ECGs requires, above all, thoroughness and care. Therefore, it is essential to develop a systematic method of reading ECGs that is applied in every case. Many of the most common mistakes are errors of omission: failure to note certain subtle but critical findings. For example, overlooking a short PR interval may result in missing the important diagnosis of the Wolff-Parkinson-White pattern. Marked prolongation of the QT interval, a potential precursor of torsades de pointes (p. 210) and sudden death, often goes unnoticed.

There are 14 points that should be analyzed on every ECG.

1. Standardization
2. Heart rate
3. Rhythm
4. PR interval
5. P wave size
6. QRS width
7. QT interval
8. QRS voltage
9. Mean QRS electrical axis
10. R wave progression in chest leads
11. Abnormal Q waves
12. ST segment
13. T wave
14. U wave

Standardization (p. 11). Make sure that the electrocardiograph has been properly calibrated so the standardization mark is 10 mm tall (1 mV = 10 mm).*

Heart rate (p. 18). Calculate the heart rate. If the rate is faster than 100 beats/min, then a tachycardia is present. A rate slower than 60 beats/min means a bradycardia is present.

Rhythm. Decide whether normal sinus rhythm (NSR) is present or whether some arrhythmia is present.

Be particularly careful not to overlook hidden P waves (seen, for example, in some cases of second- or third-degree AV block, paroxysmal atrial tachycardia [PAT] with block, and blocked PACs). Also, whenever the ventricular rate is about 150/min, always consider the possibility of atrial flutter since the flutter waves may mimic the P waves of sinus or AV junctional rhythm.

PR interval. The normal PR interval (measured from the beginning of the P wave to the beginning of the QRS complex) is 0.12 to 0.2 second. A consistently prolonged PR interval means *first-degree AV block* is present. A short PR interval (with wide QRS complex and delta wave) is seen with the Wolff-Parkinson-White syndrome. A short PR interval with a normal-width QRS may represent Lown-Ganong-Levine type of preexcitation. In contrast, a short

---

*In special cases the ECG may be intentionally recorded at ½ standardization (1 mV = 5 mm) or 2× standardization (1 mV = 20 mm).

PR interval with retrograde P waves (negative in lead II) generally indicates an ectopic atrial or AV junctional pacemaker.

P wave size. Normally, the P wave does not exceed 2.5 mm amplitude and is less than 3 mm wide in all leads. Tall peaked P waves are a sign of right atrial enlargement (P pulmonale). Wide P waves are seen with left atrial abnormality.

QRS width. Normally the QRS width is 0.1 sec or less in all leads. The differential diagnosis of a wide QRS complex is described on p. 16.

QT interval. A prolonged QT interval may be a clue to electrolyte disturbances (hypocalcemia, hypokalemia), drug effects (quinidine, procainamide), or myocardial ischemia. Shortened QT intervals are seen with hypercalcemia and digitalis effect.

QRS voltage. Look for signs of left or right ventricular hypertrophy (p. 85). Remember that thin-chested people and young adults frequently show tall voltage without left ventricular hypertrophy. Do not forget about low voltage (p. 149), which may result from pericardial effusion, myxedema, emphysema, obesity, or myocardial disease.

Mean QRS electrical axis. Estimate the mean QRS axis in the frontal plane. Decide by inspection whether the axis is normal (between $-30°$ and $+100°$) or whether left or right axis deviation is present.

R wave progression in chest leads. Inspect leads V_1 to V_6 to see if the normal increase in R waves is seen as you move across the chest. Poor R wave progression may be a sign of myocardial infarction, but it may also be seen with left ventricular hypertrophy, chronic lung disease, left bundle branch block, and other conditions in the absence of infarction.

Abnormal Q waves (Chapter 8). Abnormal Q waves in leads II, III, and aV_F may indicate transmural inferior wall infarction. Abnormal Q waves in the anterior leads (I, aV_L, and V_1 to V_6) may indicate transmural anterior wall infarction.

ST segment. Look for abnormal ST segment elevations or depressions.

T wave. Inspect the T waves. Normally they are positive (upright) in leads with a positive QRS complex. They are also normally positive in leads V_3 to V_6 in adults, negative in lead aV_R, and positive in lead II. The polarity of the T waves in the other extremity leads depends on the QRS electrical axis. (T waves may be normally negative in lead III in the presence of a vertical QRS axis.)

U wave. Also look for prominent U waves, which may be a sign of hypokalemia or drug effect (as with quinidine).

• • •

After you have analyzed these 14 points, you should formulate an overall interpretation. For example, an ECG might show sinus tachycardia, first-degree AV block, and Q waves and T wave inversions consistent with an evolving anterior wall myocardial infarction. Fig. 21-1 illustrates this systematic approach to ECG reading. Part III contains other examples for practice.

We would like to emphasize that every ECG abnormality you identify should summon up a list of differential diagnostic possibilities. The ECG is a clinical tool, and you should search for a clinical explanation for any ECG abnormality you find. For example, if the ECG shows sinus tachycardia, then the next question to ask is what caused this arrhythmia? Is the sinus tachycardia a result of anxiety, hyperthyroidism, congestive heart failure, hypovolemia, sympathomimetic drugs, or other causes? If you find ventricular tachycardia, what are the diagnostic possibilities? Is the ventricular ectopy caused by myocardial infarction or some potentially reversible cause such as hypoxemia, digitalis toxicity, toxic effects of another drug, hypokalemia, or hypomagnesemia? If you see signs of left atrial enlargement or left ventricular hypertrophy, what is the cause: valvular heart disease, hypertensive heart disease, ischemic heart disease, or cardiomyopathy? In this way, the interpretation of an ECG becomes an integral part of diagnosis and patient care.

Fig. 21-1. ECG for interpretation:

1. Standardization: normal (10 mm); mark recorded at end of leads I, V_1, and V_6 (Standardization mark need be recorded only once when taking an ECG.)
2. Heart rate: 88 beats/min
3. Rhythm: normal sinus
4. PR interval: 0.16 second
5. P waves: normal size
6. QRS width: 0.08 second (normal)
7. QT interval: 0.36 second (normal for rate)
8. QRS voltage: normal
9. Mean QRS axis: about $-30°$ (biphasic QRS complex in lead II with positive QRS in lead I)
10. R wave progression in chest leads: normal
11. Abnormal Q waves: pathologic in leads II, III, and aV_F
12. ST segments: isoelectric
13. T waves: ischemic inversions in leads II, III, aV_F, and V_6
14. U waves: normal

Impression: This ECG is consistent with an inferolateral wall MI of indeterminate age.
Comment: You cannot determine the age of an infarct from the ECG. The changes here (Q waves and T wave inversions) could have been caused by an infarct that occurred the day before or the year before.

ECG artifacts

We will conclude this section with a brief discussion of some important ECG *artifacts*. The ECG, like any other electronic recording, is subject to numerous artifacts that may interfere with accurate interpretation. Some of the most common of these are described here.

60-Hertz (cycle) interference. Interference from alternating-current generators produces the characteristic pattern shown in Fig. 21-2. Note the fine-tooth comb 60 hertz (Hz) artifacts. By switching the electrocardiograph plug to a different outlet or by turning off other electrical appliances in the room, you can usually eliminate 60 Hz interference.

Muscle tremor. Involuntary muscle tremor (Fig. 21-3) can produce undulations in the baseline that may be mistaken for atrial fibrillation or flutter.

Wandering baseline. Upward or downward movement of the baseline may produce spurious ST segment elevations or depressions (Fig. 21-4).

Poor electrode contact or patient movement. Poor electrode contact or patient movement (Fig. 21-5) can produce artifactual deflections in the baseline that may obscure the underlying pattern or be mistaken for abnormal beats.

Improper standardization. The electrocardiograph, as mentioned, should be standardized before each tracing so a 1 mV pulse produces a square wave 10 mm high (Fig. 2-5). Failure to properly standardize will result in complexes that are either spuriously low or spuriously high. Furthermore, most electrocardiographs are equipped with half standardization and double standardization settings. Unintentional recording of an ECG on either of these settings will also result in spuriously low or high voltage.

Fig. 21-2. A common ECG artifact is that produced by 60-hertz (Hz) interference. **A,** Fine oscillations of the baseline. **B,** Same pattern without the artifact.

Fig. 21-3. Another common artifact is that produced by muscle tremor. **A,** Wavy baseline resembling atrial flutter. **B,** Same pattern without the artifact showing normal P waves.

Fig. 21-4. Wandering baseline resulting from patient movement.

Fig. 21-5. Deflections simulating PVCs produced by patient movement. A 60 Hz artifact is also present.

REVIEW OF CHAPTER 21

The following 14 points should be evaluated in every ECG:
1. Standardization
2. Heart rate
3. Rhythm
4. PR interval
5. P wave size
6. QRS width
7. QT interval
8. QRS voltage
9. Mean QRS axis
10. R wave progression in chest leads
11. Abnormal Q waves
12. ST segment
13. T wave
14. U wave

Any ECG abnormality should be related to the clinical status of the patient. The ECG can also be affected by numerous artifacts, including 60 Hz interference, patient movement, poor electrode contact, muscle tremor, and so on.

PART THREE

Self-Assessment Problems

This third and final section of the text is intended for self-assessment. We have included numerous review questions and practice examples based entirely on the material covered in Parts I and II. The review begins with a number of short answer questions followed by actual ECGs for interpretation. The ECGs have been standardized so 1 mV = 10 mm, unless otherwise indicated.

QUESTIONS

1. The P wave represents _____ _____ *(two words)*.
2. The QRS complex represents _____ _____ *(two words)*.
3. The T wave represents _____ _____ *(two words)*.
4. The normal range of the PR interval in adults is between _____ and _____ second.
5. Lead V_1 is obtained by placing the chest electrode to the right of the sternum in the _____ intercostal interspace.
6. With hypocalcemia the QT interval _____ .
7. A *delta* wave is seen in what syndrome?
8. Name a drug that may prolong the QT interval.
9. Name three causes of low-voltage QRS complexes.
10. Name at least three arrhythmias that are commonly caused by digitalis toxicity.
11. A wide rSR′ complex in lead V_1 with sinus rhythm most likely indicates _____.
12. Name three ECG patterns that may be seen with acute pulmonary embolism.
13. If the P wave in lead aV_R is −2 mm and the P wave in lead aV_L is −3 mm, then what must the amplitude of the P wave in lead aV_F be?
14. Two factors that may potentiate digitalis toxicity are _____ and _____.
15. Digitalis *(increases? decreases? has no effect on?)* conduction of impulses through the AV junction.
16. With paroxysmal atrial tachycardia the atrial rate is generally between 140 and ___ beats/min.
17. Prominent U waves are often seen with what electrolyte abnormality?
18. Tall peaked P waves in leads II, III, and aV_F are suggestive of _____.
19. With normal sinus rhythm the P wave is virtually always negative in lead _____ and positive in lead _____.
20. Draw the hexaxial diagram showing the six extremity (frontal plane) leads.
21. Normally the R/S ratio in lead V_1 (in adults) is less than _____.
22. Atrial fibrillation is sometimes seen in which endocrine disorder?
23. Name the three basic ECG patterns that may be seen in cardiac arrest.
24. Name three causes of sinus tachycardia.
25. Syncope caused by complete heart block is called the _____-_____ syndrome.
26. Define ventricular tachycardia.

27. Tall, peaked T waves are characteristic of which electrolyte disturbance?
28. Name three causes of ST segment elevations.
29. A patient experiencing typical angina pectoris with exertion may show what ECG pattern as a sign of subendocardial ischemia?
30. Right bundle branch block is always a sign of serious organic heart disease *(true or false)*.
31. Atrial fibrillation is always a sign of serious organic heart disease *(true or false)*.
32. Left bundle branch block is often a sign of serious organic heart disease *(true or false)*.
33. The *early repolarization* pattern is a normal variant *(true or false)*.
34. Prinzmetal's angina is characterized by ST segment elevations *(true or false)*.
35. With an acute anterior wall infarction, leads II, III, and aV_F are likely to show ST segment _____.
36. Retrograde P waves are characteristic of _____ rhythm.
37. Draw a QS complex.
38. A wide (>0.12 sec) QS complex in lead V_1 is seen with _____.
39. Name five causes of ventricular ectopy.
40. A 20-year-old college student complaining of light-headedness and palpitations is found to have a regular tachycardia with narrow QRS complexes at a rate of 200 beats/min. The most likely diagnosis is _____.
41. A patient is found to have a pulse rate of 35 beats/min. The ECG is most likely to show one of five basic rhythms. Name them.
42. Left axis deviation is defined as an axis more negative than −_____°.
43. Name three causes of sinus bradycardia.
44. Name three causes of atrial fibrillation.
45. Persistent ST segment elevations several weeks following a transmural myocardial infarct suggest a possible _____.
46. Which of the following tachycardias is most likely to terminate abruptly following carotid sinus massage: sinus tachycardia, atrial fibrillation, paroxysmal atrial tachycardia, or ventricular tachycardia?
47. A wide biphasic P wave in lead V_1 may indicate _____.
48. Which of the following drugs may shorten the QT interval: digitalis, quinidine, procainamide, furosemide (Lasix)?
49. Normally the QRS width is equal to or less than 0._____second.
50. A qR complex is normally seen in which lead: V_1, V_6, or aV_R?

Define the Following Terms

51. "R on T" phenomenon (p. 203)
52. Ectopic beat (p. 173)
53. Current of injury (p. 104)
54. P mitrale (p. 77)
55. P pulmonale (p. 74)
56. Bifascicular block (p. 219)
57. Frontal plane leads (p. 33)
58. Horizontal plane leads (p. 34)
59. Hyperacute T wave (p. 104)
60. Vertical QRS axis, horizontal QRS axis (p. 50)

Draw the QRS-T Pattern You Would Expect to See in Lead V_6 (for nos. 61 to 65)

61. Normal pattern
62. Left bundle branch block
63. Right bundle branch block
64. Left ventricular hypertrophy with stain
65. Digitalis effect

66. Is sinus rhythm present on the ECG below?

67. What drug could have produced these ST-T changes?

68. What ventricular conduction disturbance is present here?

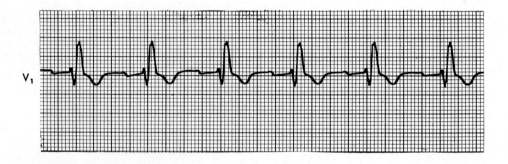

69. What is this heart rhythm?

70. What is X?

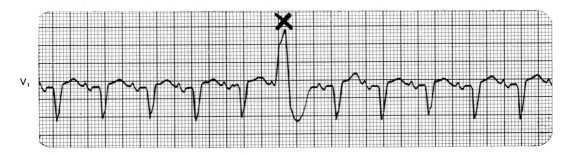

71. Calculate the mean QRS axis in *A* and *B*.

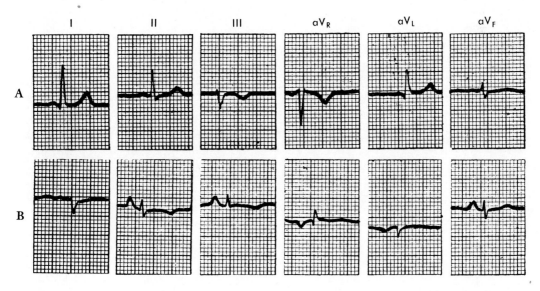

72. Calculate the mean QRS axis in these leads.

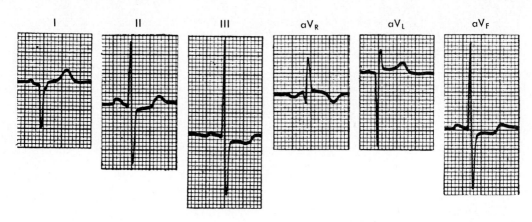

73. Is the mean QRS axis in this example normal, right, or left?

74. a. What is the major abnormality shown here?
    b. What factors can produce this abnormality?

75. What is this heart rhythm?

76. a. What is the approximate heart rate?
    b. The P wave suggests what abnormality?

77. a. What is the approximate heart rate?
    b. What arrhythmia is present here?

78. What type of AV conduction disturbance is present?

79. Identify beats A and B.

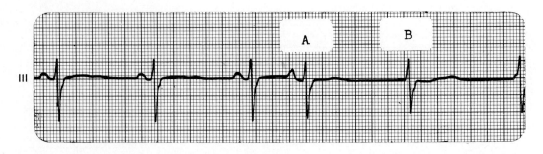

80. a. What arrhythmia is present?
    b. Of what symptom might this patient be complaining?

81. Of what symptom might the patient whose rhythm strip is shown below be complaining?

82. What type of conduction disturbance is present here?

83. What is the arrhythmia shown here?

Identify the Rhythm in Each Case
(for nos. 84 to 111)

84.

85.

86.

87.

88.

89.

90.

91.

92.

93.

94.

Monitor lead

95.

II

96.

aV_R

97.

II

98.

Monitor lead

99.

II

100.

II

101.

Monitor lead

102.

103.

104.

105.

106.

II

107.

aV_R

108.

V₁

109.

II

110.

111.

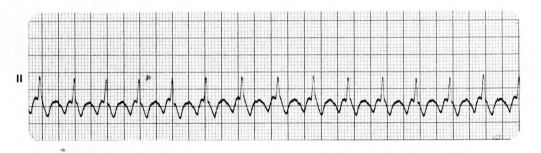

112. What two abnormalities are present here?

113. What two conduction disturbances are present?

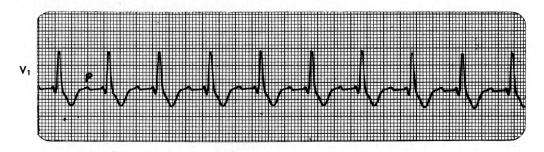

114. What three abnormalities are present here?

115. What abnormality is present here?

116. What conduction disturbance is present?

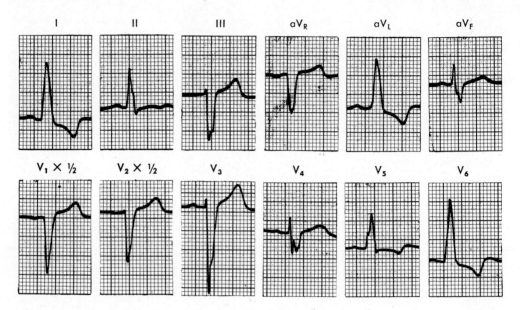

Interpret These ECGs Fully According to the Method Suggested in Chapter 21
(for nos. 117 to 121)

117.

118.

119.

120.

121.

122. What is the major ECG diagnosis here?

123. Answer these questions about the following ECG:
   a. Is it normally standardized?
   b. What is the heart rate?
   c. Is sinus rhythm present?
   d. What is the mean QRS axis?
   e. Is axis deviation present?
   f. Is the QRS voltage normal?
   g. What is the major abnormality?

124. Answer these questions about the following ECG:
    a. What is the approximate heart rate?
    b. What evidence is there of myocardial infarction?

125. The following rhythm strip shows
    a. Frequent premature atrial contraction
    b. Complete heart block
    c. 3:2 AV Wenckebach
    d. Multifocal atrial tachycardia

II

126. The following rhythm strip shows
    a. Atrial fibrillation
    b. Paroxysmal atrial tachycardia
    c. Multifocal atrial tachycardia
    d. Atrial bigeminy

127. The ECG strip below, obtained during an exercise test, shows
    a. Ventricular tachycardia
    b. ST changes consistent with acute transmural infarction
    c. ST changes consistent with Prinzmetal's angina
    d. ST changes consistent with acute subendocardial ischemia

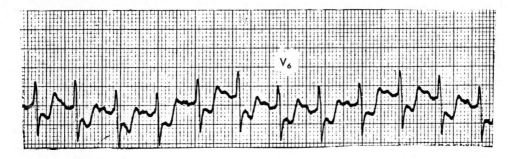

128. Answer these questions from the following ECG:
    a. What waveform is abnormally prominent here?
    b. What are the major causes for this finding?

129. What wave does the arrow in V_5 point to, and what is the significance of this wave?

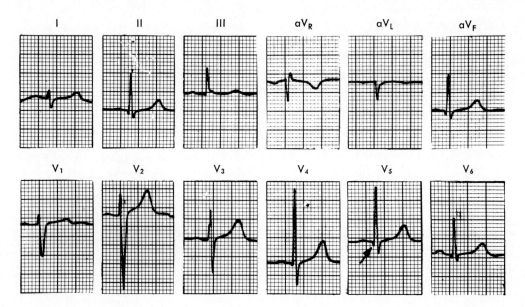

130. A patient complaining of severe chest pain had abnormally elevated cardiac enzymes. Using the ECG shown below, what is the clinical diagnosis?

131. Answer these questions about the following ECG:
    a. What is the rhythm?
    b. What conduction disturbance is present?

132. A 50-year-old man is complaining of chest pain. What is the cause of his complaint?

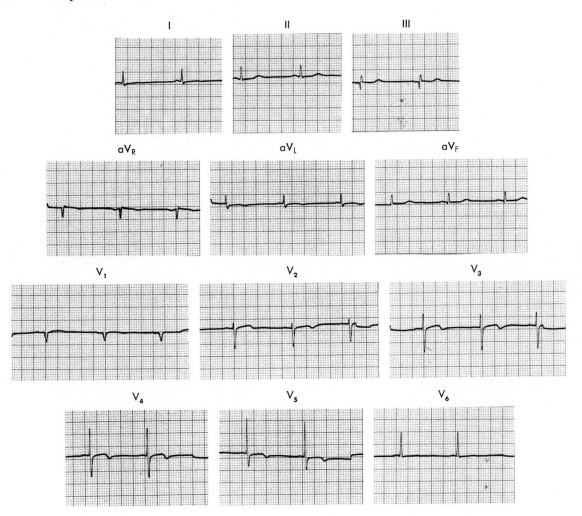

133. What is this rhythm?

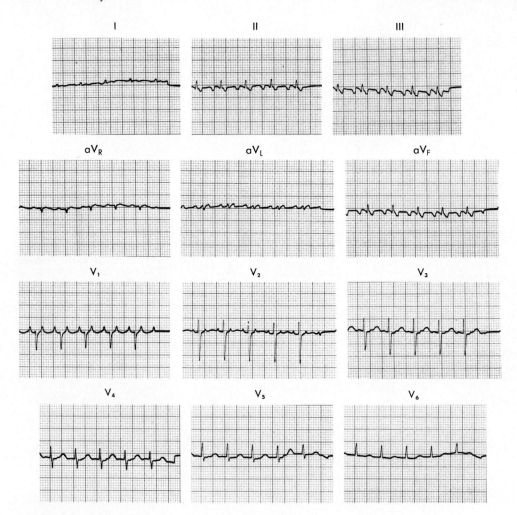

134. What arrhythmia is present here?

135. What is the major ECG diagnosis?

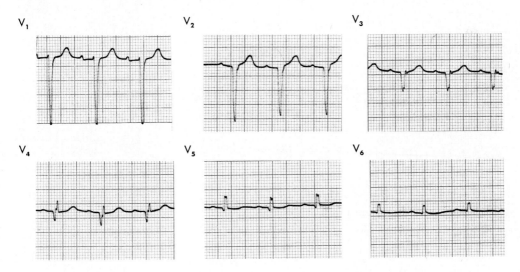

136. A patient presenting with palpitations received carotid sinus massage. What is the arrhythmia?

137. This patient's ECG was normal 3 days ago. What is the diagnosis from this repeat ECG?

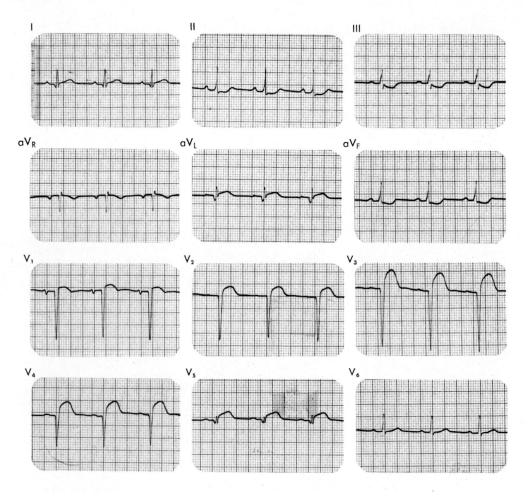

138. This lead II rhythm strip shows what four abnormalities?

139. What is this rhythm?

140. A 41-year-old man is complaining of "indigestion." What is the diagnosis?

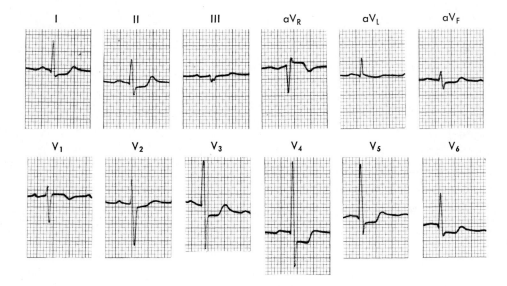

141. What is this rhythm?

Lead II: continuous

142. What is this rhythm?

V₁

143. Name the major abnormalities here.

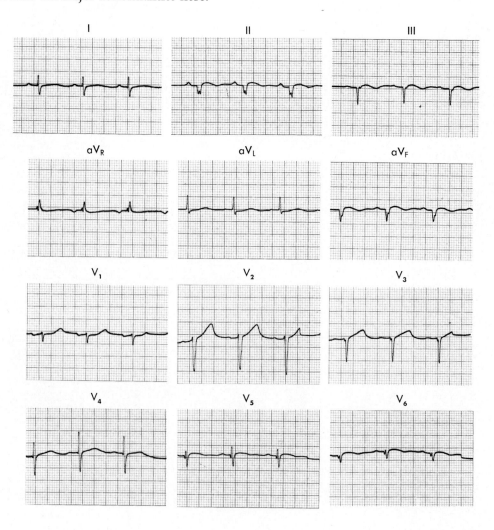

144. Name the major abnormalities here.

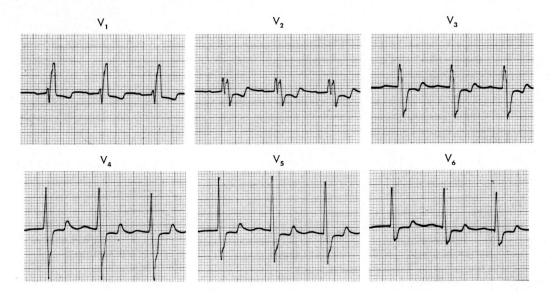

145. Name the major abnormalities here.

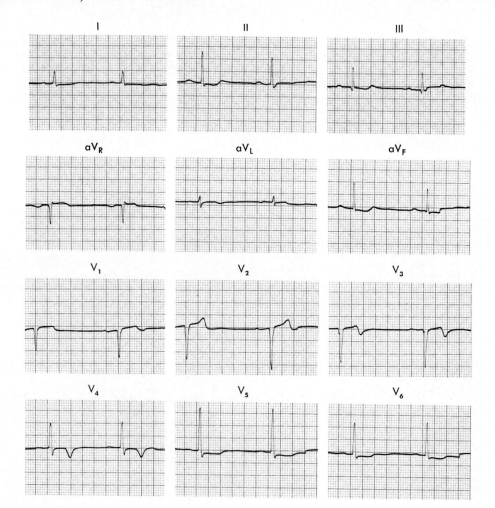

146. What is this arrhythmia?

147. What is this arrhythmia?

148. What is this rhythm?

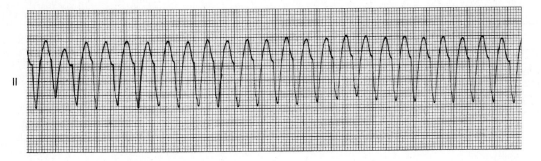

149. Following is the preoperative ECG of a 45-year-old-man. What is the diagnosis?

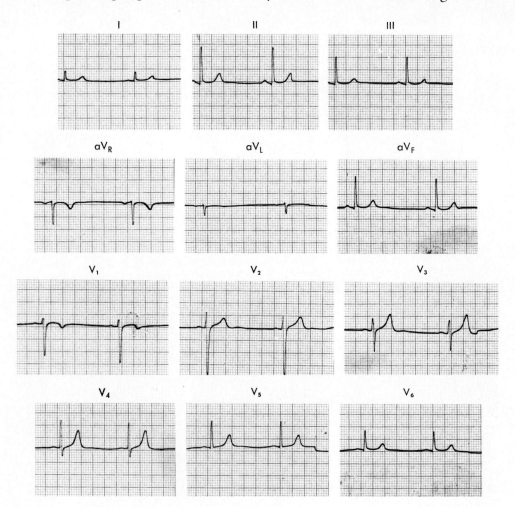

150. Following is the preoperative ECG of a 65-year-old woman. What is the diagnosis?

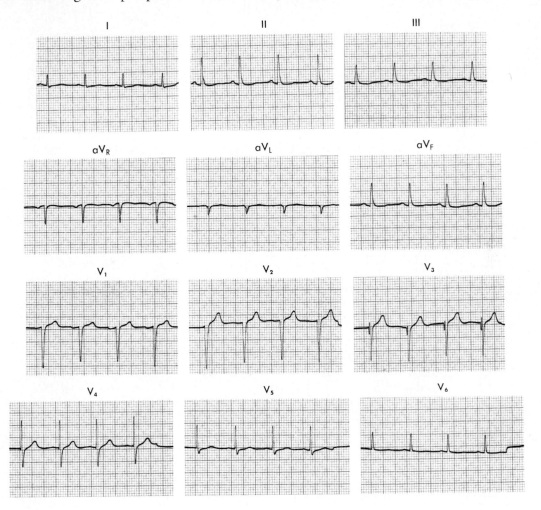

151. What caused this patient's syncope?

Monitor lead

152. The following ECG is from a 60-year-old man with hypertension. What are the findings?

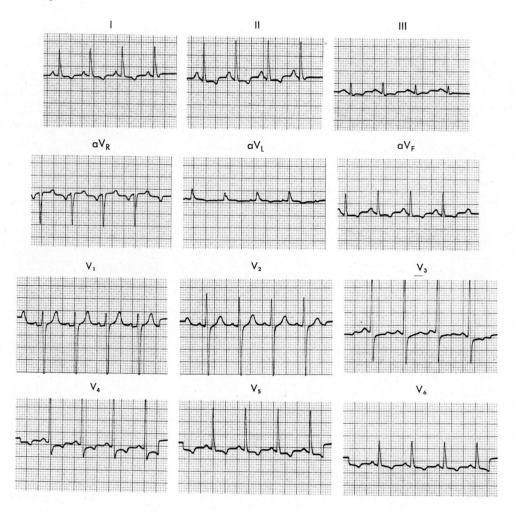

153. The following ECG is from a 24-year-old healthy male student. What is the diagnosis?

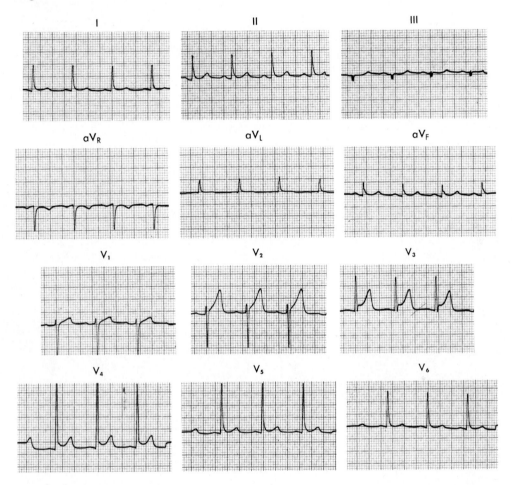

154. The following ECG is from a 50-year-old dialysis patient complaining of sharp, pleuritic chest pain. What is the cause of the complaint?

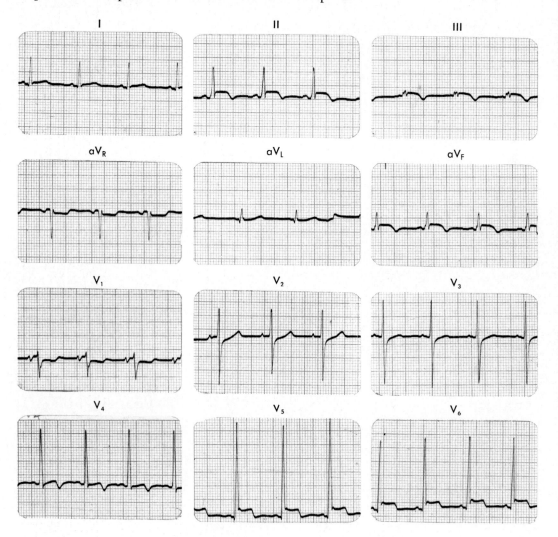

155. The following ECG is from a 62-year-old man. Describe the major abnormalities.

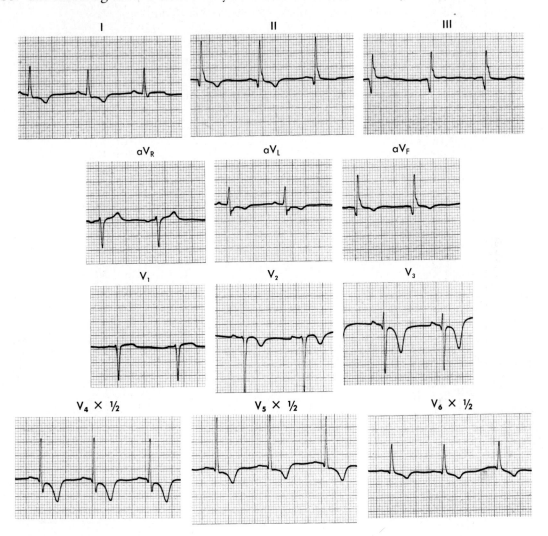

156. The following ECG is from a 40-year-old man who had been told that his ECG showed evidence of a prior "heart attack." Patient's major complaint was intermittent palpitations. What is the diagnosis?

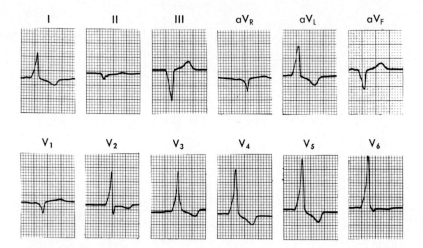

157. The following ECG is from a 59-year-old woman. Describe the major findings.

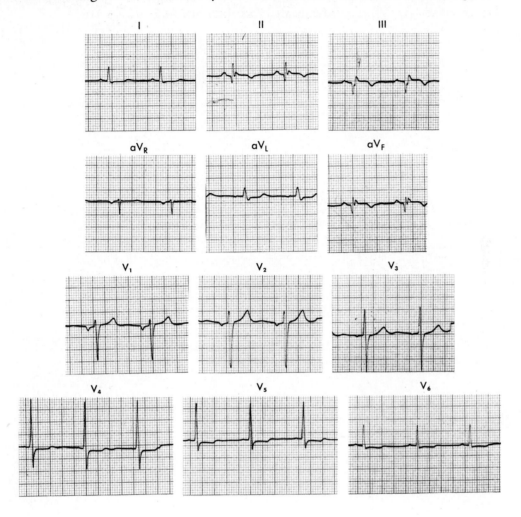

158. The following ECG is from a 50-year-old woman with suspected recurrent pulmonary emboli. What are the major ECG abnormalities?

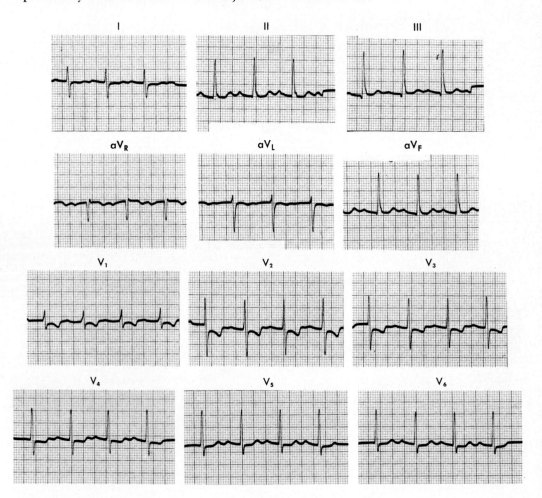

159. The following ECG is from a 20-year-old woman with chest pain. What is the diagnosis?

160. What abnormality might have caused the change from *A* to *B*?
    a. Hypocalcemia
    b. Hyperkalemia
    c. Hypokalemia
    d. Digitalis

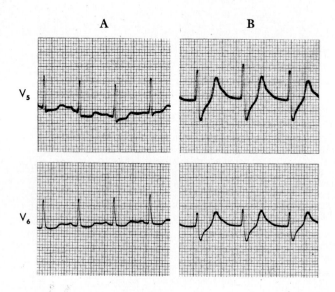

161. What is the cause of the wide QRS complexes?

162. What is this rhythm?

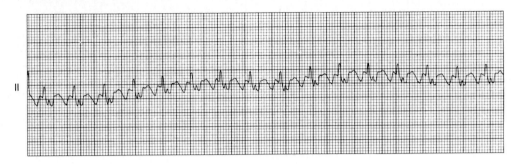

163. What are the notable findings here?

164. What is this rhythm?

165. What is this rhythm and what clinical condition do you suspect?

166. What is this rhythm and what clinical condition do you suspect?

167. What metabolic problem was corrected in this patient, accounting for the marked change on the ECG from one day, *A,* to the next, *B*?

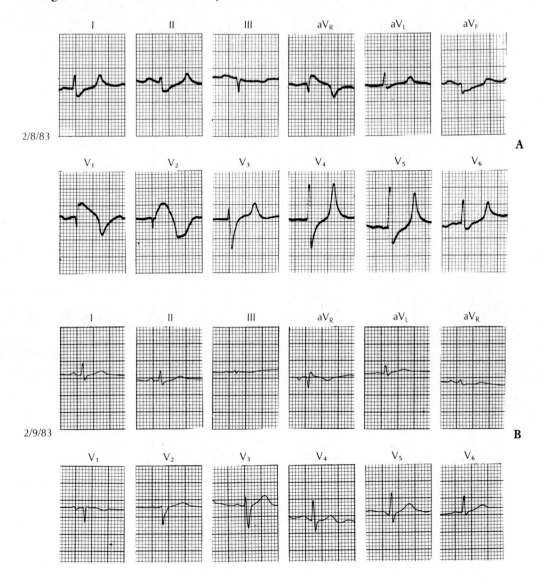

168. What type of conduction disturbance is present here?

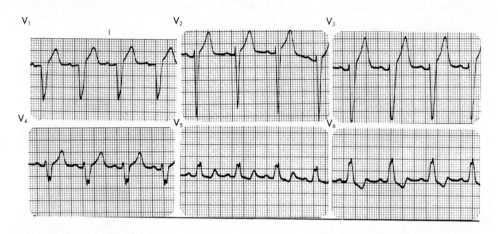

169. This patient's bradycardia is associated with what rhythm?

170. A patient with an evolving inferior infarction developed intermittent wide QRS complexes. What are these beats?

171. A 44-year-old woman with a history of intermittent atrial fibrillation complains of palpitations. What drug is she probably taking, and what is the arrhythmia?

172. This patient is being seen in the emergency room with pulmonary edema that developed over the past 2 days. What are the major ECG findings?

173. A 48-year-old man complains of intermittent palpitations. What arrhythmia does he have?

174. A 70-year-old man taking propranolol for hypertension comes to the emergency room complaining of light-headedness and weakness for the past week. What does his monitor lead rhythm strip show?

MONITOR LEAD

175. A 70-year-old man was given verapamil for treatment of angina. What does his rhythm strip show?

176. A 76-year-old woman complains that her "heart skips beats." What does her rhythm strip show?

177. A 72-year-old man develops an acute left hemiparesis. What etiology does his ECG suggest?

178. A 92-year-old man loses consciousness while eating dinner. What does his rhythm strip indicate?

179. A 54-year-old psychiatrist complains of palpitations after an argument with a "significant other." What does his ECG show?

LEAD II

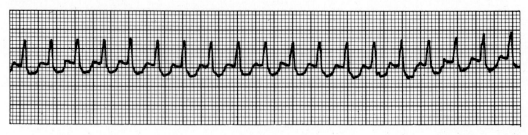

180. This ECG was initially misinterpreted as showing "accelerated idioventricular rhythm." What is the correct diagnosis?

181. A 60-year-old man is admitted with severe congestive heart failure. His ECG is identical to one recorded 6 months earlier. Cardiac enzymes are normal. What is the diagnosis?

182. A 27-year-old man is told he has "congenital heart disease." Except for some mild exertional fatigue, he feels fine. He is not cyanotic on physical examination, and a systolic ejection murmur is heard. What does his ECG show, and what is the likely clinical diagnosis?

183. A 37-year-old man with intermittent palpitations. What does his ECG show?

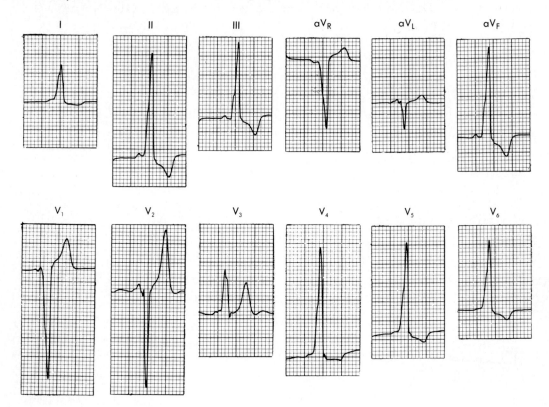

184. A 75-year-old woman treated with quinidine for atrial arrhythmias has a cardiac arrest 4 days later. This rhythm strip was obtained. What does it show?

MONITOR LEAD

185. An 80-year-old woman complained of light-headedness. The following rhythm strip was obtained in the coronary care unit. What conduction disturbance is present?

MONITOR LEAD

Answers

1. Atrial depolarization (stimulation).
2. Ventricular depolarization (stimulation).
3. Ventricular repolarization (recovery).
4. 0.12 and 0.2.
5. Fourth.
6. Lengthens.
7. Wolff-Parkinson-White syndrome.
8. Quinidine, procainamide, and others.
9. Pericardial effusion, emphysema, and obesity. Also extensive myocardial fibrosis or infiltration with substances like amyloid. Low voltage may also be a normal variant.
10. Ventricular ectopy (PVCs, ventricular bigeminy, ventricular tachycardia, ventricular fibrillation, bidirectional tachycardia), sinus bradycardia and SA block, junctional rhythms, PAT with block, and so on. (See p. 229.)
11. RBBB.
12. Right axis shift, $S_I Q_{III}$ pattern, RBBB, sinus tachycardia and other arrhythmias, right ventricular strain. (See p. 149 for other patterns.)
13. +5 mm. Recall that the voltages of the P wave, QRS complex, and T wave in leads $aV_R + aV_L + aV_F$ must equal 0.
14. Hypokalemia and renal insufficiency; also hypoxia, hypercalcemia, hypomagnesemia, old age, and others. (See p. 229.)
15. Decreases.
16. 250.
17. Hypokalemia.
18. P pulmonale (right atrial enlargement).
19. aV_R, II.
20. See p. 59.
21. One.
22. Hyperthyroidism.

23. Ventricular fibrillation (and related ventricular tachyarrhythmias), asystole (with or without escape beats), and electromechanical dissociation.
24. Fever, excitement, and congestive heart failure. (See p. 166 for other causes.)
25. Stokes-Adams.
26. Three or more consecutive PVCs.
27. Hyperkalemia.
28. Acute myocardial infarction, acute pericarditis, Prinzmetal's angina; also ventricular aneurysm.
29. ST segment depressions.
30. False. Some normal people will show an RBBB pattern.
31. False. Atrial fibrillation, although usually seen in people with organic heart disease (coronary, hypertensive, valvular, and so on), may occasionally occur in people with normal hearts.
32. True.
33. True. (See p. 149.)
34. True.
35. Depressions (reciprocal to the ST elevations seen in the anterior leads).
36. AV junctional or sometimes ectopic atrial.
37. See p. 14.
38. LBBB.
39. Myocardial ischemia, digitalis toxicity, hypokalemia, hypoxia, pulmonary embolism, and congestive heart failure. (See p. 204 for additional causes.)
40. Paroxysmal atrial tachycardia.
41. Sinus bradycardia, AV junctional rhythm, AV heart block (second or third degree) or AV dissociation, atrial fibrillation or flutter with a slow ventricular response, or idioventricular escape rhythm.

42. −30°.
43. Normal variant, drugs such as propranolol (Inderal), digitalis toxicity, increased vagal tone caused by myocardial ischemia, and so on.
44. Coronary artery disease, hypertensive heart disease, and mitral valve disease.
45. Ventricular aneurysm.

46. Paroxysmal atrial tachycardia.
47. Left atrial enlargement.
48. Digitalis.
49. 0.1 second.
50. V_6.
51-60. See pages listed.
61-65. See diagrams below.

66. No. There are no P waves visible on this rhythm strip from lead II because a junctional rhythm is present.
67. Digitalis.
68. RBBB is present with wide rSR' complexes in lead V_1. (In addition, first degree AV block is present.)
69. Sinus bradycardia.
70. Ventricular premature contraction.
71. *A.* 0°.
    B. +180°.
    In both *A* and *B,* lead aV_F shows a biphasic RS-type complex; thus the mean QRS axis must be directed at right angles to the lead axis of aV_F, which is +90°. In example *A* lead I shows a positive R wave deflection, so the axis must be pointed in that direction (at 0°). In example *B* the mean QRS axis is directed at right angles to lead aV_F, away from lead I, and toward leads III and aV_R, or at +180° (marked right axis deviation).
72. +150°. Lead II shows a biphasic RS complex; thus the mean QRS axis must be directed at right angles to the axis of lead II, which is at +60°. Therefore, the axis must be either −30° or +150°. Obviously, since lead I is negative and leads II and aV_R are mainly positive, the axis must be +150°. This indicates right axis deviation.
73. Left.
74. a. The QT interval is markedly prolonged (QT = 0.44 second with heart rate of 94/min).
    b. QT prolongation may be caused by numerous factors including hypocalcemia, hypokalemia (often with large U waves), drugs such as quinidine or procainamide, myocardial infarction (with deep T wave inversions), and so on.

75. Atrial flutter. Note the characteristic sawtooth flutter waves. The atrial (flutter) rate is approximately 300 beats/min, while the ventricular (QRS) rate is about 75 beats/min; thus 4:1 flutter is present.
76. a. 100 beats/min.
    b. Left atrial abnormality,
77. a. About 130 beats/min. (There are about 13 QRS cycles/6 sec.) (See p. 18.)
    b. Atrial fibrillation. Often, as in this case, with rapid atrial fibrillation, the fibrillation waves are not well seen. The diagnosis of atrial fibrillation is then made by finding a haphazardly irregular rhythm with no visible P waves.
78. First-degree AV block (PR interval is about 0.22 sec). Note also that the QRS complex is somewhat wide, about 0.11 sec, indicating some type of intraventricular conduction disturbance as well.
79. *A* is a premature atrial contraction (PAC). *B* is a junctional escape beat.
80. a. Complete heart block. To analyze this arrhythmia, label each P wave and each QRS complex. The ventricular rate is about 40 beats/min. Looking at the P waves (some of which are hidden by QRS complexes and T waves), you can see that the atrial rate is 90 to 100 beats/min and the PR intervals are completely variable. Therefore, complete heart block is present. The QRS complexes are abnormally wide because the ventricles are being paced by an idioventricular focus located below the AV junction.
    b. The patient complained of light-headedness and fainting spells (Stokes-Adams syndrome).

81. Angina. The ECG shows ischemic ST segment depressions.
82. RBBB.
83. Atrial fibrillation with rapid ventricular rate.
84. Normal sinus rhythm.
85. Atrial fibrillation.
86. Sinus arrhythmia.
87. Sinus rhythm with multiform PVCs.
88. Sinus tachycardia (nonspecific ST-T changes are also present).
89. Ventricular fibrillation.
90. Ventricular tachycardia.
91. Atrial fibrillation.
92. Sinus rhythm with first-degree AV block.
93. Sinus rhythm with premature atrial contractions (third, sixth, and ninth beats are PACs; therefore, this is atrial trigeminy).
94. Sinus rhythm with premature ventricular contractions (second and sixth beats are PVCs).
95. Sinus bradycardia. (Note also the abnormal ST-T segment because of left ventricular strain or ischemia.)
96. AV junctional rhythm (note the absence of visible P waves).
97. Sinus tachycardia with short burst of ventricular tachycardia. The ninth beat is also a PVC.
98. Sinus rhythm with PAC (fourth beat).
99. Atrial flutter with variable block.
100. Paroxysmal atrial (or junctional) tachycardia.
101. Ventricular bigeminy.
102. Coarse atrial fibrillation with incomplete RBBB (note the rSR′ in lead V_1).
103. Ventricular escape rhythm.
104. Atrial fibrillation with rapid ventricular response. The rate is irregular with slight undulation of the baseline.
105. Ventricular trigeminy. Every second sinus beat is followed by a PVC.
106. Coarse atrial fibrillation.
107. Junctional rhythm. Note the absence of visible P waves.
108. Paced rhythm. Note the pacemaker spike before each QRS and the nonconducted P waves (some hidden). The latter indicate underlying complete heart block.
109. Junctional tachycardia. Note the retrograde P waves in lead II.
110. Ventricular tachycardia.
111. Atrial flutter with 2:1 block (atrial rate, about 300 beats/min; ventricular rate, about 150 beats/min).
112. Lead II rhythm strip shows marked ST segment elevations (caused by acute inferior wall infarction) with junctional rhythm (note the retrograde P waves preceding each QRS complex).
113. First-degree AV block with RBBB (note the wide rSR′ complex in lead V_1).
114. a. First-degree AV block (PR interval, 0.32 sec).
    b. Abnormal Q wave caused by inferior wall infarction.
    c. Abnormally wide QRS complex (0.11 sec) from ventricular conduction disturbance.
115. Pacemaker rhythm with pacemaker malfunction. Note the pacemaker spike in the center of the strip, which is not followed by a QRS complex owing to pacemaker failure.
116. LBBB.
117. a. Analysis
    1. Standardization was normal; mark not shown.
    2. Heart rate: about 60 beats/min.
    3. Rhythm: normal sinus.
    4. PR interval: about 0.16 second (normal).
    5. P wave size: biphasic P wave is lead V_1 suggests possible left atrial enlargement, although the P waves in other leads are within normal limits.
    6. QRS width: 0.1 second (upper limits of normal).

7. QT interval: about 0.4 second (normal for rate).
8. QRS voltage: R wave in lead aV_L is abnormally tall (15 mm).
9. Mean QRS axis: about $-60°$. The R wave in lead aV_L equals the S wave in lead aV_F, so the mean QRS axis must lie between the positive pole of lead aV_L ($-30°$) and the negative pole of lead aV_F ($-90°$). Therefore, the mean QRS axis must be approximately $-60°$.
10. R wave progression in chest leads: poor with QS complexes in leads V_1 to V_3.
11. Abnormal Q waves: leads V_1 to V_3 show abnormal QS complexes. Note the bizarre W-shaped QS complex in lead V_3.
12. ST segment: there is ST elevation in lead V_2 with slight depression in leads V_3 to V_6.
13. T waves: inverted in leads I, aV_L, and V_4 to V_6, with some scooping of the ST segment in leads I and aV_L.
14. U waves: normal.

b. Interpretation

Left axis deviation consistent with left anterior hemiblock.

Abnormal QS complexes in leads V_1 to V_3 consistent with anteroseptal infarction of indeterminate age.

Left ventricular hypertrophy by voltage.

Left atrial abnormality.

Abnormal ST-T changes consistent with left ventricular strain, and/or ischemia, and possibly with digitalis effect (with scooping of ST-T in leads I and aV_L). (The ST-T changes on this ECG are somewhat complicated. As noted, the T wave inversions and slight ST depressions in leads V_3 to V_6 may reflect a combination of left ventricular strain and/or lateral wall ischemia. The scooping of the ST-T segment in leads I and aV_L may also reflect strain or ischemia but are suggestive of the classic pattern of digitalis effect as well. Finally, note the high takeoff of the ST segment in lead V_2, suggesting acute infarction. However, in cases of LVH the right precordial leads may show such ST segment elevation as a persistent finding in the absence of acute ischemia.)

118. a. Analysis
1. Standardization normal; mark not shown.
2. Heart rate: approximately 40 beats/min.
3. Rhythm: sinus bradycardia.
4. PR interval: about 0.18 second.
5. P wave size: biphasic P wave in lead V_1 suggests possible left atrial abnormality.
6. QRS width: 0.1 to 0.11 second.
7. QT interval: 0.52 second (within normal limits for rate).
8. QRS voltage: tall voltage in chest leads ($SV_1 + RV_6$ = more than 35 mm).
9. Mean QRS axis: about $+30°$; R waves of equal amplitude in leads I and II so the mean QRS axis must be directed between these leads.
10. R wave progression in chest leads: delayed R wave progression with the transition zone between leads V_4 and V_5.
11. Abnormal Q waves: none.
12. ST segments: isoelectric.
13. T waves: inversion in leads I, II, aV_L, V_5, and V_6.
14. U waves: small in leads V_2 to V_4.

b. Interpretation

Marked sinus bradycardia.

Left ventricular hypertrophy by voltage. ST-T changes are consistent with left ventricular strain and possibly ischemia.

Possible left atrial abnormality.

In this case, the left ventricular hypertrophy and atrial enlargement resulted from hypertensive heart disease. The marked sinus bradycardia was caused by one of the drugs (beta-blockers) that the patient was taking for high blood pressure.

119. a. Analysis

1. Standardization normal; mark not shown.
2. Heart rate: approximately 75 beats/min.
3. Rhythm: junctional or ectopic atrial rhythm. (Note the retrograde P waves in lead II with biphasic P waves in lead aV_R.)
4. PR interval: 0.1. (The PR interval is short because of junctional rhythm.)
5. P wave size: normal.
6. QRS width: 0.08 second.
7. QT interval: 0.35 second (normal for rate).
8. QRS voltage: tall voltage in lead aV_L (R wave = 16 mm).
9. QRS axis: approximately $-45°$. (The R wave in lead I is about equal to the S wave in lead aV_F. Therefore the mean QRS axis must lie midway between the positive pole of lead I [$0°$] and the negative pole of lead aV_F [$-90°$], making the axis $-45°$. Furthermore, by inspection, you can tell that left axis deviation is present [axis more negative than $-30°$], since lead II shows an rS

complex with the S wave deeper than the r wave is tall.) (See p. 65.)

10. R wave progression in the chest leads: delayed R wave progression with QS complexes in leads V_1 to V_3.
11. Abnormal Q waves: QS complexes in leads V_1 to V_3. Abnormally wide Q wave in lead aV_L. (Note that the Q wave in lead aV_L is 0.04 sec wide, making it abnormal even though it is not very deep.)
12. ST segments: slightly elevated in leads V_2 to V_4.
13. T waves: deeply inverted and symmetric in leads I, II, aV_L, and V_2 to V_6.
14. U waves: normal.

b. Interpretation

Abnormal ECG.

Junctional or ectopic atrial rhythm.

LVH by voltage.

Left axis deviation consistent with left anterior hemiblock.

Abnormal Q waves and T wave inversions consistent with evolving anterior wall infarction. The exact age of the infarct cannot be deduced from the ECG. In this case it was 1 week old.

120. a. Analysis

1. Standardization normal; mark shown in lead V_1.
2. Heart rate: approximately 75 beats/min, with slight irregularity.
3. Rhythm: normal sinus, with both premature atrial contractions (in leads I, aV_F, V_2, and V_6) and premature ventricular contractions (third beat in lead V_1).
4. PR interval: 0.12 second (lower limits of normal).

5. P wave size: biphasic P wave in lead V_1 (suggesting left atrial abnormality).
6. QRS width: 0.12 to 13 second. (The RSR' in lead V_1 suggests RBBB.)
7. QT interval: 0.36 second (normal for rate).
8. QRS voltage: normal.
9. Mean QRS axis: $+90°$ (Note the phasic RS wave in lead I.)
10. R wave progression in chest leads: normal.
11. Abnormal Q waves: wide Q waves in leads II, III, and aV_F.
12. ST segments: normal.
13. T waves: slight inversion in leads II, III, and aV_F.
14. U waves: normal.

b. Interpretation
Abnormal ECG.
Sinus rhythm with atrial and ventricular ectopy.
RBBB.
Left atrial abnormality.
Inferior wall infarct of indeterminate age.

121. a. Analysis
1. Standardization normal; mark not shown.
2. Heart rate: 55 to 60 beats/min.
3. Rhythm: sinus bradycardia.
4. PR interval: 0.16 second.
5. P wave size: normal.
6. QRS width: 0.08 second.
7. QT interval: 0.4 second (normal for rate).
8. QRS voltage: upper normal limits.
9. QRS axis: $+30°$
10. R wave progression in chest leads: normal.
11. Abnormal Q waves: none.
12. ST segments: isoelectric in the extremity leads; slightly elevated J point in leads V_2 and V_3.

13. T waves: normal.
14. U waves: normal.

b. Interpretation
Normal electrocardiogram. The ST elevation in the chest leads represents a normal "early repolarization" variant.

122. Major finding is ST segment elevations and hyperacute T waves in anterior chest leads (V_1 to V_5) with reciprocal ST segment depressions in leads II, III, and aV_F. (This patient was having an acute anterior wall infarction.)

123. a. Yes. (Note that the standardization mark in lead I is 10 mm tall.)
b. 60 beats/min.
c. Yes.
d. $+30°$.
e. No.
f. Yes.
g. Ischemic T wave inversions in leads I, aV_L, and V_2 to V_6. (Clinically the patient had an evolving MI.)

124. a. 60 beats/min.
b. Prominent Q waves in leads II, III, and aV_F with ST segment elevations in those leads and reciprocal ST depressions in leads I, aV_L, and V_2 to V_3; deep T wave inversions in leads II, III, aV_F, and V_4 to V_6. (This pattern is consistent with evolving inferolateral infarct.)

125. c.
126. c.
127. d.
128. a. Prominent U waves.
b. The two major causes are hypokalemia and drug effect (particularly, quinidine, procainamide, disopyramide [Norpace]). (This patient was hypokalemic. Patients on quinidine who develop markedly prolonged repolarization with large U waves may, in addition, be at risk of developing torsades de pointes [p. 209].)

129. This is a normal "septal" q wave, representing left-to-right spread of septal depolarization forces. (Note the low amplitude and short duration [less than 0.04 sec] of this q wave.)

130. Subendocardial infarction. (Note the diffuse, marked ST depressions (I, II, III, aV$_F$, and V$_3$ to V$_6$) with reciprocal ST elevation in aV$_R$. These changes indicate actual subendocardial ischemia or infarction.)

131. a. Sinus tachycardia.
    b. Left anterior hemiblock. Note marked left axis deviation, with normal duration QRS.

132. ECG showing abnormal T wave inversions in aV$_L$ and V$_3$ to V$_5$, suggesting myocardial ischemia, with or without actual infarction.

133. Atrial flutter with 2:1 AV conduction. (The atrial rate is about 300/min, and the ventricular rate is about 150/min. Note the positive flutter waves in V$_1$ and the negative flutter waves in lead II. The classic sawtooth configuration may not be seen in all leads [for example, V$_1$ here]. Low voltage in the limb leads is also present.)

134. Atrial bigeminy.

135. Prior anterior wall MI. (Note the loss of normal R wave progression, with pathologic Q waves in V$_2$ to V$_5$.)

136. Paroxysmal atrial tachycardia (PAT) converting abruptly to normal sinus rhythm. (Note the sudden slowing of heart rate and appearance of P waves.)

137. Acute anterior wall MI. (Note the pathologic Q waves in V$_1$ to V$_5$ and aV$_L$, with ST segment elevations in these leads and reciprocal ST depression in II, III, and aV$_F$.)

138. a. Left atrial abnormality (enlargement).
    b. First-degree AV block (PR = 0.24 sec).
    c. One PVC.

    d. Axis deviation. (Note the RS complex in lead II with S wave > R wave. Therefore, the axis must be more negative than −30° or more positive than +150°. You need two frontal plane leads to know if the axis is markedly leftward or rightward.)

139. PAT with 2:1 block. Note the two P waves for every QRS, with atrial rate of about 190/min and ventricular rate of about 95/min. This patient was suffering from digitalis toxicity.

140. Diffuse subendocardial ischemia. (Note the horizontal or downward sloping ST segment depression, best seen in leads I, II, aV$_F$, and V$_3$ to V$_6$, with ST elevation only in lead aV$_R$.)

141. Isorhythmic AV dissociation. (Atrial and ventricular rates are about equal, with P waves moving "in" and "out" of the QRS.) (See p. 221.)

142. Sinus tachycardia with atrial quadrigeminy (that is, every fourth beat is a PAC).

143. a. Prior inferior and anterolateral MIs, with Q waves in leads II, III, and aV$_F$, as well as the left chest leads, with T wave inversions.
    b. Borderline first-degree AV block PR is about 0.2 sec).
    c. QT prolongation (QT interval is 0.4 sec, which is long for a heart rate of about 77/min. The patient was taking quinidine, a drug that may prolong the QT interval.)
    d. Left axis deviation.

144. a. RBBB.
    b. First-degree AV block.
    c. Nonspecific ST-T abnormalities. Note that with "pure" RBBB one expects to see T wave inversions in leads with an rSR' complex, so-called secondary ST-T changes. However, the ST segments here are also abnormally depressed in leads I, II, aV$_F$, and V$_3$

to V_6. These "primary" ST-T changes are nonspecific and could have been caused by ischemia, digitalis effect, or other conditions.

145. a. Evolving anterior wall MI with Q waves in V_1 to V_3 and deep T wave inversions in V_3 and V_4. (The ST-T changes in the inferolateral leads are also suggestive of ischemia.)
    b. First-degree AV block.
    c. Probable left atrial abnormality (enlargement) with a broad, biphasic P wave in lead V_1.

146. Complete heart block. Note the independent atrial and ventricular complexes, with an atrial rate of about 100/min and a ventricular rate of 43/min.

147. Accelerated idioventricular rhythm (AIVR). The first three beats are sinus beats, followed by a run of wide QRS complexes at a rate of about 110/min. Note that the fourth QRS is actually a fusion beat resulting from simultaneous occurrence of a sinus beat and an idioventricular beat. AIVR is commonly observed during acute MI and is usually self-limited.

148. Ventricular tachycardia.

149. Normal ECG. (Note, however, that a "normal" ECG does not exclude significant underlying heart disease.)

150. Prior anteroseptal infarction. Note abnormal Q waves in leads V_1 to V_3

151. Complete heart block. (Note the independent atrial and ventricular complexes, with the ventricle being paced by a slow idioventricular pacemaker [wide QRS]. The combination of heart block and syncope is called the Stokes-Adams syndrome.)

152. LVH with strain. (Note the prominent chest lead voltage [S_{V_1} and R_{V_5} greater than 35 mm] with "strain" pattern. P waves are prominent, broad, and notched in lead III [consistent with left atrial abnormality]. Note also the relatively peaked P waves in lead II. In some cases left atrial abnormality causes tall P waves simulating right atrial enlargement, the so-called "pseudo–P pulmonale pattern.")

153. Normal variant "early repolarization." (Note the ST segment elevations [without reciprocal ST depressions] in leads V_2 to V_4.)

154. Acute pericarditis. (Note the ST elevations in leads I, II, III, aV_F, and V_4 to V_6, with T wave inversions in most of these leads. Diffuse distribution of ST elevations [present in I, II, and III] supports the clinical diagnosis of pericarditis. Note also the LVH by voltage with left atrial abnormality. The patient was hypertensive as a result of chronic renal disease and had uremic pericarditis.)

155. a. Inferior wall MI of indeterminate age with Q waves in leads II, III, and aV_F and T wave inversions.
    b. Anterior wall MI of indeterminate age with loss of R waves in V_1 to V_3 and Q waves in V_3 to V_5, as well as deep ischemic T wave inversions in I, aV_L, and V_2 to V_6.
    c. LVH. (Note the very prominent precordial voltage, with V_4 to V_6 recorded at one-half standardization.)

156. Wolff-Parkinson-White (WPW) preexcitation pattern. (Note the triad of short PR interval, wide QRS, and delta wave [slurring of the upstroke of QRS in V_2 and V_4 to V_6]. Q waves in the inferior leads were caused not by infarction but by abnormal ventricular activation [so-called pseudo-infarct Q waves]. Patients with WPW preexcitation are particularly susceptible to atrial tachyarrhythmias. A Holter monitor in this patient revealed runs of PAT as the cause of the palpitations.)

157. a. Prior inferior wall MI.
    b. Probable left atrial abnormality.
    c. Nonspecific ST-T changes in V_4 to V_6 (consistent with ischemia or other causes).

158. a. First-degree AV block.
    b. Right axis deviation. (Note the R wave in lead III greater than in lead II.)
    c. Right ventricular hypertrophy with strain. (Note the tall R wave in V_1 with T wave inversions in the right chest leads.)

159. Acute pericarditis. (Note the diffuse ST segment elevations in leads I, II, aV_F, and V_4 to V_6. This pattern differs from ST elevations of acute MI, which are more localized [anterior or inferior] with reciprocal changes. This pattern also differs from normal variant "early repolarization" [Fig. 10-10], which does not usually produce such marked ST elevations in V_5 and V_6 as are seen here. With normal variant early repolarization, the ST elevations are most prominent in V_3 and V_4.)

160. b. Hyperkalemia. (Note the widening of QRS, peaking of T waves, and loss of P waves [junctional rhythm].)

161. Wolff-Parkinson-White pattern. (Note the triad of short PR interval, wide QRS, and slurring on the QRS upstroke [delta wave].)

162. Atrial flutter with 2:1 conduction (block). Flutter waves at a rate of about 300/min (*arrows* in ECG below).

163. Sinus tachycardia and P pulmonale (right atrial enlargement).

164. AV junctional rhythm. Retrograde P waves following the QRS.

165. Multifocal atrial tachycardia (MAT), which is most commonly associated with chronic obstructive lung disease.

166. Paroxysmal atrial tachycardia (PAT) with 2:1 AV block. Note the P waves sitting on the T waves. (This arrhythmia is often, but not always, associated with digitalis toxicity.)

167. Severe hyperkalemia. The serum potassium was markedly elevated (8.1 mEq/L), and the ECG showed tall peaked T waves. (ST elevations in V_1 and V_2 may also be seen in this setting.) By the next day the serum potassium was normal (4.4 mEq/L).

168. Left bundle branch block.

169. Wandering atrial pacemaker. (Note the subtle change in P waves.)

170. Accelerated idioventricular rhythm (AIVR).

171. The ST-T changes are consistent with digitalis effect, and the rhythm is atrial bigeminy.

172. Evolving pattern of anterior wall infarction and right bundle branch block. Left atrial abnormality is also seen (V_1).

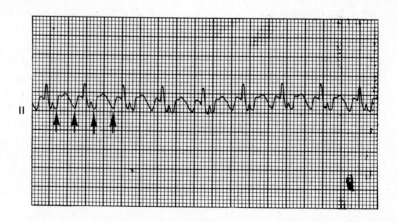

173. Atrial flutter with spontaneous conversion to sinus rhythm. Initially there is atrial flutter with 2:1 conduction. The degree of block increases just before conversion.

174. Sinus rhythm with 2:1 AV block. Because the QRS is of normal duration here, this arrythmia probably represents a Mobitz type I (Wenckebach) mechanism and not a Mobitz type II, which is usually associated with a wide QRS.

175. Sinus rhythm with AV Wenckebach. Nonconducted P waves are present on the T wave of the third and eighth QRS-T complexes. AV Wenckebach may be caused by a variety of factors, including drug toxicity (for example, digitalis, beta-blockers, and, in this case, verapamil).

176. Sinus rhythm with frequent premature atrial contractions (PACs) at the end of the strip. This type of rhythm may lead to sustained multifocal atrial tachycardia (MAT) or atrial fibrillation.

177. Atrial fibrillation may lead to left atrial thrombus formation and eventual embolization. An embolic-type cerebrovascular accident is therefore suggested. (Note that with rapid atrial fibrillation, fibrillatory waves may be hard to detect. The changes in QRS complexes here from one beat to the next may reflect variability in ventricular conduction due to the fast rate.)

178. Complete heart block. Note the independence of atrial (sinus) P wave activity (with a rate of about 88/min) and ventricular (QRS) complexes (at a rate of about 33/min). The combination of high-degree heart block and syncope is sometimes referred to as the Stokes-Adams syndrome. (This patient was treated with a permanent pacemaker.)

179. Paroxysmal atrial (or AV junctional) tachycardia (PAT).

180. Intermittent left bundle branch block. The first four beats are conducted with a left bundle branch block pattern, the last four with a normal QRS. In this case the bundle branch block was *rate related*. When the heart rate exceeded a critical value, the bundle branch block appeared. (Note that all the beats are preceded by a P wave with a constant PR interval. Therefore the rhythm could not be accelerated idioventricular.)

181. Sinus rhythm, left axis deviation, and an intraventricular conduction delay (QRS duration = 0.12 sec). The major abnormality is extensive anterior wall infarction with pathologic Q waves in leads aV_L and V_1 to V_6. In addition, the ST segments are elevated in these leads. Persistent ST segment elevation following infarction suggests a *ventricular aneurysm*, which was the cause of the patient's heart failure in this case.

182. The ECG shows right bundle branch block and right axis deviation. This pattern, given the patient's history and physical examination findings, is most suggestive of an atrial septal defect (p. 260).

183. Wolff-Parkinson-White (WPW) pattern. The triad of short PR interval, wide QRS, and slurring of the QRS upstroke (delta wave) is best seen in leads II, III, aV_F, and V_4 to V_6. WPW is often associated with supraventricular tachycardias (in particular, PAT), which may have been the source of this patient's chief complaint of palpitations.

184. The classic pattern of *torsades de pointes,* a form of ventricular tachycardia characterized by oscillations in QRS amplitude and axis in the same lead. This potentially fatal arrhythmia is usually seen in the setting of abnormally prolonged ventricular repolarization, evidenced by a long QT interval or prominent U wave. Drugs such as quinidine may cause the arrhythmia (quinidine syncope). (See p. 210 for other causes.)

185. There is underlying sinus bradycardia with a 2.4-second pause following the third beat. This pause is almost exactly twice the underlying PP interval. Therefore, this probably represents 2:1 SA block. In contrast to 2:1 AV block (in which a P wave is not followed by a QRS), in 2:1 SA block an entire P-QRS cycle is "dropped". The patient had "sick sinus syndrome" and required a permanent pacemaker.

Bibliography

Chapters 1 to 7

Goldberger, E.: Unipolar lead electrocardiography and vectorcardiography, ed. 3, Philadelphia, 1953, Lea & Febiger.

Klein, R.C., et al.: Electrocardiographic diagnosis of left ventricular hypertrophy in the presence of left bundle branch block, Am. Heart J. **108**:502, 1984.

Lipman, B.S., et al.: Clinical electrocardiography, ed. 7, Chicago, 1984, Year Book Medical Publishers, Inc.

Marriott, H.J.C.: Practical electrocardiography, ed. 7, Baltimore, 1983, The Williams & Wilkins Co.

Chapters 8 and 9

Goldberger, A.L.: Myocardial infarction: electrocardiographic differential diagnosis, ed. 3, St. Louis, 1984, The C.V. Mosby Co.

Goldberger, A.L.: Recognition of ECG pseudoinfarct patterns, Mod. Conc. Cardiovasc. Dis. **49**:13, 1980.

Goldberger, E.: Treatment of cardiac emergencies, ed. 4, St. Louis, 1985, The C.V. Mosby Co.

Chapter 10

Goldberger, A.: A specific ECG triad associated with congestive heart failure, PACE **5**:593, 1982.

Goldberger, E.: How to interpret electrocardiograms in terms of vectors, Springfield, Ill., 1968, Charles C Thomas, Publisher.

Goldman, M.J.: Principles of clinical electrocardiography, ed. 11, Los Altos, Calif., 1982, Lange Medical Publications.

Spodick, D.H.: Electrocardiographic responses to pulmonary embolism, Am. J. Cardiol. **30**:695, 1972.

Surawicz, B.: Relationship between electrocardiogram and electrolytes, Am. Heart J. **73**:814, 1967.

Chapters 11 to 21

Beller, G.A., et al.: Digitalis intoxication: a prospective clinical study with serum level correlations, N.Engl. J. Med. **284**:989, 1971.

Bellet, S.: Clinical disorders of the heart beat, ed. 3, Philadelphia, 1971, Lea & Febiger.

Chung, E.K.: Principles of cardiac arrhythmias, ed. 3, Baltimore, 1983, The Williams & Wilkins Co.

DeSilva, R.A., et al.: Cardioversion and defibrillation, Am. Heart J. **100**:881, 1980.

Goldberger, E.: Treatment of cardiac emergencies, ed. 4, St. Louis, 1985, The C.V. Mosby Co.

Josephson, M.E., and Kastor, J.A.: Supraventricular tachycardia: mechanisms and management, Ann. Intern. Med. **87**:346, 1977.

Josephson, M.E., and Wellens, H.J.J., editors: Tachycardias—mechanisms, diagnosis, treatment, Philadelphia, 1984, Lea & Febiger.

Kastor, J.A.: Atrioventricular heart block. I and II, N. Engl. J. Med. **292**:462, 572, 1975.

Ludmer, P.L., and Goldschlager, N.: Cardiac pacing in the 1980's, N. Engl. J. Med. **311**:1671, 1984.

Mancini, G.B.J., and Goldberger, A.L.: Cardioversion of atrial fibrillation: consideration of embolization, anticoagulation, prophylactic pacemaker, and long-term success, Am. Heart J. **104**:617, 1982.

McIntyre, K.M., and Lewis, A.J., editors: Textbook of advanced cardiac life support, Chicago, 1981, American Heart Association.

Moses, H.W., et al.: A practical guide to cardiac pacing, Boston, 1983, Little, Brown & Co.

Natural history of "high risk" bundle-branch block: final report of a prospective study. N. Engl. J. Med. **307**:137, 1982.

Smith, W.M., and Gallagher, J.J.: "Les torsades de pointes": an unusual ventricular arrhythmia, Ann. Intern. Med. **93**:578, 1980.

Standards and guidelines for cardiopulmonary resuscitation (CPR) and emergency cardiac care (ECC), J.A.M.A. **244**:453, 1980.

Wellens, H.J.J., et al.: The value of the electrocardiogram in the differential diagnosis of a tachycardia with a widened QRS complex, Am. J. Med. **64**:27, 1978.

Zipes, D., and Duffin, E.G.: Cardiac pacemakers. In Braunwald, E.B., editor: Heart disease: a textbook of cardiovascular medicine, ed. 2, Philadelphia, 1984, W.B. Saunders Co.

Index

A

Aberrant conduction, 250-253
Accelerated idioventricular rhythm (AIVR), 208-209
Adams-Stokes syndrome; *see* Stokes-Adams syndrome
AIVR; *see* Accelerated idioventricular rhythm
Alcohol, 152, 191, 260
Ambulatory ECG monitoring, 36, 255, 260
Amyloid, cardiac, 149
Aneurysm, ventricular, 117, 118, 132, 260
Angina pectoris, 124, 125
    ECG patterns with, 125, 131, 132
    Prinzmetal's variant, 130, 131, 132
Anterior myocardial infarction, 103, 104, 105, 108-111;
    see also Myocardial infarction
Anterolateral myocardial infarction, 95, 110, 111; *see also*
    Myocardial infarction
Anteroseptal myocardial infarction, 109; *see also*
    Myocardial infarction
Aortic regurgitation, 83
Aortic stenosis, 83, 260
Arrhythmias, 169, 170
    differential diagnosis of, 244-256
Artifacts, ECG, 279-280
    with external cardiac massage, 237-238
Asystole, 235, 236, 237
    in cardiac arrest, 235, 236, 237
    straight-line pattern with, 236, 237
Athletes, arrhythmias in, 167, 246n
Atria, 3, 9, 19
    depolarization of, 9, 13, 19
    repolarization of, 9, 20, 147
Atrial bigeminy, 174, 175
Atrial enlargement, 74-77
Atrial fibrillation, 186, 189-194, 244, 245, 247, 249, 260
    causes of, 191
    complete heart block with, 193, 194
    digitalis toxicity with, 227, 228, 229, 244, 246
    electrical cardioversion of, 192, 254
    with rapid ventricular rate, 189, 190, 247-249, 251, 252
    with slow ventricular rate, 193, 194, 228, 229, 244,
        246

Atrial fibrillation—cont'd
    treatment of, 192-194, 254, 255
    with Wolff-Parkinson-White syndrome, 251, 252
Atrial fibrillation-flutter, 194
Atrial flutter, 186-189, 244, 247, 248, 249, 261
    causes of, 188
    electrical cardioversion of, 189, 254
    treatment of, 188, 189, 254, 269
Atrial pacing, 189, 264, 268-270
Atrial septal defect, 75, 91, 260
Atrial tachycardia; *see* Paroxysmal atrial tachycardia (PAT)
Atrioventricular block; *see* AV heart block
Atropine, 166, 219, 237
Automatic atrial tachycardia, 182
Automaticity, cardiac, 5
AV dissociation, 221, 222, 261
    differentiation from complete heart block, 222, 261
    isorhythmic, 221
    in ventricular tachycardia, 252
AV heart block, 214-222
    complete (third-degree), 19, 217-219, 222
        digitalis toxicity causing, 194, 228
    first-degree, 214
    incomplete, 217
    Mobitz type I (Wenckebach), 215-217, 262
        with digitalis toxicity, 228
        with inferior wall infarction, 217
    Mobitz type II, 217, 271
        second-degree, 214-217
        treatment with pacemaker, 218, 219, 269
AV junction, 3-5
AV junctional escape beats, 5, 179
AV junctional premature contractions, 173, 179, 180
AV junctional rhythms, 5, 177-182, 227
AV junctional tachycardia, 179, 181, 182, 247, 248
AV Wenckebach; *see* AV heart block, Mobitz type I
    (Wenckebach)
Axis; *see* QRS electrical axis

B

Bidirectional ventricular tachycardia, 227
    with digitalis toxicity, 227
Bifascicular block, 219-221

---

n indicates footnote.